PHYSICAL FITNESS AND WELLNESS

PHYSICAL FITNESS AND WELLNESS

Jerrold S. Greenberg
University of Maryland

George B. Dintiman
Virginia Commonwealth University

Barbee Myers Oakes
Wake Forest University

Allyn and Bacon

Boston   London   Toronto   Sydney   Tokyo   Singapore

Senior Series Editor: Suzy Spivey
Vice President and Publisher, Social Sciences: Susan Badger
Editorial Assistants: Jennifer Strada, Sarah L. Dunbar
Development Editor: Cheryl Marconi
Marketing Manager: Anne Harvey
Production Administrator: Susan McIntyre
Editorial-Production Service: Colophon
Text Designer: Wendy LaChance/*By Design*
Cover Administrator: Linda Knowles
Prepress Buyer: Linda Cox
Manufacturing Buyer: Megan Cochran

Copyright © 1995 by Allyn & Bacon
A Simon & Schuster Company
Needham Heights, MA 02194

Library of Congress Cataloging-in-Publication Data
Greenberg, Jerrold S.
    Physical fitness and wellness / by Jerrold S. Greenberg, George B. Dintiman,
Barbee Myers Oakes.
        p.   cm.
    Includes bibliographical references and index.
    ISBN 0-205-15389-5
    1. Physical fitness. 2. Health. 3. Exercise. I. Dintiman, George B. II. Myers Oakes,
Barbee. III. Title.

RA781.G799   1994
613.7—dc20   94-16503
                                                             CIP

Printed in the United States of America
10 9 8 7 6 5 4 3 2   99 98 97 96 95

Contents

**10 STRESS MANAGEMENT AND
PHYSICAL FITNESS 205**

9 EXPLORING WEIGHT CONTROL 181

14   WOMEN AND PHYSICAL FITNESS   299

15   DESIGNING A PROGRAM UNIQUE FOR YOU: A LIFETIME OF FITNESS   329

GIVEN THE EXISTENCE of numerous books on physical fitness, one might reasonably ask, "Why another?" The answer to this question lies within this book's unique features. We were frustrated in our attempts to find a fitness textbook that responded to the diverse readers one might expect to be interested in reading such a book. Given that concern, we made sure to incorporate all the usual fitness content but in a way that was sensitive and appreciative of the diversity of readers.

Certainly we discuss topics one might expect to be discussed in a book on physical fitness. There are chapters on principles of exercise, cardiorespiratory fitness, muscular strength and endurance, flexibility, and the like. In other words, there is an array of valid information about physical fitness in this book sufficient for you to become physically fit or maintain your present state of fitness if it is adequate.

APPROACH

We have recognized, though, that physical fitness is but one component of wellness and not an isolated one. Therefore, we discuss physical fitness in a larger context we describe as wellness, which views physical fitness as related to health and well being. That is why we also discuss topics such as nutrition, weight control, stress and stress management, chemicals and drugs, heart disease and cancer, and exercise injuries. To be fit without being healthy and well is not to have finished the journey toward a full life.

UNIQUE FEATURES

In addition to these more traditional approaches to the topic of physical fitness, we added information unique to this book. For example, recognizing that researchers have found knowledge of physical fitness insufficient in itself to motivate people to become fit and to maintain adequate lifelong levels of physical fitness, we included a whole chapter on Behavioral Change and Motivational Strategies. These well-researched strategies are further described throughout the text in examples of how they might be used to overcome barriers to fitness. Most chapters have a **Behavioral Change and Motivational Strategies** box that describes obstacles specific to that chapter's content that can interfere with achieving fitness, and behavioral change strategies that can be employed to overcome these obstacles.

We also know that changing behavior can be easier if role models exist to encourage changes. That is why we have provided fitness role models in each chapter in a feature entitled **Fitness Heroes**. These boxes describe people who have achieved high levels of fitness and wellness in spite of obstacles. These models are designed to expand readers' perceptions of their capabilities in the face of whatever fitness obstacles they might experience; for example, being overweight or previously sedentary, having a physical disability, being uncoordinated, or lacking muscular strength.

We were also exasperated by the misconceptions about fitness encountered. Given the popularity of this topic and an array of fitness gurus that are not adequately trained nor qualified to teach about physical fitness, too often misconceptions and inaccurate information are passed along as valid. For this reason we included a **Myth and Fact Sheet** box in each chapter. These boxes present general misconceptions related to the content of the chapter and correct these myths with factual information.

Perhaps the most important features of this book are the **Diversity Issues** boxes and the chapter on "Women and Physical Fitness." Both of these features are designed to celebrate the diversity of our readers. The Diversity Issues boxes present issues specific to the content of the chapter but also have ethnic, racial, cultural, gender, age, and/or physical capability implications. This feature directs attention throughout the book to the existence of and the value in our differences and our similarities. We refrain from grouping everyone into the majority cultural norm and we recognize our diversity as a strength rather than an interference.

The chapter on "Women and Physical Fitness" is another example of the fact that everyone is not the same. The U.S. National Institutes of Health (NIH) was so appalled by the lack of research studies that included women subjects and, therefore, the inability to generalize results from these studies to women, that they created the Office of Research on Women's Health. That office reviews proposed research to be funded by NIH to ensure it includes female subjects, and it funds other studies concerned with female health issues such as breast cancer. Similarly, there has been a lack of adequate attention to issues specific to women and physical fitness. To correct this oversight, and to have sufficient space to discuss the issues fully, we devoted a whole chapter to this topic.

We have presented the information needed to engage in a physical fitness program, we have provided techniques that can be used to motivate and encourage continued participation in this program, and we have done so in a manner that recognizes the diversity of our readers. The use of this book to achieve physical fitness, health, and high-level wellness is now up to each reader. We will feel no greater satisfaction than if we have succeeded in improving the lives of our readers throughout the country by having written this book. Make our days—Become physically fit!

SUPPLEMENTS

Instructor's Manual and Test Bank with Transparency Masters and Video Guide

This comprehensive supplement provides everything a fitness instructor will need to teach from this exciting new text. Included in the Instructor's Manual section are chapter outlines, objectives and summaries, key terms and concepts, lecture and lab activity outlines, discussion questions, suggested student activities, supplementary readings, and supplementary videos and other media materials. The Test Bank provides 50 questions for each chapter with multiple choice, true-false, fill-in, and essay type questions to choose between. A computerized version of the test bank is available to adopters in both IBM and Macintosh formats.

Video Material

Through an exclusive arrangement with Cable News Network (CNN), a new, specially edited videotape culled from relevant CNN programs provides an exciting means for enhancing classroom discussion. This unique videotape includes segments on such relevant topics as eating disorders, yoga, disabled aerobics, a wellness dorm, men's nutrition, and osteoporosis exercises. A video user's guide can be found in the Instructor's Manual that provides a description of each video segment, suggested classroom use for each segment, tie-ins with the text material, and discussion questions for each segment.

Acknowledgments

WE WOULD LIKE to thank the following reviewers for the thoughtful criticism and valuable suggestions they provided: Harry Duval, University of Georgia; Coach Michael Manley, Anderson University; Joseph T. Lopour, Southern Utah University; Larry Durstine, University of South Carolina; Joe Smith, University of Alabama; Robert Case, Sam Houston State University; Dr. Mary Mahan, Miami Dade Community College; Peggy McDonald, Central Piedmont Community College; Andrew Paterna, Manchester Community Technical College; Carol Christensen, San Jose State University; Dr. Christine L. Wells, Arizona State University; Robert Rothstein, Miami Dade Community College; Dr. Pat Vehrs, University of Houston; and Linda Halbert, University of North Carolina, Charlotte.

In addition, we owe a debt of gratitude to the people at Allyn and Bacon who committed themselves to the careful review, editing, and production of this book. In particular, we wish to thank Suzy Spivey, Senior Series Editor; Cheryl Marconi, Development Editor; and Susan McIntyre, Production Administrator. They provided us with valuable insight and guidance in all phases of the creation of this book, from the first written word to the last details of organization, design, illustration, and production.

Finally, our families provided us with the support that all authors need. They were there to bounce ideas off of, to console and to cajole (whichever happened to be needed at the time), and to provide a haven of love to which we could retreat. Although we have come to expect these things from our families, we nevertheless would like to take this opportunity to acknowledge that we probably do take them for granted too often and announce loudly for all to hear: Thanks for being there!

PHYSICAL FITNESS, HEALTH, AND WELLNESS

Chapter Objectives

By the end of this chapter, you should be able to:

1. Define and differentiate between physical fitness, health, and wellness.
2. Describe the benefits of being physically fit.
3. Discuss the relationship between physical fitness and self-esteem.

INEZ WAS A college athlete. Her basketball team always had a winning record, and she was a major reason they were so good. Still, that was long ago. Today Inez is in her 50s and an automobile accident has left her without the use of her legs. But she still participates in sports. She plays wheelchair basketball in her leisure time and coaches a community center soccer team on the weekends. She may not be able to run a mile, but she certainly can shoot foul shots. She may not be able to demonstrate a soccer kick, but she sure can motivate the girls she coaches.

Several years had passed—five to be exact—since Rodney and I last saw each other. I was looking forward to catching up on old times. When I asked the standard, "How have you been?" Rodney replied that he had never felt better. He had taken up jogging and was now running 50 miles a week. He had given up cigarette smoking, become a vegetarian, and had more confidence than ever.

In spite of his reply, I needed further assurance. He looked like death warmed over. His face was gaunt; his body emaciated. His clothes were baggy, creating a sloppy appearance. He had an aura of tiredness about him.

"How's Cynthia?," I asked.

"Fine," Rodney replied. "But we are no longer together. She just couldn't accept the time I devoted to running, and her disregard for her own health was getting on my nerves. She is still somewhat overweight, you know, and I started viewing her differently when I became healthier myself."

You may know an Inez, a Rodney, or someone like them. Are they healthy? This is a complicated question, one that this chapter explores, first by defining physical fitness, health, and wellness and then by differentiating among them.

Physical fitness is defined differently by different people. In this text, it is defined as the ability to meet life's demands and still have enough energy to respond to unplanned events. There are five basic components of physical fitness: cardiorespiratory endurance, muscular strength, muscular endurance, flexibility, and body composition. Participation in sports activities that can improve these fitness components often requires certain motor skills. Consequently, motor skills (such as agility, balance, coordination, power, speed, and reaction time) are often included in physical fitness programs. It *is* possible to develop the five basic components of physical fitness without proficiency in these and other motor skills. That is why someone who is not a natural athlete can still be extremely fit.

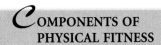

COMPONENTS OF PHYSICAL FITNESS

Elsewhere in this book we will discuss developing the five basic components of physical fitness. First, however, we must define these components.

Cardiorespiratory Endurance

To engage in physical activity, even breathing, requires oxygen. Without oxygen, it would be impossible to burn the food you need for energy. To supply

---

Muscular strength The amount of force a muscle can exert for one repetition.

Muscular endurance A muscle's ability to continue submaximal contractions against resistance.

Flexibility The range of motion around a joint or the ability to move limbs gracefully and efficiently.

Fat weight The weight of your body fat.

Percent body fat The percentage of your body weight made up of fat.

Lean body mass The nonfatty component of your body.

Body composition The relationship between your fat weight and your lean body mass.

---

oxygen to the various parts of the body requires a transport system. The body's transport system consists of lungs, heart, and blood vessels. When you breathe, you inhale air that contains oxygen into the lungs. The lungs absorb oxygen into their blood vessels and transport it to the heart where it is pumped out through other blood vessels to all parts of the body. The more efficiently and effectively you transport oxygen, the greater your cardiorespiratory endurance (*cardio* for heart and *respiratory* for lungs and breathing), the ability to supply and use oxygen, over a period of time and in sufficient amounts, to perform normal and unusual activities.

Muscular Strength and Endurance

The maximal pulling force of a muscle or a muscle group is called **muscular strength**. The ability of a muscle to contract repeatedly or to sustain a contraction is called **muscular endurance**. Lifting a load or moving an object depends on muscular strength. Doing that repeatedly over time requires muscular endurance. In spite of tremendous cardiovascular endurance, without sufficient muscular strength or endurance you may not be able to do the things you wish to do.

Muscular Flexibility

The range of motion around a joint, or more simply the degree to which you can move your limbs with grace and efficiency, is **flexibility**. Flexibility is important in performing exercise efficiently, safely, and enjoyably. Without adequate flexibility you might not be able to stretch far, might overstress a muscle or ligament, and might even feel uncomfortable moving. Flexibility is probably the component of physical fitness that is most overlooked; yet the consequences of ignoring flexibility can be injury, pain and discomfort, and poor health.

Body Composition

Your body contains some parts that are made up of fats and others that are not. The fat component is usually referred to as **fat weight**, and fat in relation to the body as a whole is referred to as **percent body fat**. The nonfatty component is called **lean body mass**. **Body composition** is the relationship between these two components. In the past, people relied on height-weight charts to evaluate body composition. We now realize that someone can weigh many more pounds than a chart based on height says is appropriate but still have good body composition. This can happen

Diversity Issues

Paralympics

In 1992, just after the Olympic games concluded in Barcelona, 4,000 elite athletes competed in the ninth Paralympic games. The first of these games was held in Rome in 1960 and was limited to athletes with spinal-cord injuries. In 1976, any athlete who had some form of physical impairment was allowed to compete.

The following 15 sports make up the Paralympics:

1. **General athletics:** Participants compete in track, throwing, and jumping events; the pentathlon; and the marathon.
2. **Basketball:** Participants move about in wheelchairs as they pass and shoot and otherwise play basketball as usual. Games last 40 minutes and baskets are at the same height as they are for regular basketball.
3. **Bocce:** This game, which is a combination of bowling and shuffleboard, is played by athletes with cerebral palsy. Participants roll a ball that fits in the hand toward other balls rolled by competitors, attempting to get the closest to a middle circle.
4. **Cycling:** Participants are divided into three groups based on disability—cerebral palsy, visual impairment, or impaired mobility—and race against competitors from within their group.
5. **Fencing:** In wheelchairs fixed to the floor, competitors attempt to hit their opponents with a fencing foil while avoiding getting hit themselves.
6. **Seven-a-Side soccer:** Similar to regular soccer, this sport is played by athletes with cerebral palsy.
7. **Goalball:** This sport, which is like football, is played by blind athletes. The balls contain small bells so athletes can determine where the ball is and when it is approaching.
8. **Weight lifting and power lifting:** Paraplegics, amputees, and athletes with polio sequelae and cerebral palsy compete in two adapted versions of the bench press.
9. **Judo:** Athletes with visual impairments follow regular rules governing judo.
10. **Swimming:** Participants in this sport are divided by gender and two disability groupings—blind athletes and those with other disabilities.

Accommodations are made for the physical condition of the athlete. For instance, blind swimmers have their heads gently touched when they approach the pool wall.

11. **Tennis:** Moving about the court in wheel chairs, players are allowed to let the ball bounce twice before it must be returned. Athletes compete in men's and women's singles and doubles.
12. **Table tennis:** Divided into two groups, wheelchairs and standing, athletes compete against each other in standard table tennis, or ping pong.
13. **Archery:** Standing and in wheelchairs, competitors shoot arrows toward a target. The competitions are divided into men's and women's events.
14. **Shooting:** Standing and in wheelchairs, athletes compete in rifle and pistol, air and 22-caliber events. Competitions are divided into men's, women's, and mixed-gender events.
15. **Volleyball:** Seated in wheelchairs and standing, players must return a volleyball hit onto their side of the court before it bounces twice.

In addition to the above considerations, ramps are located throughout the Paralympic village to make it easy for the athletes to get around.

The next Paralympic games will be held in 1996 in Atlanta, Georgia, just after the next Olympic games. To learn more about sports for physically challenged athletes, contact

1. National Handicapped Sports, 451 Hungerford Drive, Rockville, MD 20850; (301) 217-0960.
2. National Wheelchair Athletic Association, 3595 E. Fountain Boulevard, Colorado Springs, CO 80910; (719) 574-1150.
3. U.S. Association for Blind Athletes, 33 N. Institute, Colorado Springs, CO 80903; (719) 630-0422.
4. U.S. Cerebral Palsy Athletic Association, 34518 Warren Road, Westland, MI 48185; (313) 572-1399.
5. Dwarf Athletic Association of America, 3725 W. Holmes Road, Lansing, MI 48911; (313) 231-1235. ✦

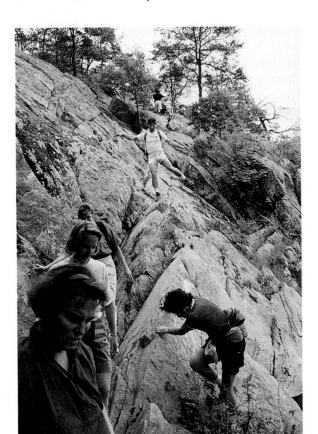

Exercising outdoors is an invigorating way to enhance spiritual health while at the same time improving physical health. (Photo Courtesy of the Aspen Hill Club.)

because the person is muscular and has a good deal of lean body mass. Conversely, someone at just the right weight according to a height chart could in actuality be overweight because of too much fatty tissue and not enough lean body mass.

HEALTH AND WELLNESS

What do you mean when you think of health? If someone told you Aaron was really healthy, what picture of Aaron would you have in your mind? If you were asked to elaborate on your health, what would you say? We will help you answer that question, but first try listing five ways in which you could improve your health.

We are willing to bet you listed ways to improve your physical health. You probably listed ways to prevent contracting heart disease such as eating less fatty foods or exercising more or ways to prevent cancer by not smoking cigarettes and getting regular checkups. Yet physical health is not the total picture; there are

other components of health that are just as important. These include:

1. **Social health** This is the ability to interact well with people and the environment, to have satisfying interpersonal relationships.

2. **Mental health** This is the ability to learn and grow intellectually. Life's experiences as well as more formal structures (for example, schools) enhance mental health.

3. **Emotional health** This is the ability to control emotions so that you feel comfortable expressing them and you can express them appropriately. Conversely, it is the ability to not express emotions when it is inappropriate to do so.

4. **Spiritual health** This is a belief in some unifying force, which will vary from person to person but will have the concept of faith at its core. Faith is a feeling of connection to other humans, of a purpose to life, and of a quest for meaning in life.

So health is not just caring for your body. It concerns your social interactions, mind, feelings, and spirit. Often we decide to give up health in one area to gain greater health in another. For example, when you decide you're just not up to exercising today, you may choose to improve your emotional health (to seek relaxation) at some expense to your physical health. When you decide to study instead of spending time with your friends, you may be choosing mental over social health. We make decisions like these about our health all the time even though we do not express them in these terms.

To identify the strengths and weaknesses of the components of your health, complete Lab Activity 1.1: Identifying Your Health Strengths and Weaknesses at the end of this chapter.

Now you can appreciate that physical fitness is just one component of health. In fact, it is just one component of physical health, which, in turn, is a component of overall health. **Health** then is an individual's total physical, social, emotional, mental, and spiritual status, and health is separate and distinct from illness (see Figure 1.1).

In Figure 1.1 the continuum is a dotted, rather than a solid, line. Each dot is made up of the five health components (see Figure 1.2), and therefore everyone has some degree of health no matter where they are located on the continuum.

Imagine that each health dot, as depicted in Figure 1.2, is a tire on the vehicle in which you travel

Figure 1.1 ✦ The Health-Illness Continuum

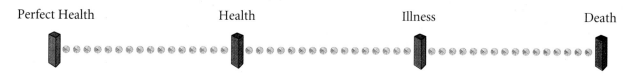

Perfect Health   Health   Illness   Death

through life. If the tire is properly inflated, you will have a smooth ride; if it is not, the ride will be bumpy. The same is true for your *health tire.* If you do not pay enough attention to your health and all its components, improving (inflating) them when you can, you will experience conditions that make life more difficult and dissatisfying. For example, if you do not exercise frequently enough or properly, you may become fatigued easily or susceptible to various illnesses.

If you overdo any one component of health at the expense of the others, you may wind up with a tire like the one in Figure 1.3. That tire is *out of round* and will not provide a smooth ride. That health tire has expanded physical health to the detriment of the other aspects of health. Here is where Rodney, introduced at the beginning of this chapter, comes to mind. He expanded his physical health but was no longer married and looked terrible. He had no time for friends (social health), reading (mental health), or enjoying nature or participating in religious traditions (spiritual health). Even though he was more physically fit, he was not arguably healthier. Further-

more he did not possess a very high level of wellness. We refer to **wellness** as having your health tire in round, that is, having the components of health adequately inflated and balanced, paying attention to and improving all aspects of health without exaggerating any one. Inez, the other person we introduced at the beginning of this chapter, did not have the use of her legs, but she did participate in physical activity at the level at which she was capable. She even learned about soccer so she could coach a community center team. Inez probably possessed a higher level of wellness than did the physically advantaged Rodney. That is why you need to focus on your social, mental, emotional, and spiritual health as you read about physical fitness in this book. We will help you do that by regularly presenting the health and wellness implications of the content discussed.

Figure 1.2 ✦ A Single Health-Illness
Continuum Dot

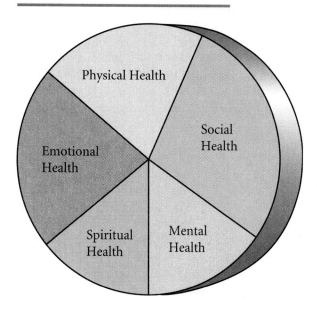

Figure 1.3 ✦ An Asymmetrical Dot on
the Health-Illness Continuum

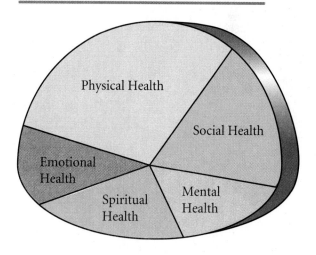

Health The total of your physical, social, emotional, mental, and spiritual status.

Wellness Having the components of health balanced and at sufficient levels.

Figure 1.4 ✦ Comparison of Causes of Death, 1900 and Today

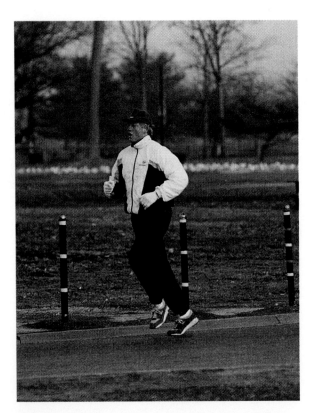

Health Objectives for the Nation

Figure 1.4 compares the major causes of death in 1900 and today. Heading the 1900 list are diseases that are passed from one person to another or that are the result of unsanitary practices (tuberculosis, pneumonia, influenza). The incidence of these diseases has, for the most part, been drastically reduced through the development of proper waste disposal and sewage systems, quarantine, and other community actions to prevent their spread through increased knowledge that led to legislation.

The killers of today do not lend themselves to such remedies. These conditions (heart disease, cancer, and stroke) are more the result of lifestyle than of a microorganism. In a democratic society, we cannot legislate lifestyle. For significant decreases to occur in these diseases, people must voluntarily change unhealthy behaviors (cigarette smoking, lack of regular physical activity, lack of proper amounts of sleep, abuse of alcohol and other drugs, eating foods high in saturated fats, and so forth). Medical researchers estimate that 20 percent of the risk for heart disease, cancer, and stroke can be attributed to heredity, another 20 percent to environmental factors, 10 percent to inadequate health care, and an alarming 50 percent to unhealthy lifestyles.

Recognizing the need to encourage the adoption of healthy lifestyles, the Surgeon General of the United States developed health goals for the nation. The first national health goals were distributed in 1979 and 1980. More recently, goals for the year 2000 have been announced. Although many of the national health objectives are related to physical fitness and wellness, we list those *directly* related to physical fitness in Table 1.1.

To assess the risk of ill health associated with your lifestyle decisions, complete Lab Activity 1.2: Assessing Your Health Risk at the end of this chapter.

Exercise is something that we all need to fit into our schedules. If President Clinton, who works more than 15 hours a day, can find time to run, perhaps you can too! (Photo Courtesy of The White House.)

Table 1.1 ✦ National Health Objectives Specific to Physical Fitness and Wellness

The following are objectives related to physical fitness and wellness. The objective and the baseline condition, the status of the behavior or condition when the objective was written, are presented here.

OBJECTIVE	BASELINE
1. Reduce coronary heart disease deaths to no more than 100 per 100,000 people.	135 per 100,000
2. Reduce overweight to no more than 20 percent of people aged 20 and older and no more than 15 percent of adolescents aged 12 through 19.	26 percent for people aged 20 through 74 and 15 percent for adolescents aged 12 through 19
3. Increase to at least 30 percent the proportion of people aged 6 and older who engage in light to moderate physical activity for at least 30 minutes per day.	22 percent of people aged 18 and older are active at least 30 minutes five or more times per week and 12 percent are active seven or more times per week
4. Increase to at least 20 percent the proportion of people aged 18 and older and to at least 75 percent the proportion of youths aged 6 through 17 who engage in vigorous physical activity that promotes the development and maintenance of cardiorespiratory fitness three or more days per week for 20 or more minutes per occasion.	12 percent for people aged 18 and older and 66 percent for youth aged 10 through 17
5. Reduce to no more than 15 percent the proportion of people aged 6 and older who engage in no leisure-time physical activity.	24 percent for people aged 18 and older
6. Increase to at least 40 percent the proportion of people aged 6 and older who regularly perform physical activities that enhance and maintain muscular strength, muscular endurance, and flexibility.	None available
7. Increase to at least 50 percent the proportion of overweight people aged 12 and older who have adopted sound dietary practices combined with regular physical activity to attain an appropriate body weight.	30 percent of overweight women and 25 percent of overweight men for people aged 18 and older
8. Increase to at least 50 percent the proportion of children and adolescents in first through twelfth grade who participate daily in school physical education.	36 percent
9. Increase to at least 50 percent the proportion of school physical education class time that students spend being physically active, preferably engaged in lifetime physical activities.	27 percent
10. Increase the proportion of worksites offering employer-sponsored physical activity and fitness programs.	Worksite with 50 to 99 employees, 14 percent; with 100 to 249 employees, 23 percent; with 250 to 749 employees, 32 percent; with more than 749 employees, 54 percent
11. Increase community availability and accessibility of physical activity and fitness facilities.	Hiking, biking, and fitness trails—1 per 71,000 people; public swimming pools—1 per 53,000 people; park and recreation open space—1.8 per 1,000 people
12. Increase to at least 50 percent the proportion of primary care providers who routinely assess and counsel patients regarding the frequency, duration, type, and intensity of physical activity practices.	Counseling routinely provided for 30 percent of sedentary patients

Source: U. S. Department of Health and Human Services, *Healthy People 2000: National Health Promotion and Disease Prevention Objectives.* Washington, DC: U.S. Government Printing Office, 1991, DHHS Publication No. (PHS) 91-50212.

Fitness Heroes

In 1993, Evander Holyfield became the third heavyweight fighter in history to regain his title by defeating the man who dethroned him. Holyfield is known for his disciplined and dignified behavior, in a sport marked by questionable conduct.

Holyfield was born on October 19, 1962, in Alabama. He was the youngest of eight children being raised by a single mother. He and his brothers went to the boys club almost every afternoon to escape the run-down, inner-city neighborhood in which they lived.

At the age of eight, Evander took an interest in boxing after watching a boxer work out on a speed bag at the boys club gym. He competed in this first boxing match at the age of nine.

In 1983, Holyfield won the National Sports Festival boxing title, making him a leading contender for a spot on the 1984 Olympic team. At the 1984 Olympic Games, he was awarded a bronze medal. He turned professional in 1984, and began intense weight training in order to qualify for the heavyweight class. He defeated George Foreman in April 1991, Larry Holmes in 1992, and, finally, lost his title to Riddick Bowe in 1992. In 1993, he agreed to a return bout with Bowe and subsequently won.

While Evander Holyfield is a fitness hero in his own right, he has never forgotten where he came from. He now supports his mother, his ex-wife, and his four children, and he gives financial assistance to the boys club that he frequented as a boy. He is still a frequent visitor there. ✦

WHAT PHYSICAL FITNESS CAN DO FOR YOU

As we have discussed, physical fitness can make you healthier and help you to achieve high-level wellness. And, as you will soon see, it can even help you feel better about yourself and be more self-assured.

The Benefits of Physical Activity

A friend of ours likes to kid that he gets his exercise serving as a pallbearer at the funerals of his jogger friends. Aside from just being contentious, he is expressing an important point. Exercise itself will not guarantee a long life. Heredity sets limits on how long you will live, but within these limits is a range. Regular physical activity of sufficient duration and intensity can help you reach your upper limits. This is demonstrated in the studies of Harvard alumni by Paffenbarger and colleagues (1986). Paffenbarger found that mortality rates were lower for physically active alumni. By age 80, the amount of additional life attributed to adequate exercise, compared to sedentariness, was between one and two plus years. The multiple risk factor intervention trial (MRFIT) study involved over 12,000 men and also found that the men most physically active lived longer than the least physically active (Leon and Connett, 1991). Furthermore, the MRFIT study indicated that *any* activity (not just vigorous activity) of 30 minutes, five times a week, decreased the risk of coronary heart disease, although more exerting physical activity was more protective. Blair and associates (1989) found that death rate increased as fitness level decreased. Two of the major reasons for lower death rates in exercisers can be explained by our knowledge that exercise can help prevent coronary heart disease (Donahue et al., 1988) and cancer (Krucoff, 1992), the first and second leading causes of death in the United States. Researchers have found an increase in natural killer (NK) cell activity among people who exercised as seldom as once per week (Kusaka, Kondou, and Morimoto, 1992). NK cells help prevent cancer.

Physical activity can both prevent illness and disease and help rehabilitation. In this way, it enhances physical health. Since we will discuss the relationship between physical activity and health in more detail elsewhere in this book, suffice it to say here that among the illnesses and diseases that physical activity can help prevent are the nation's leading killers: heart disease, cancer, and stroke. And this sort of activity can help prevent, and serve as a treatment for, hypertension (high blood pressure), itself a major cause of heart disease and stroke.

One reason that physical activity is so helpful in preventing and treating various conditions is that it helps people control their weight. Overweight, obesity, and malnutrition are implicated in numerous states of ill health. These conditions are also related to the amount of cholesterol in the blood (serum cholesterol) that can clog arteries leading to the heart or brain, thereby resulting in a heart attack or stroke. Some cholesterol, however, is actually helpful since it picks up blood fats and deposits them outside of the body. This *good* cholesterol is called high-density lipoprotein (HDL). Exercise increases the amount of HDL in the blood (Shepard, 1989). It also decreases the amount of bad cholesterol (low-density lipoprotein [LDL]) that accumulates on the blood vessel walls and can eventually block the flow of blood to the heart and other body parts.

In addition, regular exercise can be an extremely effective means of managing stress. In this way, it improves emotional health. As we will discuss in chapter 10, stress changes the body so it is prepared to respond to a threat. It is geared up for some physical reaction. Exercise uses the built-up stress byproducts and the body's preparedness to do something physical. The result is a sense of stress relief. Exercise also enhances the production of brain neurotransmitters (endorphins) that make you feel better and less stressed.

The rehabilitative benefits of exercise are almost notorious. It wasn't too long ago that people needing surgery or women giving birth were restricted to a hospital bed for days, sometimes weeks. That is no longer the case. The benefits of physical activity in recuperating from many conditions are now well recognized. Take the case of an individual who had a triple bypass operation in which three of the blood vessels supplying the heart were found to be obstructed. The obstructed sections were bypassed with blood vessels grafted from his legs. Shortly after the operation, the patient was expected to get out of bed and walk around. Although he was nervous at first,

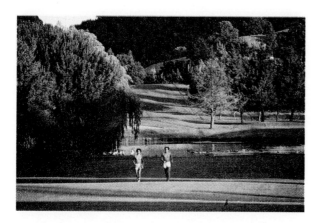

Enjoying your surroundings should become a part of your regular fitness routine. Whether you are exercising in a gym or outdoors, you are more likely to continue your exercise routine if the surroundings are appealing to you. (Photo Courtesy of The National Cancer Institute.)

he soon learned that physical movement helped him get back to his regular routine. His muscular strength returned sooner then he expected, his blood circulation was enhanced by muscular contractions forcing pressure on the blood vessel walls, and his mood improved dramatically.

Physical activity can even help elderly people live longer (Rakowski and Mor, 1992) and postpone the effects of aging. As people get older, they become susceptible to conditions that can restrict their activities, even to the extent that they become dependent on others to tie their shoes, transport them, and buy them food. A life of regular physical activity can postpone this dependency by providing elders with the necessary muscular strength and endurance, cardiorespiratory endurance, and flexibility to manage their own affairs. Several national health objectives speak to the needs of the elderly. The baseline figures that follow refer to the state of affairs that existed at the time the objectives were written. The national health objectives specific to the elderly include:

Objective	*Baseline*
1. Increase the years of healthy life to at least age 65.	Overall, 62 years; African Americans, 56; Hispanics, 62; people aged 65 and older, 12.
2. Reduce to no more than 90 per 1,000 people the proportion of all people aged 65 and older who have difficulty performing two or more personal care activities, thereby preserving independence.	111 per 1000.
3. Reduce the proportion of people aged 65 and older who engage in no leisure-time physical activity to no more than 22 percent.	43 percent.

Physical activity has additional benefits that are often overlooked. For example, several researchers have found that workers who are physically fit are absent from the job less frequently (Steinhardt, Greenhow, and Stewart, 1991; Tucker, Aldana, and Friedman, 1990). In addition, people who are physically fit are less apt to experience depression and are more likely to feel in control of their lives (Brandon and Loftin, 1991).

Myth and Fact Sheet

Myth	Fact
1. When we speak of health, we mean physical health.	1. Health consists of more than just physical health. It includes social, emotional, mental, and spiritual health as well.
2. Wellness is synonymous with health.	2. Wellness means having the five components of health in balance. No one component should be exaggerated at the expense of any other.
3. Someone who can run a long distance is physically fit.	3. Someone who can run a long distance may not possess upper body muscular strength or muscular endurance or may not be flexible enough.
4. Because the leading killers are the result of unhealthy lifestyles, there is little the U.S. government can do to make people healthier.	4. The U.S. government developed national health objectives to encourage individuals to adopt healthier lifestyles and thereby live longer, better quality lives.
5. There is not much you can do about how you feel about yourself, your self-esteem.	5. If you become physically fit, you will feel better about yourself, and your self-esteem will improve.

Physical activity can also improve spiritual health. For example, when you are exercising outdoors, you have the opportunity to experience nature and all its wonders—to feel the rush of air on your face and the heat of the sun on your skin, to hear the sound of the birds and of the wind rustling through the leaves, and to sense the exhilaration of your body performing physical movement. In this way, you can feel connected—body, mind, and spirit—to a unifying force. And if you engage in physical activity with other people, you improve your social health while improving all the other components of health.

Self-Esteem and Physical Activity

Physical activity also has the potential of giving you more confidence and making you feel better about yourself. We call this **self-esteem**. These benefits occur for several reasons. First, regular exercise helps

maintain body weight and develop a desirable body image. Feeling good about how your body looks and feels will translate into feeling good about yourself.

Second, physical activity often provides challenges that are faced and overcome. That is one of the advantages of competitive sports activities. Being

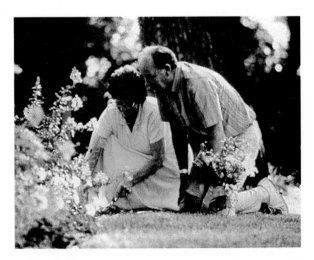

While gardening may not be the key exercise for improving cardiorespiratory fitness, it contributes to other components of fitness and can enhance social and spiritual health. (Photo Courtesy of the American Heart Association.)

Self-esteem The amount of regard you hold for yourself, the amount of value you place on yourself.

successful at these challenges will give you confidence to face other challenges in your life. And yet not all challenges are mastered. Physical activity also allows you to fail to meet the challenge but recognize that life goes on. You have probably heard someone say that you cannot hit a home run if you do not step up to the plate. When you bat, however, you can also strike out. So what? Striking out, or trying and failing, can be a more effective learning and growth experience than succeeding. After all, if you succeed, by definition you were able to do whatever it was anyhow. Only when you fail can you learn what you need to adjust to become better.

Lastly, physical activity improves endurance and strength. This allows you to perform activities more effectively and for longer periods of time. Being able to perform in this way can make you more confident and less likely to avoid events that are physically challenging. The result will be greater self-esteem and, as a result, better emotional health.

YOUR PERSONAL PHYSICAL FITNESS PROFILE

The first step in achieving the benefits of physical fitness is to assess where you begin. What level of physical fitness are you at now? Which components of physical fitness do you want to maintain and which do you want to improve? We help you perform such an assessment in the next chapter. In addition, throughout this book we include questionnaires, scales, physical tests to evaluate components of fitness, and even measures of psychosocial factors (such as self-esteem) related to decisions to exercise. We also provide lab activities in each chapter that are designed to help you learn more about yourself and about physical fitness. By the time you finish reading this book, you will have enough information about yourself to plan an effective fitness program, one that is based on your personal fitness profile and will meet your personal fitness goals.

SUMMARY

Physical Fitness

Physical fitness encompasses cardiorespiratory endurance, muscular strength, muscular endurance, muscular flexibility, and body composition. It also includes the motor skills of agility, balance, coordination, power, speed, and reaction time.

Health and Wellness

Health consists of five components: physical, social, mental, emotional, and spiritual. Physical fitness is but one component of physical health, albeit an important one.

Wellness is maintaining the components of health in sufficient amounts and in balance with one another. An ideal state of wellness is one in which no one component of health is emphasized at the expense of any other component.

In the past, the conditions causing the deaths of the most people in the United States were passed from one person to another or were the result of unsanitary practices. Tuberculosis and pneumonia are examples. The federal and state governments

responded by passing legislation that eliminated these unsafe practices and effectively reduced deaths from these conditions. Today, most deaths are the result of lifestyle practices such as cigarette smoking, lack of exercise, inadequate sleep, and poor nutrition. Changes in these practices are up to individuals; governments cannot legislate these changes.

The federal government has developed national health objectives, however, to publicize and encourage healthier lifestyles and attempt to reduce death and disability from lifestyle diseases and illnesses. Several of these objectives are specific to physical fitness and physical activity, and numerous others are tangentially related.

What Physical Fitness Can Do for You

Physical activity can improve physical health by decreasing LDLs (bad cholesterol) and increasing HDLs (good cholesterol), by preventing or reducing high blood pressure, by helping to maintain desirable weight and lean body mass, and by preventing some cancers.

Physical activity can also improve emotional health by helping to manage stress, spiritual health by focusing on nature and bodily sensations, and social health by exercising with other people. In addition, physical activity can help diminish and postpone the effects of aging and aid in recuperation from illnesses and medical procedures. Furthermore, physical activity can make you feel more confident and thereby improve your self-esteem. It can also improve self-esteem by helping to maintain recommended body weight and a desirable body image, and by providing challenges that develop confidence and the realization that, even if the challenges are not successfully overcome, significant learning occurs. Self-esteem is also enhanced when endurance and strength are developed so you can perform daily activities effectively and for longer periods of time.

REFERENCES

Blair, Steven N., Kohl, Harold W., Paffenbarger, Ralph S., Clark, Debra G., Cooper, Kenneth J., and Gibbons, Larry W. (1989). Physical fitness and all-cause mortality: A prospective study of healthy men and women. *Journal of the American Medical Association* 262: 2395–2401.

Brandon, Jeffrey E., and Lofton, J. Mark. (1991). Relationship of fitness to depression, state and trait anxiety, internal health locus of control, and self-control. *Perceptual and Motor Skills* 73: 563–568.

Donahue, Richard P., Abbott, Robert D., Reed, Qwayne M., and Yano, Katsuhiko. (1988). Physical activity and coronary heart disease in middle-aged and elderly men: The Honolulu heart program. *American Journal of Public Health* 78: 683–685.

Krucoff, Carol. (1992). Exercise and cancer: Moderate activity may help reduce risk of some tumors. *Washington Post Health* January 14, 1992, p. 16.

Kusaka, Yukinori, Kondou, Hiroshi, and Morimoto, Kanehisa. (1992). Healthy lifestyles are associated with higher natural killer cell activity. *Preventive Medicine* 21: 602–615.

Leon, Arthur S., and Connett, John. (1991). Physical activity and 10.5 year mortality in the multiple risk factor intervention trial (MRFIT). *The International Journal of Epidemiology* 20: 690–697.

Paffenbarger, Ralph S., Hyde, Robert T., Wing, Alvin L., and Hsieh, Chung-Cheng. (1986). Physical activity, all-cause mortality, and longevity of college alumni. *New England Journal of Medicine* 314: 605–613.

Rakowski, William, and Mor, Vincent. (1992). The association of physical activity with mortality among older adults in the longitudinal study of aging. *Journal of Gerontology* 47: M122–M129.

Shepard, Roy J. (1989). Nutritional benefits of exercise. *Journal of Sports Medicine* 29: 83–90.

Steinhardt, Mary, Greenhow, Linda, and Stewart, Joy. (1991). The relationship of physical activity and cardiovascular fitness to absenteeism and medical care claims among law enforcement officers. *American Journal of Health Promotion* 5: 455–460.

Tucker, Larry A., Aldana, Steven G., and Friedman, Glenn M. (1990). Cardiovascular fitness and absenteeism in 8,301 employed adults. *American Journal of Health Promotion* 5: 140–145.

Lab Activity 1.1

Identifying Your Health Strengths and Weaknesses

INSTRUCTIONS: *On this chart, list your strengths and weaknesses for each of the five components of health. Once you have done that, develop a plan for maximizing your strengths and minimizing your weaknesses. This means that you should find ways to use your strengths to make them even more influential on your health and to eliminate health weaknesses or decrease their negative effects on your health. Once you put your plan into action, you will become healthier and achieve a higher level of wellness.*

COMPONENT	STRENGTHS	WEAKNESSES
Mental health		
Physical health		

COMPONENT	STRENGTHS	WEAKNESSES
Social health		
Spiritual health		
Emotional health		

Lab Activity 1.2

Assessing Your Health Risk

INSTRUCTIONS: *The U.S. government developed this questionnaire to help people assess their health behavior and risk of ill health. Notice that this questionnaire has six sections. Complete one section at a time by circling the number corresponding to the answer that describes your behavior. Then add the numbers you have circled to determine your score for that section. Write your score at the line provided at the end of each section.*

✦ Cigarette Smoking

	Almost Always	Sometimes	Almost Never
1. I avoid smoking cigarettes.	2	1	0
2. I smoke only low-tar and low-nicotine cigarettes, or I smoke a pipe or cigars only.	2	1	0

Your Cigarette Smoking Score: _____

✦ Alcohol and Drugs

	Almost Always	Sometimes	Almost Never
1. I avoid drinking alcoholic beverages, or I drink no more than one or two a day.	4	1	0
2. I avoid using alcohol or other drugs (especially illegal drugs) as a way of handling stressful situations or my problems.	2	1	0
3. I am careful not to drink alcohol when I am taking certain medicines (for example, medicine for sleeping, pain, colds, and allergies).	2	1	0
4. I read and follow the label directions when I use prescribed and over-the-counter drugs.	2	1	0

Your Alcohol and Drugs Score: _____

◆ Eating Habits

	Almost Always	Sometimes	Almost Never
1. I eat a variety of foods each day, such as fruits and vegetables, whole grain breads and cereals, lean meats, dairy products, dry peas and beans, and nuts and seeds.	4	1	0
2. I limit the amount of fat, especially saturated fat, and cholesterol I eat (including fats in meats, eggs, butter, cream, shortenings, and organ meats such as liver).	2	1	0
3. I limit the amount of salt I eat by not adding salt at the table, avoiding salty snacks, and making certain my meals are cooked with only small amounts of salt.	2	1	0
4. I avoid eating too much sugar (especially frequent snacks of sticky candy or soft drinks).	2	1	0

Your Eating Habits Score: _____

◆ Exercise and Fitness

	Almost Always	Sometimes	Almost Never
1. I maintain a desired weight, avoiding overweight and underweight.	3	1	0
2. I do vigorous exercise for 15 to 30 minutes at least three times a week (examples include running, swimming, and brisk walking).	3	1	0
3. I do exercises that enhance my muscle tone for 15 to 30 minutes at least three times a week (examples include yoga and calisthenics).	2	1	0
4. I use part of my leisure time participating in individual, family, or team activities that increase my level of fitness (such as gardening, bowling, golf, or baseball).	2	1	0

Your Exercise and Fitness Score: _____

Lab Activity 1.2 *(continued)*
Assessing Your Health Risk

◆ **Stress Control**	Almost Always	Sometimes	Almost Never
1. I enjoy the school or other work I do.	2	1	0
2. I find it easy to relax and express my feelings freely.	2	1	0
3. I recognize early, and prepare for, events or situations likely to be stressful for me.	2	1	0
4. I have close friends, relatives, or others with whom I can talk about personal matters and call on for help when it is needed.	2	1	0
5. I participate in group activities (such as church/synagogue or community organizations) or hobbies that I enjoy.	2	1	0

Your Stress Control Score: _____

◆ **Safety**	Almost Always	Sometimes	Almost Never
1. I wear a seat belt while I am riding in a car.	2	1	0
2. I avoid driving while I am under the influence of alcohol and other drugs. I also avoid getting in a car with someone driving who is under the influence of alcohol or other drugs.	2	1	0
3. I obey the traffic rules and the speed limit when I am driving and ask others to do so when I am a passenger in a car with them.	2	1	0
4. I am careful when I am using potentially harmful products or substances (such as household cleaners, poisons, and electrical devices).	2	1	0
5. I avoid smoking in bed.	2	1	0

Your Safety Score: _____

✦ Your Health Score

After you have totaled your score for each of the six sections, circle the number in each column below that matches your score for that section of the test.

CIGARETTE SMOKING	ALCOHOL AND DRUGS	EATING HABITS	EXERCISE AND FITNESS	STRESS CONTROL	SAFETY
10	10	10	10	10	10
9	9	9	9	9	9
8	8	8	8	8	8
7	7	7	7	7	7
6	6	6	6	6	6
5	5	5	5	5	5
4	4	4	4	4	4
3	3	3	3	3	3
2	2	2	2	2	2
1	1	1	1	1	1
0	0	0	0	0	0

✦ Interpreting Your Score

Scores of 9 or 10 are excellent! Your answers show you are aware of the importance of this area to your health. More important, you are putting your knowledge to work by practicing good health habits. Even so, you may want to consider areas where your health habits can be improved.

Scores of 6 to 8 indicate that your health practices in this area are good, but that there is room for improvement. Look again at the items you answered with "sometimes" or "almost never." What changes can you make to improve your score?

Scores of 3 to 5 mean your health risks are showing! You should ask your instructor for more information about the health risks you are facing. Your instructor will probably be able to help you decrease these risks. An exception is the cigarette smoking section for which a score of 3 to 4 is excellent. Review your responses to the cigarette smoking items to better interpret their meaning.

Scores of 0 to 2 for all sections except the cigarette smoking section mean you may be taking serious, unnecessary risks with your health. Maybe you are not aware of the risks and what to do about them. Consult with a health expert or your instructor to improve your health. For the cigarette smoking section, scores of 0 to 1 mean you may be taking unnecessary risks with your health. Review your responses to these items to better interpret their meaning.

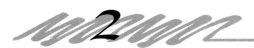

ASSESSING YOUR PRESENT LEVEL OF FITNESS

Chapter Objectives

By the end of this chapter you should be able to:

1. Indicate when it is appropriate to obtain a medical examination prior to beginning an exercise program or test.

2. List the components of a good medical evaluation.

3. List the major components of a fitness appraisal.

4. Measure and analyze your cardiorespiratory endurance, muscular strength and endurance, flexibility, nutrient intake, and body composition.

KIM'S EXCUSE FOR avoiding a regular exercise program is one that is voiced by many university students: "I get enough exercise in my part-time job at the department store and my daily routine. I'm already fit. Why should I use my valuable time exercising more?" Unfortunately, there are few, if any, active occupations, including that of a university student, that develop cardiorespiratory endurance, muscular strength, muscular endurance, flexibility, and control body weight and fat. One way for Kim to find out if she is physically fit is to complete the test battery described in this chapter to see if she can score in the average or above-average category on each item.

𝒯HE MEDICAL EVALUATION

There is an abundance of literature regarding the need for medical evaluation before beginning a program of regular exercise. There are also a number of areas of disagreement among experts concerning the components of such a medical evaluation, who should receive one, and even whether an evaluation is necessary at all. These viewpoints will be presented as objectively as possible to help you make a decision about your need for such an examination.

The Need for a Medical Evaluation

Most physicians indicate that a physical examination is necessary for individuals over the age of 40, those with symptoms of heart disease or other medical ailments, and those who have previously been sedentary. Some physicians favor a comprehensive exam; others prefer only general screening.

The recommendations of the American College of Sports Medicine (ACSM) provide sound information related to the health, status, and age of the participant (see Table 2.1). They classify individuals who may undergo exercise testing into three categories:

1. **Apparently healthy** Those who appear to be in good health and have no major coronary risk factors

2. **Individuals at higher risk** Those who have symptoms suggestive of heart disease, pulmonary or metabolic disease, or at least one major coronary risk factor

3. **Individuals with disease** Those with known cardiac, pulmonary, or metabolic diseases

The National Heart, Lung and Blood Institute (NHLBI) advises that most people under 60 years of age do not need a medical examination prior to beginning a gradual and sensible exercise program. Their rationale is based on the realization that sedentary living is a far more dangerous practice than exercising without a physician's approval, that many people will not take the time to secure an examination, and that a recommended medical exam is nothing more than another excuse to avoid exercise.

Certainly it is desirable for everyone to have a complete medical examination before their physical fitness evaluation and the start of a new exercise program to increase safety and aid in the exercise prescription. It is also a generally accepted fact that certain categories of people face some risk when en-

Table 2.1 ✦ Guidelines for Exercise Testing

	APPARENTLY HEALTHY		HIGHER RISK*		
	Younger ≤ 40 years (men) ≤ 50 years (women)	Older	No symptoms	Symptoms	With Disease†
Medical exam and diagnostic exercise test recommended prior to					
Moderate exercise‡	No§	No	No	Yes	Yes
Vigorous exercise#	No	Yes**	Yes	Yes	Yes
Physician supervision recommended during exercise test					
Sub-maximal testing	No	No	No	Yes	Yes
Maximal testing	No	Yes	Yes	Yes	Yes

*Persons with two or more risk factors or symptoms.
†Persons with known cardiac, pulmonary, or metabolic disease.
‡Moderate exercise (exercise intensity 40 to 60% VO_{2max})—Exercise intensity well within the individual's current capacity and can be comfortably sustained for a prolonged period of time, i.e., 60 minutes, slow progression, and generally non-competitive.
#Vigorous exercise (exercise intensity > 60% VO_{2max})—Exercise intense enough to represent a substantial challenge and which would ordinarily result in fatigue within 20 minutes.
§The "no" responses in this table mean that an item is "not necessary." The "no" response does not mean that the item should not be done.
**A "yes" response means that an item is recommended.

Source: American College of Sports Medicine, *Guidelines for Exercise Testing and Prescription,* 4E (Philadelphia: Lea & Febiger, 1991), p. 7.

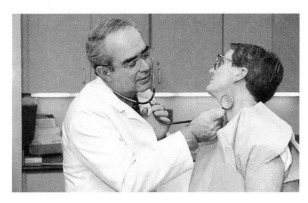

A medical evaluation may be necessary before beginning an exercise program. (Photo Courtesy of the George Washington University Medical Center.)

gaging in fitness programs without a medical examination.

Components of the Ideal Medical Evaluation

Although the exact contents of the ideal evaluation depends on the history and symptoms of each individual, common areas include a medical history that asks questions about your own and your family's history of diabetes and coronary heart disease and associated risk factors such as hypertension, stress, smoking, eating habits, current activity level, and physical disabilities. If symptoms indicate the need, the examination may also include measurement of blood pressure, listening to the sounds of the heart and lungs, determining resting pulse rate, chest X-ray, **blood lipid analysis**, a resting **electrocardiogram (ECG)**, and a **graded exercise test (stress test)**.

The results of this medical evaluation should be discussed with the patient, and any restrictions on physical activity or fitness testing should be identified

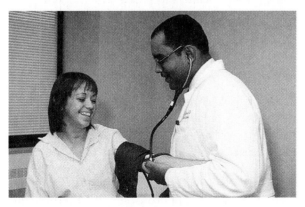

Blood pressure screening may be part of a medical evaluation. (Photo Courtesy of the George Washington University Medical Center.)

at that time. Remember that the fact that your physical activity may have limits does not mean you should avoid exercise. This book provides you with a number of sound exercise choices that will meet your fitness needs without endangering your health.

THE FITNESS APPRAISAL

In addition to the medical evaluation, it is also important to appraise your present level of physical fitness, to monitor your body's response to exercise, to determine your initial fitness level, to prepare your individualized program, and to monitor your progress. You can easily assess each major component of fitness: cardiorespiratory endurance, muscular strength and endurance, flexibility, and body composition.

During your fitness appraisal, stop any test immediately if you begin to feel chest pains, faintness, or dizziness; develop an excruciating headache; or cannot get enough air. If you notice any other disturbing sensations, do not complete the test. If any of these signs appear, consult a physician to determine their causes. It may be that your fitness level is just so low that your body cannot handle strenuous activity, or a medical problem may exist. To avoid endangering your health and eliminate worry, it is important to have the problem diagnosed.

Cardiorespiratory Assessment

All sound exercise programs place primary emphasis on cardiorespiratory endurance. The publicity surrounding the benefits of exercise for the nation's leading killer (heart disease), whether justified or not, is probably responsible for the emphasis on improving the functioning of the heart, circulatory system, and lungs. Exercise that overloads the **oxygen-transport system** (aerobic activity) leads to an increase in car-

Blood lipid analysis Examination and study of the fats present in the blood.

Electrocardiogram (ECG) A tracing of the electrical currents involved in the cycles of a heart beat.

Graded exercise test (stress test) Test designed to monitor the electrical activity of the heart; it is performed by walking on a treadmill that is slowly being elevated to increase the work load.

Oxygen-transport system The ability of the body to take in and use oxygen at the tissue level during physical activity.

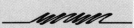

Myth and Fact Sheet

Myth	Fact
1. Fitness testing will make me too sore to function the next day.	1. When sedentary people complete tests that require maximum effort, they do experience considerable soreness the next day. The areas of soreness show which muscles you have not been using. Many college instructors eliminate the problem of soreness by using a two- to three-week preconditioning program before performing any maximum effort fitness testing.
2. I know enough about my fitness level already and do not need to be tested.	2. You may have a good feel for some aspects of your physical fitness. On the other hand, standardized tests may be just what you need to compare yourself to others of your age and to highlight the areas in which you need the most improvement. Test results often provide strong motivation for individuals to begin an exercise program.
3. The 1.5-mile test for cardiorespiratory endurance is too dangerous.	3. The test is not dangerous if it is performed properly. If you have been inactive for more than a year or have never engaged in aerobic exercise, you have several choices. First, you can skip the 1.5-mile test, assume that your cardiorespiratory fitness rating is poor, and choose a beginner's aerobic exercise program that allows you to progress slowly and safely to higher levels. Secondly, you can undertake a two- to three-week preconditioning program of walking and jogging to prepare yourself for the 1.5-mile test. Finally, you can choose to stop and walk during any or all of the test as long as you provide your best effort.
4. I'm fit enough. Too much exercise will cause athlete's heart and jeopardize my health.	4. "Athlete's heart," or "sporterz," is a term used by a Swedish researcher who detected enlarged heart muscles among skiers in 1899. As the years passed, the term gained momentum and was used incorrectly to refer to an abnormally large heart brought on by exercise. Because of this myth, some people actually became concerned that exercise would damage their hearts and result in disability or death. Aerobic exercise does develop the heart muscle more fully and cause it to become heavier and larger. It also causes the heart to pump more blood per beat (stroke volume) and per minute (cardiac output) and to become a more efficient organ. Cardiac changes that occur from aerobic exercise are both natural and healthy, and it is highly unlikely that proper aerobic exercise would cause damage to a healthy heart.

diorespiratory endurance and the muscular strength and endurance of some large muscle groups.

The 1.5-Mile Test You can assess your cardiorespiratory endurance using the 1.5-mile run either indoors or outdoors. It is relatively simple to measure off a 1.5-mile course on a track or other flat area where you can run or walk. Your objective is to complete the distance as quickly as possible by running,

walking, or the combination of the two. Consult Table 2.2 to determine your cardiorespiratory fitness rating based on your time. Record both your time and rating in Lab Activity 2.1: Your Physical Fitness Profile sheet at the end of this chapter.

The Harvard Step Test This test provides an alternate assessment method that accurately identifies your cardiorespiratory fitness level. Since test results are

Table 2.2 ✦ 1.5-Mile Run Test (time in minutes)

Fitness Category		13–19	20–29	30–39	40–49	50–59	60+
				AGE (YEARS)			
I. Very poor	(men)	> 15:31	> 16:01	> 16:31	> 17:31	> 19:01	>20:01
	(women)	> 18:31	> 19:01	> 19:31	> 20:01	> 20:31	> 21:01
II. Poor	(men)	12:11–15:30	14:01–16:00	14:44–16:30	15:36–17:30	17:01–19:00	19:01–20:00
	(women)	16:55–18:30	18:31–19:00	19:01–19:30	19:31–20:00	20:01–20:30	21:00–21:31
III. Fair	(men)	10:49–12:10	12:01–14:00	12:31–14:45	13:01–15:35	14:31–17:00	16:16–19:00
	(women)	14:31–16:54	15:55–18:30	16:31–19:00	17:31–19:30	19:01–20:00	19:31–20:30
IV. Good	(men)	9:41–10:48	10:46–12:00	11:01–12:30	11:31–13:00	12:31–14:30	14:00–16:15
	(women)	12:30–14:30	13:31–15:54	14:31–16:30	15:56–17:30	16:31–19:00	17:31–19:30
V. Excellent	(men)	8:37–9:40	9:45–10:45	10:00–11:00	10:30–11:30	11:00–12:30	11:15–13:59
	(women)	11:50–12:29	12:30–13:30	13:00–14:30	13:45–15:55	14:30–16:30	16:30–17:30
VI. Superior	(men)	< 8:37	< 9:45	< 10:00	< 10:30	< 11:00	< 11:15
	(women)	< 11:50	< 12:30	< 13:00	< 13:45	< 14:30	< 16:30

Note: < means *less than*; > means *more than*.

Source: From *The Aerobics Program for Total Well Being* by Kenneth H. Cooper, M.D., M.P.H. Copyright © 1982 by Kenneth H. Cooper. Used by permission of Bantam Books, a division of Bantam Doubleday Dell Publishing Group, Inc.

based on accurate resting and exercise heart rates, it is important to improve your skill in this area by completing Lab Activity 2.2: Determining Your Resting and Exercise Heart Rate. To complete the test, secure a sturdy 18-inch bench or stool and a wrist watch with a second hand and then follow these procedures:

1. Step on the bench first with one foot and then the other until you are standing erect with the knees unbent. Then step down with one foot followed by the other to return to the starting position.

2. Step at a cadence that will result in 30 such repetitions each minute (one every 2 seconds) for 4 (females) or 5 (males) minutes.

3. At the end of the 4- or 5-minute period, sit down.

4. After waiting exactly 1 minute, take your pulse or have a partner take your pulse for 30 seconds, and record that number.

5. Wait an additional 30 seconds before taking your pulse once again for a 30-second period, and record that number.

6. Repeat step 5 in 30 seconds. You will now have taken your pulse between 1 and 1-1/2 minutes, 2 and 2-1/2 minutes, and 3 and 3-1/2 minutes after completing the step test.

7. Using the total of the three pulse counts, compute the formula:

$$\text{index} = \frac{\text{duration of exercise in seconds} \times 100}{2 \times \text{sum of the 3 pulse counts in recovery}}$$

8. Determine your cardiorespiratory fitness level from the scale below:

Below 55	Poor
55–64	Low average
65–79	Average
80–89	Good
90 and above	Excellent

Record your appraisal on the Lab Activity 2.1: Your Physical Fitness Profile sheet.

Muscular Strength Assessment

In the laboratory, muscular strength, the absolute maximum force that a muscle can generate, is measured using elaborate and expensive equipment. Dynamometers, cable tensiometers, and force transducers and recorders have all been used this way. One problem with such methods is the need to test numer-

1.5-mile test Field test designed to measure cardiorespiratory endurance (aerobic fitness).

Harvard step test Test designed to measure cardiorespiratory endurance (aerobic fitness).

Diversity Issues

Exercise for Everyone

Physical fitness takes on considerably more importance in some cultural or ethnic groups than it does in others. In Spanish cultures, this difference has been much more dramatic in the past as regular exercise such as jogging and sports participation for women was actually discouraged.

In Puerto Rico in the 1960s, for example, the sight of a woman jogging, walking, or exercising in public was extremely rare. In fact, the few women who did exercise were viewed as eccentric and were ridiculed. Part of the problem in Puerto Rico involved customs and morals about dress. Shorts and other workout gear were commonplace among boys and men, but they were not acceptable attire for girls and women. Unfortunately, this practice limited the development of women's sports in Puerto Rico and increased health risks.

Puerto Rico has made great strides in women's athletics and in the general area of health-related fitness. Both the public schools and the university system have contributed to the fitness movement for women by expanding and improving their programs in physical education and athletics. In addition, the government continues to turn on the lights until late at night at local baseball, football, and soccer fields; track and workout areas; and basketball courts throughout the island seven days a week. Organized programs are now in place for women as well as men in public schools, universities, and local recreation programs. Olympic development programs for women have also been initiated in numerous sports that Puerto Rico focuses on. Puerto Rico has come a long way in the past few decades toward providing equal opportunity and giving equal importance to men and women in the area of health-related fitness. ✦

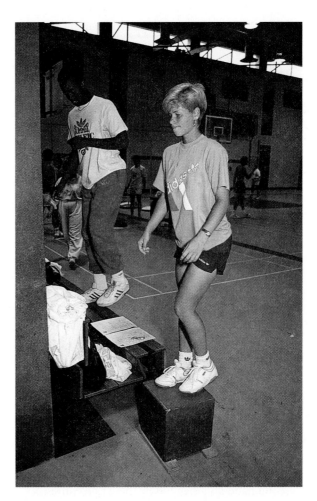

The Harvard Step Test is one way to determine your cardiorespiratory endurance. It involves stepping up and down repeatedly and then measuring the pulse rate to determine how fast the heart recovers. (Photo Courtesy of the United States Tennis Association.)

ous muscle groups to obtain an accurate measure in the legs, the abdomen, and the arms. These muscles cover such diverse body parts, however, that you can safely assume their levels of muscular strength are representative of total body strength.

You can also measure the strength and endurance of practically any muscle group by using free weights or a variety of weight machines. In some cases, you can test yourself; in others, such as the 1-RM testing using barbells, you will need a *spotter* to assist you throughout the movement.

1-RM (Repetitions Maximum) Testing Free weights are commonly used to determine your **1-RM** (maximum amount of weight you can lift one time) for a particular muscle group.

The *bench press* and *shoulder press* will accurately measure the strength of your triceps, pectoralis, and deltoid muscles; the *arm curl* measures bicep muscle strength, and the *leg press* will determine the strength of the quadriceps muscle group. For each test, a weight is selected that can be lifted comfortably. Additional weight is then added in subsequent trials until the weight is found that can be lifted correctly just one time. If the weight can be lifted more than

Table 2.3 ✦ Optimal Strength Values for Various Body Weights (based on the 1-RM test)

Body weight (lb)	BENCH PRESS		SHOULDER PRESS		BICEPS CURL		LEG PRESS	
	Male	*Female*	*Male*	*Female*	*Male*	*Female*	*Male*	*Female*
80	70	60	55	40	40	30	160	120
100	85	70	70	50	50	35	200	150
120	105	85	80	60	60	40	240	180
140	125	100	95	65	70	50	280	210
160	145	115	110	75	80	60	320	240
180	160	125	120	85	90	65	360	270
200	180	140	135	95	100	70	400	300
220	200	155	150	105	110	75	440	330
240	225	170	160	115	120	85	480	360

Note: Data in pounds; obtained on Universal Gym apparatus; applicable ages 17 to 30.

Source: Reprinted with the permission of Macmillan College Publishing Company from *Health and Fitness Through Physical Activity* by Michael Pollock, Jack Wilmore, and Samuel Fox III (New York: Macmillan College Publishing Company, 1978). All rights reserved.

once, additional weight is added until a true 1-RM is determined. Approximately three trials with a two- to three-minute rest interval between each are needed to determine the 1-RM for each muscle group. Since the resistance to be overcome in 1-RM testing is heavy, it is important to use one or two spotters to protect you from injury by taking over the barbell should you be unable to complete the lift. See Chapter 6 for an explanation of the proper technique for these tests.

Record your scores on the Lab Activity 2.1: Your Physical Fitness Profile sheet. You can also use Table 2.3 to compare your strength to others of similar age in the bench press, shoulder press, biceps curl, and leg press.

Muscular Endurance Assessment

There is a great difference between muscular endurance and muscular strength, and therefore among the kinds of tests that apply to these components. Strength tests determine the maximum amount of weight that can be moved one time whereas endurance tests measure continuous work by determining the total number of times a specific weight can be moved. It is important to evaluate the muscular endurance of your arms, shoulders, and abdominal area by completing the *pull up* or *bar dip* (men), *flexed-arm hang* (women), and the *sit up* (men and women). After completing these tests, remember to record your scores on the Lab Activity 2.1: Your Physical Fitness Profile sheet.

Abdominal Endurance Testing Although it is difficult to obtain a pure, isolated measurement of the abdominal region, the 60-second *bent-knee sit-up test* is one of the best tests available. To test yourself, assume a supine position with arms folded across your chest, knees bent at a 90-degree angle with both feet flat on the floor and in front of your buttocks. The feet should be anchored by a partner who grasps your ankles. You may do several practice sit ups prior to the official testing session. At the "go" command, begin a series of rapidly executed bent-knee sit ups. Your partner will count each correct repetition, eliminating those containing any procedural infraction such as failing to reach the vertical sitting position, lifting the feet from the floor, or not returning to the starting position with the middle of the back touching the floor. Consult Table 2.4 on page 26 to evaluate your performance.

Arm and Shoulder Muscular Endurance You can complete the *pull-up test* for men by grasping an adjustable horizontal bar with your palms facing away from the body. Now raise your body until your chin clears the top of the bar, then slowly lower yourself to a full hang without any pause as many times as you can. Your body must return to a stretch position (elbows locked) each time. Deliberate swinging, resting,

1-RM The maximum amount of weight that can be lifted at one time.

Table 2.4 ✦ Norms for the 60-Second Bent-Knee Sit-Up Test

COLLEGE FEMALES	PERFORMANCE STANDARDS	COLLEGE MALES
51 or above	Excellent	60 or above
46 to 50	Good	50 to 59
33 to 45	Average	34 to 49
21 to 32	Low	26 to 33
0 to 20	Poor	0 to 25

or leg kicking is not permitted. Table 2.5 will help you evaluate the strength and endurance of your arms and shoulders.

The *modified pull up* for women closely resembles the pull up for men. An adjustable horizontal bar is grasped with your palms facing away from the body at a level that is just even with the base of the sternum (breastbone). Your body is now placed under the bar until a 90-degree angle is formed at the point where the arms and the chest join. Only the heels support the weight of the lower body. One point is scored each time your chin is pulled over the bar and the body returns to the support position with the arms fully extended.

The *bar dip test* is used to determine the strength and endurance of the triceps and shoulder girdle. Using parallel bars, begin in a straight-arm support position close to the bar ends. The idea is to lower your body slowly until your arms form a 90-degree bent-arm position. After reaching this position, attempt to straighten your arms until you return to the starting position.

Flexibility Assessment

Flexibility is an important component of fitness. It involves the ability to move the body throughout a range of motion and stretch the muscles and tissues around skeletal joints. The *shoulder reach, trunk flexion,* and *trunk extension* tests provide an excellent indication of body flexibility. Use Table 2.6 to help evaluate your flexibility.

Shoulder Reach Standing against a pole or a projecting corner, raise your right arm and reach down behind your back as far as possible. At the same time, reach up from behind with the left hand and try to overlap the palm of the right hand. Have a partner measure, in inches, how much the fingers on your right hand overlap the fingers of the left hand. If you overlap, place a plus sign in front of the amount of overlap on the Lab Activity 2.1: Your Physical Fitness Profile sheet; if the fingers of your right and left hand do not touch, place a minus sign in front of the amount of the gap. If the fingers of one hand just barely touch those of the other, give yourself a score of zero. Repeat this test with the arms reversed; that is, the arm that first reached down over the shoulder will now reach up from behind the back.

Trunk Flexion To measure the ability to flex your trunk and to stretch the back of your thigh muscles, remove your shoes and sit with your legs straight and your feet flat against a box positioned against a wall. Place a ruler on top of the box. Place one hand on top of the other so the middle fingers are together and the same length. While your partner keeps your knees from bending, lean forward and place your hands on top of the box. Slide your hands along the measuring scale as far as possible without bouncing and hold that position for at least three seconds. Repeat the test two more times and record your highest score to the nearest inch on the Lab Activity 2.1: Your Physical Fitness Profile sheet. Your score is the number of inches beyond the edge of the box you can stretch (use a plus sign in front of that value) or the number of inches short of the edge of the box you can reach (use a minus sign in front of that value). If you can reach only to the edge of the box, give yourself a score of zero.

Trunk Extension To determine the flexibility of your back, lie on the floor face down with a partner applying pressure on your upper legs and buttocks.

Table 2.5 ✦ Scoring of Pull Ups, Modified Pull Ups, and Dips

PERFORMANCE STANDARDS	PULL UPS (NO.)	MODIFIED PULL UPS (NO.)	BAR DIPS (NO.)
Excellent	13 or above	30 or above	20 or above
Good	10 to 12	25 to 29	15 to 19
Average	5 to 9	16 to 24	7 to 14
Poor	0 to 4	0 to 15	0 to 6

Table 2.6 ✦ Flexibility Interpretations

	SHOULDER REACH (RUP/LUP)	TRUNK FLEXION	TRUNK EXTENSION
For men			
Above average	6+/3+	11+	15+
Average	4–5/0–2	7–10	8–14
Below average	Below 4/below 0	Below 7	Below 8
For women			
Above average	7+/6+	12+	23+
Average	5–6/0–5	7–11	15–22
Below average	Below 5/below 0	Below 7	Below 15

Clasp your hands behind your neck, raise your head and chest off the ground as high as possible, and hold that position for three seconds. Ask your partner to measure the distance to the nearest inch between your chin and the floor. Enter this value on the Lab Activity 2.1: Your Physical Fitness Profile sheet.

Nutritional Assessment

Numerous IBM- and Apple/ Macintosh-compatible software programs are available to analyze your dietary intake accurately over a three- to seven-day period. Regardless of the software program you choose, it will be necessary to record your dietary intake (food and drink) carefully over a three- to seven-day period, making note of portion sizes, brand names of products whenever they are available, specific fast food products, and other specific information that you will code later according to the specifications of the software manual. It is also possible to provide a fairly accurate analysis of your nutritional habits by completing Lab Activity 8.2: Do You Meet the U.S. Government Dietary Recommendations at the end of chapter 8. This lab activity will also help you identify major food and fluid intake problems as well as factors contributing to your control of body weight and fat.

Body Composition Assessment

Numerous tests are available to measure your body's composition. Height-weight charts, discussed in chapter 9, are perhaps the least accurate method of providing an indication of associated health risks except for the very obese individual. Three practical tests provide an accurate assessment of your body composition and the associated health risks based on body fat content. Record your scores on the Lab Activity 2.1 sheet.

Fitness Heroes

John Fitzgerald Kennedy had a strong interest in physical fitness. It started with touch football games on the lawn of the Kennedy estate in Massachusetts and continued throughout his life. When he was elected president in 1960, he made physical fitness an American concern. His article, "The Fat American," appeared in the *Journal of the National Association for Health, Physical Education, and Dance* and attracted national attention. He formed the President's Council on Youth Fitness and appointed its first director. Within a very short time, standardized fitness testing was implemented throughout the United States in elementary, middle, and secondary schools. Test results revealed a tremendous need for regular exercise designed to improve strength and endurance in the arms, shoulders, and abdominal area; improve cardiorespiratory endurance; and lower the percent of body fat. The new emphasis on fitness was a much needed shot in the arm for school-based physical education programs and for the health of our nation. This council remains in existence today and plays a major role in the promotion of physical fitness in U.S. schools.

When President Kennedy was assassinated, the nation lost a great leader and the world of fitness lost the single highest official of all time who finally realized the importance of fitness to the health of a nation. No president has focused similar attention on the importance of physical fitness since. ✦

Behavioral Change and Motivational Strategies

Roadblock	Behavioral Change Strategy
Like many other men and women, you may not like undergoing a medical examination. The setting may make you feel so uncomfortable and embarrassed that you will do almost anything to avoid it.	These feelings are quite natural. Fortunately, there are ways to make the experience less traumatic. Consider calling your physician and say that you want to begin an exercise program and would feel better knowing that there are no medical contraindications. Your physician may know enough about your medical history to give you the green light over the phone. If not, make an appointment with your physician to have the tests you want completed, and make it clear that these are the only tests you need at this time and that you are not interested in other examination procedures.

You may detest running and would never choose that form of aerobic exercise. In fact, the mere thought of running 1.5 miles to complete the aerobic test may be a turn-off and destroy your motivation to begin a program.

Many people dislike running as a form of exercise. Fortunately, there are other valuable aerobic choices as beneficial as jogging or running. You also can assess your cardiorespiratory endurance without running. Review the Harvard Step test described in this chapter. Find a bench and complete the test in your gym. Many step classes at fitness centers use this method as a complete workout. You can complete the test alone. If you dislike physical tests, avoid both the 1.5-mile and Harvard Step tests, and select an aerobic exercise program that has a beginner's level and slowly progresses toward more advanced fitness.

You are self-conscious about the amount of fat on your body and do not want anyone to measure you with skinfold calipers.

This is a common concern, and you have the right to avoid such tests of body composition. Consider some options that will still provide you with some type of assessment.

1. Borrow a skinfold caliper for an hour or two and ask a relative or a close friend to take the measurements.

2. Find equipment to perform hydrostatic (underwater) weighing. A school physical education or biology department might have this kind of equipment. Then you need only put on a bathing suit and submerse yourself in water.

3. Avoid any specific test of body composition, and apply your own *pinch an inch* method to various body parts. If you are pinching an inch, you are now aware that you possess too much fat in that area. If this occurs in more than two areas, it is an indication that your total body fat is too high.

List other roadblocks you are experiencing that seem to be reducing the effectiveness of the fitness assessment phase of your program.

Now list the behavior change strategies that can help you overcome these roadblocks. Read ahead in chapter 3 for help with behavior change and motivational techniques.

1. _____

2. _____

3. _____

1. _____

2. _____

3. _____

Figure 2.1 ✦ Nomogram for BMI

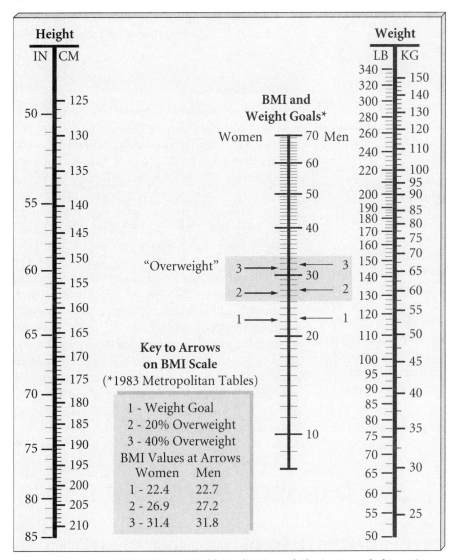

Source: B.T. Burton and W.R. Fosters, Health Implications of Obesity, *Journal of Amercian Dietetic Association* (1985) 85: 1117–1121. ©1988. Metropolitan Life Insurance Company. All rights reserved. Reproduced by permission.

1. **Body mass index (BMI)** provides a more sensitive indicator of body composition and health risks than body weight. You can determine your BMI using Figure 2.1 by placing a "dot" at your exact height in inches in the column to the left and another dot at your exact weight in pounds in the column to the right, drawing a straight line to connect the two dots, and recording the number where the line intersects the vertical column in the middle. Keep in mind that weights and heights are determined without clothing.

   Example: A college woman five feet, six inches tall and weighing 185 pounds will have a BMI of 29.82. Table 2.7 on page 30 provides an interpretation of this score along with values to categorize men and women as underweight, acceptable in weight, overweight, severely overweight, and morbidly obese.

2. **Waist-to-hip ratio** provides an indication of the way you store fat. Obese people who tend to store large amounts of fat in the abdominal area, rather than around the hips and thighs, are at higher risk for coronary heart disease, high blood pressure,

> **Body mass index (BMI)** A method of determining overweight and obesity by dividing body weight (in kilograms) by height (in meters) squared; this method is considered superior to height/weight table ranges.

Table 2.7 ✦ BMI Values for Men and Women

	Men	Women
Underweight	< 20.7	< 19.1
Acceptable weight	20.7 to 27.8	19.1 to 27.3
Overweight	27.8	27.3
Severe overweight	31.1	32.3
Morbid obesity	45.4	44.8

Source: From the 1983 Metropolitan Life Insurance Company tables, designed by B.T. Burton and W.R. Foster, Health Implications of Obesity, an NIH Consensus Development Conference, *Journal of the American Dietetic Association* (1985) 85: 1117–1121. Copyright © 1983. Metropolitan Life Insurance Company. All rights reserved. Reproduced by permission.

congestive heart failure, strokes, and diabetes. To provide an accurate and practical indicator, the waist-to-hip ratio test was devised by a panel of scientists appointed by the National Academy of Sciences and the Dietary Guidelines Advisory Council for the U.S. Departments of Agriculture and Health and Human Services. If the waist-to-hip ratio is 1.0 or higher in men or .85 or higher in women, the panel recommends weight loss.

Example: John has a 40" waist and a 38" hip. His ratio of 1.05 (40 ÷ 38) is indicative of increased risk for disease.

3. **Skinfold measures** at various sites on the body provide an accurate indicator of your percent of body fat. The four-site skinfold test described in chapter 9 is designed for both college men and women.

Conclusion

Your fitness profile is complete. You can now evaluate your physical fitness in absolute terms (Are you satisfied with your levels of each component?) or in relative terms (Are you happy with how you compare with others?). Wellness requires information. Where are you now? Where do you want to be? How can you get there? Now that you have identified your current fitness level, you can decide on what goals you need to set for yourself. For example, if you are not satisfied with your cardiorespiratory fitness, read the remainder of this book with a view toward improving that component. You can do the same for muscular strength and endurance, flexibility, or body composition. This book contains the means for you to be successful at enhancing your level of physical fitness. All you need to do is apply them. Always keep in mind that improving one aspect of your health or fitness should not result in the decline of another component. It is important to strive for a balance in all components of physical fitness.

$\mathcal{S}$UMMARY

The Medical Evaluation

Not all experts agree whether everyone starting an exercise program should obtain a medical evaluation. Even when there is agreement in this area, experts may disagree concerning exactly what the examination should entail. We recommend that a medical examination is necessary after the age of 45 and at any age when identifiable risk or disease is present. The contents of the evaluation depend on the age of the patient and the symptoms present and may include taking a medical history, measurement of blood pressure, listening to the sound of the heart and lungs, determining resting pulse rate, having a chest X-ray, administering a resting ECG and a graded exercise test, and administering blood tests for blood fats and the ratio between high- and low-density lipoproteins. We also feel that all readers should decide whether they need a medical examination before they start exercise testing and an exercise program based on their knowledge of their personal health, present physical fitness level, and medical history.

The Fitness Appraisal

The ideal physical fitness appraisal should include measures of cardiorespiratory endurance, muscular strength and endurance, flexibility, and body composition. Specific tests are available that allow the individual to obtain an accurate assessment in each of these areas: cardiorespiratory endurance can be measured by the 1.5-mile test or the Harvard Step test; muscular strength by the bench press, arm curl, and leg press; muscular endurance by sit ups, bar dips, and pull ups or the flexed-arm hang; flexibility by the shoulder reach, trunk flexion, and trunk extension tests; nutritional analysis through the use of numerous software programs or by manually recording and analyzing dietary intake; and body composition by determining your BMI, waist-to-hip ratio, or skinfold measures at four specific sites. For an accurate evaluation of your level of physical fitness, it is important to give your best effort on each test, while staying alert to physical signs of overexertion. See Tables 2.8 and 2.9 for sample assessments.

Table 2.8 ✦ An Assessment Example: 42-Year-Old Bill

Bill has been sedentary for most of his adult life. Now, approaching the coronary-prone years, he has decided that an ounce of prevention is worth a pound of cure. Consequently, Bill spoke with his physician about beginning a regular program of exercise. His physician classified Bill in the C category of the American College of Sports Medicine's guidelines for exercise testing because Bill was over 35 years old, physically inactive, and was without coronary heart disease or its risk factors. As a result, Bill needed a complete medical exam. Bill related his medical history as part of this examination: There was little CHD in his family; there were a few cases of hypertension, but most family members had lived well into their eighties. He was not currently ill or taking any medication, did not smoke, and had no physical disabilities of which he was aware. His physician tested Bill's blood pressure (135/85), took his pulse (80), listened to his lungs and heart, took a chest X-ray, tested his blood for blood fats and for the ratio of high- and low-density lipoproteins, and administered a resting electrocardiogram and a stress test. All these procedures determined Bill to be within normal limits.

Bill's physician then recommended he consult with a fitness expert and gave him the telephone number of the local university physical education department. Bill was referred to the fitness program conducted at the university, and an appointment was made for him to be screened.

The screening consisted of Bill's completing a 1.5-mile run/walk on the track to determine his cardiorespiratory endurance; several weight-lifting one-repetition maximum tests to determine his muscular strength; sit ups and pull ups to determine his muscular endurance; shoulder reach, trunk flexion, and trunk extension tests to determine his degree of flexibility; skinfold tests to determine his degree of body fat; and the Illinois agility run to determine how much agility he possessed. The results of these tests were as follows:

1. **Run/walk:** 14 minutes, 10 seconds (fair)
2. **1-RM tests**

   Bench press: 130 pounds (below average)

   Standing press: 90 pounds (below average)

   Curl: 65 pounds (below average)

   Leg press: 325 pounds (average)
3. **Sit ups:** 30 (below average)
4. **Pull ups:** 2 (below average)
5. **Shoulder reach:** 2/0 inches (below average)
6. **Trunk flexion:** 5 inches (below average)
7. **Trunk extension:** 6 inches (below average)
8. **Skinfold:** 18% (average body fat)
9. **Agility:** 19.5 seconds (average)

Based on these results, Bill's exercise program emphasized cardiorespiratory endurance (by beginning a walking program, progressing to run/walks, and leading up to jogging), development of greater upper body strength (with bench press, standing press, and curl exercises with low weights progressing to greater weights), muscular endurance (sit ups beginning with just the head and shoulders lifting off the ground and progressing to the whole upper body lifting, with increasing repetitions, and pull ups beginning with flexed-arm hangs), and flexibility (with hamstring, shoulder and chest, and spine and waist stretches).

Source: From Jerrold S. Greenberg, *Physical Fitness: A Wellness Approach* (Englewood Cliffs, NJ: Prentice-Hall, 1989).

Table 2.9 ✦ An Assessment Example: 66-Year-Old Joan

Joan was older than Bill, and her fitness profile differed in some respects. Her physician classified Joan in the D category of the American College of Sports Medicine's guidelines for exercise testing because she was asymptomatic, physically inactive, had no coronary diseases, but did have a high cholesterol level and elevated blood pressure readings. Joan's medical history was without incident except for her 20-year-old cigarette smoking habit, and her screening revealed only the concern for her hypercholesteremia and hypertension.

She too was put in touch with the local university's physical fitness program. When tested, her results were:

1. **Run/walk:** 21 minutes (poor)
2. **Sit ups:** 31 (below average)
3. **Shoulder reach:** 3 inches (average)
4. **Trunk flexion:** 8 inches (average)
5. **Trunk extension:** 16 inches (average)
6. **Skinfold:** 32% (above-average fat)

It was determined to withhold the muscular strength testing at this time, since the concern was to devise a program to respond to the hypercholesteremia and the hypertension. Consequently, an aerobic exercise program would be needed, and to develop one required a determination of Joan's present endurance fitness. It was decided to test flexibility as well, since the program the fitness experts had in mind had a tendency to decrease flexibility.

The analysis of Joan's fitness testing concluded she needed to develop cardiovascular and muscular endurance and decrease her body fat. Her flexibility was fine.

Based on these findings, a program was developed to get Joan jogging. Jogging has a tendency to burn up calories, strengthen muscles, improve the ratio of high- and low-density lipoproteins, and decrease blood pressure. Since Joan's run/walk test placed her in the poor category, she was instructed to walk 4 days a week for a distance that did not exhaust her (perhaps 1.5 miles initially) and gradually work up to a slow jog after several weeks or months. When she could begin jogging would be determined by how Joan felt walking and her heart rate response.

Prior to jogging, however, Joan was instructed to walk some and jog some of her route. The program then progressed gradually from walking, to walking some and jogging some, to jogging. Joan was told that even if she stayed at the walking stage and could do that while maintaining her target heart rate, she would be benefitting physically.

In addition to the walk/run program, Joan was instructed on which stretches to do before and after each exercise session to maintain a satisfactory level of flexibility.

Since it has been found that regular exercisers tend not to smoke cigarettes, it was hoped that Joan would give up her habit. In particular, aerobic exercise is incompatible with cigarette smoking. However, to be assured to be responding to Joan's high cholesterol and blood pressure, her physician recommended she enroll in a stop-smoking program and put her in touch with a registered dietitian who would develop a diet for her.

All things considered, Joan was well on her way to taking greater control of her health. With the support of loved ones, the fitness program personnel, the dietitian, the stop-smoking staff, and her physician, we can expect that Joan's health will soon improve—especially if she is committed to that goal.

Source: From Jerrold S. Greenberg, *Physical Fitness: A Wellness Approach* (Englewood Cliffs, NJ: Prentice-Hall, 1989).

Lab Activity 2.1

Your Physical Fitness Profile

INSTRUCTIONS: *As you complete each test, place your score where indicated. Consult the tables on standards for each test, and check the appropriate rating in the column to the right. Summarize your fitness profile by completing section VII.*

✦ **I. Cardiorespiratory fitness**

    A. 1.5-mile test

        Score _____

        Rating (check one)

        _____ Very poor

        _____ Poor

        _____ Fair

        _____ Good

        _____ Excellent

        _____ Superior

    B. Harvard step test

        Index _____

        Rating (check one)

        _____ Poor

        _____ Low average

        _____ Average

        _____ Good

        _____ Excellent

✦ **II. Muscular strength**

    A. Bench press

        Amount lifted _____

        Rating (check one)

        _____ Optimal

        _____ Above optimal

        _____ Below optimal

B. Standing press

Amount lifted _____

Rating (check one)

_____ Optimal

_____ Above optimal

_____ Below optimal

C. Curl

Amount lifted _____

Rating (check one)

_____ Optimal

_____ Above optimal

_____ Below optimal

D. Leg press

Amount lifted _____

Rating (check one)

_____ Optimal

_____ Above optimal

_____ Below optimal

✦ III. Muscular endurance

A. Abdominal

Number of sit ups _____

Rating (check one)

_____ Excellent

_____ Good

_____ Average

_____ Low

_____ Poor

B. Arm and shoulder

Number of pull ups or dips _____

Rating (check one)

_____ Excellent

_____ Good

_____ Average

_____ Poor

✦ IV. Flexibility

A. Shoulder reach

Score in inches _____

Rating (check one)

_____ Above average

_____ Average

_____ Below average

Lab Activity 2.1 *(continued)*
Your Physical Fitness Profile

B. Trunk flexion

Score in inches _____   Rating (check one)

_____ Above average

_____ Average

_____ Below average

C. Trunk extension

Score in inches _____   Rating (check one)

_____ Above average

_____ Average

_____ Below average

✦ **V. Nutrition**

A. List the deficiency areas identified:

✦ **VI. Body composition**

A. Body mass index (BMI) _____   Rating (check one)

_____ Underweight

_____ Acceptable weight

_____ Overweight

_____ Severe overweight

_____ Morbid obesity

B. Waist-to-hip ratio _____   Rating (check one)

_____ High; weight loss indicated

_____ Normal

C. Percent of body fat _____

Rating (check one)

_____ Very low fat

_____ Low fat

_____ Ideal fat

_____ Above ideal fat

_____ Over fat

_____ High fat

◆ **VII. Summary**

A. List those components of physical fitness for which you rated

1. Above average

2. Average

3. Below average

Lab Activity 2.2

Determining Your Resting and Exercise Heart Rate

INSTRUCTIONS: *Resting and exercise heart rate can often provide useful information about your fitness level and training method. It is therefore important to learn how to obtain these measures accurately by use of these steps.*

1. Lie down for 15 minutes in a comfortable place. Be sure not to eat or drink for at least 3 hours before starting this activity. If you have not given up smoking, do not smoke for at least 30 minutes prior to starting this activity.

2. After the rest period and while you are still lying down, take your pulse at the carotid artery on either side of the neck or use the radial pulse at the thumb side of your wrist. Since your thumb has its own pulse and will cause inaccurate readings, use only the fingers to find and count the pulse. Count for an entire minute. The resulting number is your resting heart rate.

3. To determine your postexercise heart rate, stop at the end of your next aerobic workout and take your carotid or radial pulse for only 6 seconds. Add a 0 to determine the number of beats per minute. The 30- and 60-second pulse count should not be used at the end of a workout since the heart slows down rapidly during that lengthy period.

4. Record your resting and postexercise pulse below.

Date_____   Date_____

Resting heart rate _____   Resting heart rate _____

Postexercise heart rate_____   Postexercise heart rate_____

Date_____   Date_____

Resting heart rate _____   Resting heart rate _____

Postexercise heart rate_____   Postexercise heart rate_____

5. Repeat this activity each month to measure your progress. Your resting heart rate will continue to decline as you become more aerobically fit. This is a direct result of an increase in both stroke volume (more blood pumped per beat) and cardiac output (more blood pumped per minute). Later you can use the postexercise method to determine whether your aerobic workout is elevating your heart rate above the target level.

3

BEHAVIORAL CHANGE AND MOTIVATIONAL TECHNIQUES

Chapter Objectives

By the end of this chapter, you should be able to:

1. Discuss the importance of psychosocial lifestyle factors such as locus of control, social support, and self-esteem in deciding on a fitness program.

2. Describe several techniques that researchers have demonstrated to be effective in helping people achieve their fitness goals.

3. List several means of improving the chances of maintaining a physical fitness program once one has been started.

4. Modify a physical fitness program in the face of obstacles so it need not be interrupted.

THE COMEDIAN HENNY Youngman tells of a man who told his psychiatrist, "Doc, I have a guilt complex," to which his doctor replied, "You ought to be ashamed of yourself!" We do not want to shame you into regularly engaging in physical activity. That would be dysfunctional, something like a physical education instructor who makes physical activity so distasteful that students are repelled by exercise for the remainder of their lives. Instead we want you to appreciate the benefits of being physically fit and then to decide for yourself whether to engage in regular exercise. If you decide to do that, we can show you how to begin a program and the best way to continue participating in it over an extended period of time.

PSYCHOSOCIAL FACTORS TO CONSIDER

To plan an exercise program you need to know something about yourself: about your motivations, about your perceptions of the amount of control you have over your life, about the degree to which you associate with other people, and about the confidence you have in yourself. This chapter makes the importance of this information clear.

Locus of Control

Some people believe they can control events in their lives. This construct is called one's **locus of control.** People who believe this construct possess an internal locus of control or internality. People who do not believe in the construct possess an external locus of control or externality.

Externals believe that the course of their lives are a matter of luck, fate, or chance or of what powerful others do. This is more than merely an academic distinction. If you do not believe you control events in your life, you are apt to adopt a laissez faire attitude. Relative to physical fitness, you might believe that whether you are in good shape is a function of luck or of genetic makeup. There is no sense in engaging in an exercise program if you do not control your fitness level.

Internals believe that what they get is, for the most part, a result of what they do. Therefore internals will probably learn a good deal about exercise and physical fitness and plan a program in which they can participate. An internal locus of control is very important if you are serious about becoming physically fit and maintaining that level of fitness. Complete Lab Activity 3.1: Locus of Control Assessment at the end of this chapter to determine your locus of control. If you score as an external, make a list of the parts of your life that you influence. Then read that list daily to change your focus. In addition, take some measures before beginning an exercise program (for example, your pulse rate and weight) and measure those variables again after engaging in exercise for several weeks. The change will reinforce the notion that you can influence your body rather than resigning yourself to being a victim of your habits or of your genetic makeup.

Social Isolation

We all need to interact with other people. Researchers have found that the social support we have actually helps prevent us from getting ill and enhances the quality of our lives. Conversely, not having significant others with whom to share our joys and sorrows causes ill health or **social isolation**. Refer to Lab Activity 3.2: Alienation Assessment at the end of the chapter for a social isolation scale that will help you determine whether this is a problem for you.

If you find you need to improve your social network, structure your fitness program accordingly. Consider joining an exercise club, a health spa, the YMCA or YWCA, or Jewish Community Center. You might meet people there with whom you can become friendly. Participation in organized sports (at levels suited to your skill and experience) can also provide an opportunity to meet people. Playing in leagues and tournaments (team as well as individual) is another avenue for alleviating social isolation. You should not ignore your social self when structuring your fitness program. To do so is to endanger your health and wellness.

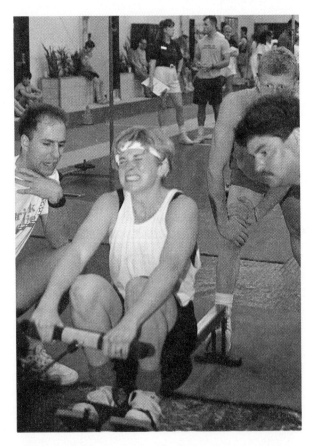

Having friends who encourage you can be an important part of achieving your fitness goals. (Photo Courtesy of the Aspen Hill Club.)

Self-Esteem

What you think of yourself, no matter whether that perception is accurate, influences your fitness, health, and wellness. If you do not think well of yourself, you might not believe you can become fit. You may lack confidence, think you are genetically inferior, or think you have so far to go that beginning a fitness program is futile.

In particular, what you think of your body, your bodily self-esteem (sometimes called **body cathexis**) will affect your health and fitness. Lab Activity 3.3: Body Self-Esteem Assessment at the end of this chapter is a scale to help you determine your bodily self-esteem.

There are parts of your body with which you are satisfied and parts with which you are dissatisfied. Be proud of those parts about which you scored 4 or 5 in Lab Activity 3.3: Body Self-Esteem Assessment. Let others know how proud of them you are, but not in a boastful way. Do not fret about those parts of your body to which you assigned a 1 or 2 value. You can improve them, at least many of them, and thereby feel better about yourself. For example, if you are dissatisfied with your waist, there are exercises you can do to strengthen the muscles in your waist. We discuss these in the chapter on muscular strength and endurance. There are even strategies that are useful for those body parts you assigned a 1 or 2 value that cannot be changed, such as your nose. These are body parts about which you need to become more accepting. One effective way of doing this is to recognize that things could be worse. Volunteering for an organization that caters to the needs of the physically challenged or the socioeconomically disadvantaged can help you put your concern about your nose, for example, in proper perspective.

STRATEGIES FOR ACHIEVING YOUR FITNESS GOALS

There is a good deal of research identifying effective ways of achieving your fitness goals. Before the appropriate techniques can be applied, however, you must first identify the goals.

Goal Setting

In determining your fitness goals, adhere to these guidelines.

Diversity Issues

Self-Esteem and Exercise

Diversity exists among people in all communities with regard to self-esteem. A person's self-esteem and self-perception is affected by all aspects of his or her life, including culture, upbringing, education, and life experiences.

Self-esteem plays a big role in physical fitness. People with very low self-esteem, for instance, may feel that exercising is futile and that they have no control over their bodies. They may compare themselves with others and feel that they do not measure up. People with high self-esteem, however, might consider themselves good at sports and coordinated or might be happy with their body structure. They understand that while some of their peers have certain abilities, those abilities may not be any more impressive than their own.

While it might be difficult for people with low self-esteem to begin a fitness program, they will find, in most cases, that a fitness program will improve their self-esteem. Whether the goal is to lose weight, build muscle, or just feel healthy, fitness can help to achieve these goals. When goals are achieved, self-esteem is improved. ✦

Be Realistic Jorge was playing tennis with a friend one pleasant summer day. The sun was out; the birds were chirping; and the water in the creek alongside the tennis court was gently caressing the rocks as it moved downstream. You couldn't ask for a better day, that is, unless you were Jorge. His game was off. "Enough is enough," Jorge thought when he netted still another backhand. Before anyone realized what was happening, his tennis racket flew over the fence,

Locus of control The degree to which you believe you are in control of events in your life.

Social isolation The lack of other people with whom to discuss important matters relevant to your life.

Body cathexis Physical self-esteem, how highly you regard your physical self.

above the trees beyond, and landed in the middle of the creek. When last seen, the racket was heading downstream, never again to be used.

Some of you may know a Jorge or you may be one. The problem is in being realistic. Some of us are has-been athletes expecting to perform at the level we could when we were younger and practiced daily. Others of us are never-beens with grand delusions and dreams that will never be fulfilled. Do not fall into either trap when setting your fitness goals. Be realistic in what you can attain and about the time it will take you to attain it. If your goals are unobtainable, you will become frustrated and give up on physical fitness altogether.

In fact, it is wise in the beginning to set goals that are easy to achieve. In that way, when you do attain them, you will reinforce fitness behavior and be more likely to achieve subsequent goals.

Periodically Assess Once you decide on your fitness goals, periodically assess how you are meeting those goals. If you conclude that you are making progress in an appropriate amount of time, keep doing what you are doing. If your assessment indicates problems meeting your goals, it is time to make adjustments. Maybe you need to exercise longer, more intensely, or more frequently. Without periodically assessing your program, you will not identify changes that are needed to help you achieve your fitness goals.

Behavioral Change Techniques

Among the more effective techniques you can employ in meeting your fitness goals are the use of social support, contracting, reminder systems, gradual programming, tailoring, chaining, and covert techniques.

Social Support This is just another way of saying you need other people to encourage and help you. It is much easier to adopt a habit of regular exercise, or any habit for that matter, if you are encouraged by others. If you can get someone else to exercise with you, to ask you daily whether you have exercised, or to buy you a piece of exercise clothing or equipment periodically, you will be more apt to stick with your regimen. To begin, make a list of people you think would be willing to assist you and discuss with them how they can help.

Contracting One way to use social support is to develop a contract to achieve a certain exercise goal and to have it witnessed by someone else. If that person then helps you periodically to assess your progress, you will be more likely to be successful. Figure 3.1 is a sample of an effective contract. It identifies the *behavior goal*, the *date* when it should be achieved (and assessed), and the *reward* for achieving the goal as well as the *punishment* for not achieving it. Rewards can be

Figure 3.1 ✦ Fitness Contract

I _____ desire to improve my physical fitness
        (your name)
because _____ .
                          (the reason)
I have decided I intend to _____
                                    (your goal)
by _____ . If I achieve this goal, I will reward myself
      (date)
by _____ . If I do not achieve my
                  (the reward)
goal, I will punish myself by _____ .
                                    (the punishment)

_____   _____
      (your signature)   (today's date)

_____   _____
      (witness signature)   (today's date)

going to the movies, buying something you have wanted for a long time, or a night free of school work. Punishments might include not watching television for a week or not eating your favorite snack for several days. Although rewards are more effective than punishments in controlling behavior, punishments have a place as well. Although contracts have been found to work best when there is a witness, they can also be effective if you merely contract with yourself.

Reminder Systems One way to remember things is to make a note of them. Reminder notes will help you remember to exercise, especially if you leave the notes in places where you cannot miss them, for example, on the doors of bathrooms and refrigerators or on the bathroom mirror. You can also use notes in appointment books and calendars as reminders.

Gradual Programming Too often people, who have never exercised regularly or who have not exercised regularly for some time, expect to be able to run a mile in under four minutes. Less obvious, but no less unrealistic for many people, is the goal of exercising every other day when they have been sedentary for years or that of exercising intensely when they have not done so for a while. Giving up the sedentary life *cold turkey* may be extremely difficult. If it is, do not fret. Instead use a graduated plan in which you start slowly and gradually increase both frequency and intensity. In fact, to prevent injury, fitness experts recommend graduated plans even for those who are already highly fit. For example, runners are warned not to increase their distance by more than 10 percent a week, and weight trainers not to increase the weight they lift by more than 5 percent. You can even use graduated plans to study more, to change your eating habits, or for other behaviors you have been meaning to change.

Tailoring No two people are alike. This is not the most provocative of statements, yet we sometimes act as though we do not know this simple fact. When you adopt a wholesale exercise program designed for a group, without adjusting that program to your own needs and circumstances, you are increasing the likelihood you will soon stop exercising regularly. Some people are free to exercise in the mornings, others in the evenings. Some people are in better physical condition than others. People vary in their choice of meal times. Some are more committed to exercise than others. We could go on and on, but the point is that any program of regular exercise must be tailored to the individual. We will present exercise activities in

later chapters, but you must choose which ones to do and when, how frequently, and how intensely to do them for your program to be successful.

Chaining In chaining, one behavior is linked to a previous one and that to a previous one, and so on like links in a chain. You can use chaining to help you achieve your fitness goals. To adopt a behavior, such as exercising regularly, you want to have as few links as possible between the decision to exercise and actually engaging in a fitness activity. To demonstrate, let us look at two people, U.R. Wrong and I.M. Right.

U.R. Wrong decides to exercise at about 5:30 in the afternoon. So U.R. rushes home and starts gathering exercise clothes. In one drawer are gym shorts and socks. In another drawer is a shirt. Sneakers are under the bed in another room. Then U.R. looks for the car keys since he needs to drive to the track to jog. The track is 10 minutes away. On the way there, U.R. realizes the car needs gas and stops to get some. Finally, U.R. arrives at the track and is ready to exercise.

I.M. Right decides to exercise at the same time of day. However, I.M. prepares beforehand. All the clothes needed for later are left on the bed in the morning. I.M. decides to run around the neighborhood instead of the track, so that all that is required at 5:30 P.M. is to come home, dress, step outside the front door, and exercise.

If we consider each behavior needed to exercise as a link in a chain, we see that U.R. Wrong has many more links. The more links, the more difficult it is to exercise, and the more likely it is not to happen. The trick is to decrease the links for a behavior you want to adopt and to increase the links for a behavior you want to give up (for example, cigarette smoking).

Covert Techniques Some people are so inactive or busy that it is difficult for them to engage in regular exercise. Three techniques can help these people change behavior without requiring them to do anything physically. These are called *covert techniques*.

1. **Covert rehearsal** This procedure requires that you imagine yourself exercising regularly. Your image must be extremely vivid; notice all the details (what you are wearing, the weather, the location), smell the atmosphere, feel the bodily sensations, and so on. Being able to imagine yourself exercising makes it more likely that you will actually exercise. You will have desensitized yourself to the image of you exercising so that seeing yourself exercising will not seem foreign to you.

2. **Covert modeling** For some of us, even imagining ourselves exercising is difficult. It is just not us. If that is the case with you, there is still hope. First identify someone else you *can* envision exercising. Next imagine, as vividly as you can, that person exercising. Once that image is clear in your mind, substitute yourself for that person. Model the image of you exercising after the image of that person exercising. After a while, it will be easier for you to think of yourself as a potentially regular exerciser, and it will be more likely that you will actually become one.

3. **Covert reinforcement** When you can imagine yourself exercising, it is a good idea to reward yourself for it. The use of another image as a reward is called *covert reinforcement*. Usually a pleasant image is used as a reward (a day at the beach, a calm lake) and is allowed to surface and be focused on only after the goal image is successfully accomplished.

MAINTAINING YOUR FITNESS PROGRAM

Once you have begun a regular program of exercise, the trick is to maintain it. In addition to the methods already described, here are additional suggestions for keeping at it.

Material Reinforcement

Behavior that is rewarded tends to be repeated. Consequently, if you want to exercise regularly, reward yourself when you do. Material rewards can take many forms. For example, you might treat yourself to a trip to the beach to show off your newly toned body. Or you might buy yourself an article of clothing you have been eyeing for some time.

Social Reinforcement

Peer group pressure need not be limited to negative influences. We can use such pressure to encourage and reward desirable behavior. Take a moment to list five people whose opinions you value. Then enlist them as social reinforcers to inquire about your exercise behavior and to pat you on the back if you report exercising regularly. After a while, exercise will become part of your lifestyle, and you will no longer need to be rewarded for continuing.

Join a Group

One of the reasons Weight Watchers, Inc. is so effective in helping people lose weight is that it employs group support and positive peer pressure. It is often easier to accomplish your goals if you are working with others. You can join a health club, a local YMCA or YWCA, or a Jewish Community Center. Or you

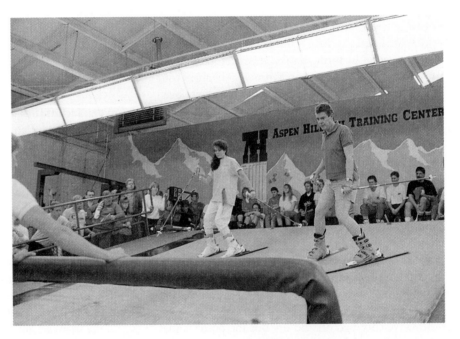

If you really want to exercise, nothing can stop you! These resourceful exercisers are training indoors for downhill skiing. (Photo Courtesy of the Aspen Hill Club.)

can organize a group of friends to exercise together at a predetermined time. You can even enroll in an exercise class at a local university or community college, or in a community program. Any group involvement will increase the likelihood of your maintaining a fitness program.

Boasting

Many people, while they were students, have had the experience of having two tests returned the same day, one on which they did well and the other on which they did not. They complained about the poor grade for days, while ignoring the test on which they did well. Many of us react this way. We relive negative experiences by repeatedly thinking about them, by being embarrassed about them over and over again, or by feeling inadequate in other ways. For positive experiences, such as getting an "A" on a test, we exhibit false modesty and say, "It was nothing." We would do better to learn from our mistakes and let them go and to relive our positive experiences and even boast about them. Of course, you do not want to be obnoxious or to be perceived of as being conceited. Yet if you run three miles daily and someone asks how far you usually run, rather than say, "Only three miles," you might say, "I'm proud to say that I run three miles regularly." Boasting in this way will help reinforce your exercise behavior.

Self-Monitoring

This is the process of observing and recording your own behavior. It is helpful to know that your fitness program is having a positive effect, that it is moving toward your goal. Remember not to expect immediate dramatic results. Assuming your exercise goal is realistic, accept small gains. Do not expect more rapid change than is warranted by the general effects of exercise and training on the body. Eventually, with persistence, you will successfully attain your goal. When you see slow but steady progress toward your goal, you will be encouraged to maintain the program.

Making It Fun

If the fitness program you designed is not fun, you selected the wrong activities. If it is not fun at least most of the time, you will not continue it for very long. We have presented so many options in this book that you should be able to find activities that accomplish your goals while providing enjoyment.

All you need to do is be selective. Think about your choices carefully, and seek help from others when that is necessary.

EXERCISING UNDER DIFFICULT CIRCUMSTANCES

If you maintain a fitness program long enough, you will undoubtedly encounter obstacles. We have selected five such obstacles to demonstrate how, if you are serious about training, your program need not be interrupted. These obstacles are traveling, being confined to a limited space, being injured, being busy, and having visitors.

Traveling

If you travel often, you should consider that when you develop your program. For example, rather than joining a local health club, you would be wise to join one with facilities throughout the country so you can exercise when you are in other cities. YMCAs and YWCAs, Jewish Community Centers, and some nationally franchised health clubs have facilities throughout the United States. In addition, select activities that take regular travel into account. You would be better off jogging, for example, than playing tennis. Jogging requires little by way of equipment or facilities and does not involve obtaining a partner. To summarize: The factors to consider if you travel often are equipment, facilities, and dependence on other people.

Being Confined to a Limited Space

If there are times when you are confined to a limited space (for example, if you are a student studying for final examinations and seldom leaving your dormitory room), you need not abandon your physical fitness program. If you have access to an exercise room, you might be fortunate enough to have treadmills, steppers, ski machines, stationary bikes, or rowers at your disposal. Since that is unlikely, you can exercise without ever leaving your office or room. For example, you can run around the room. Be sure not to run in one place since that might cause too much strain on your legs and knees. Running around the room can respond to your need for cardiorespiratory endurance. Alternatively, you can purchase a jump rope and use it in your room. You can even do some of the flexibility exercises described in chapter 7 or

Fitness Heroes

In 1984, Joan Benoit Samuelson was a world-class marathoner. She held world records and was anticipating breaking another one in the Boston Marathon, and she was preparing to run in the upcoming Olympic trials. Unfortunately, Joan was having knee problems and needed arthroscopic surgery 17 days before the trials. When her lifelong dream of winning an Olympic medal evaporated, Joan became more determined than ever. She believed that she could train for the trials by substituting another aerobic activity for the running she was unable to do, so she arranged an exercise bike so that it could be pedaled by hand. Lying on her back, Joan pedaled that exercise bike every day to get the workout she needed. When the Olympic trials were completed two weeks later, Joan stood proudly as its winner; when the Olympic medals were awarded for the first-ever women's marathon, Joan Benoit Samuelson collected a gold. ✦

perform isometric muscular strength activities. **Isometric contractions** consist of exerting a force that is equal to, or less than, that required to move an object. Therefore, the object does not move, there is no movement in the joint, and there is no change in the length of the muscle. For example, if you push against a wall, that is an isometric contraction. You can also do isotonic activities. **Isotonic contractions** consist of movement at the joint and changes in the length of the muscle. For example, if you lift weights, you are engaged in isotonic contractions. It needn't be a barbell or other weight-lifting equipment that you use. Lifting any object of sufficient weight to offer resistance will suffice. You might also be able to find someone else who also feels confined, to exercise with you. For example, rather than pushing against a

Isometric contraction Force applied to an immovable object that does not result in muscle shortening.

Isotonic contraction Shortening of the muscle in the positive phase and lengthening during the negative phase of an action.

Figure 3.2 ✦ Improving Muscular Strength with a Partner

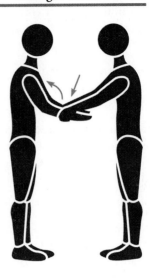

wall, you might be able to push against each other and thereby create the resistance you require (see Figure 3.2).

Being Injured

If you exercise long enough, you will inevitably experience an injury of some sort. As with any other obstacle, you can always use such an injury as an excuse not to exercise. On the other hand, you can almost always find a way to exercise around the injury. For example, injury to your leg may preclude jogging but not swimming, and one to your shoulder may eliminate a regular racquetball game but not jogging. For most injuries, common sense will dictate what you can and cannot do. For more serious fitness injuries, however, consult a professional for advice. By doing so you might prevent further damage or prolonged recovery.

Being Busy

"I don't have time to exercise. I'm too busy," sounds out like a battle cry from some people. Yet when even busy schedules are dissected, there is always enough time for participation in fitness activities. The problem is that people decide to use this time for other activities, such as watching television, partying, or talking on the telephone. It may make sense to use your time in this way. But you must realize that is your decision to make, and as with all decisions, you can change it if you so choose.

Myth and Fact Sheet

Myth	Fact
1. There are some situations in which you really have no control.	1. You have some control in all situations, even if it is only control over your own feelings and reactions.
2. Some people are born to value physical activity and others to abhor it.	2. Everyone can find some physical activity that they enjoy and that can be the basis of an effective fitness program.
3. The reason people do not achieve their fitness goals is because they do not work hard or long enough.	3. People may not achieve their fitness goals because their goals are unrealistic or unobtainable.
4. When trying to change a behavior, it is best to work at changing by yourself so you do not embarrass yourself in front of other people.	4. It is a good idea to involve other people to help you change a behavior because they can provide both support and peer pressure so you are more likely to be successful.

It seems self-destructive to say you value health and fitness but to take a long lunch instead of a short lunch and a short workout or to meet your friends at the local watering hole instead of exercising. You can find time to exercise if you really value health and fitness. In fact, exercise can rejuvenate you, make you more efficient, and provide just the break you need, both physically and mentally.

We do not mean to imply that no adjustments are necessary during particularly busy times. The operative word here, however, is *adjustment*. With the proper adjustment, you can maintain your program

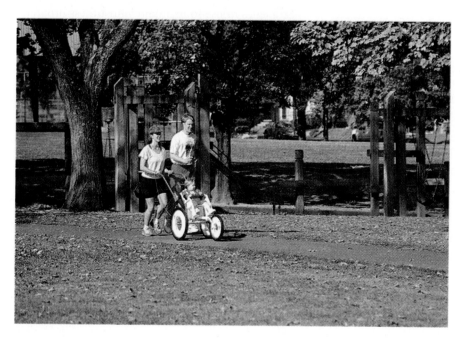

Maintaining a fitness program is possible, even in the face of obstacles. This couple is using a special stroller to take their baby on a jog. (Photo Courtesy of RunAbout, Inc.)

and resume your normal activities when the busy period passes.

Having Visitors

Suppose a friend comes to stay with you. What happens to your fitness program? Although visits from friends or relatives can encourage fitness, especially if they also exercise regularly, such visits usually interfere with your exercise program. There are several strategies you can use to maintain training during visits. If visitors are regular exercisers, there is no problem. Just exercise at the same time they do. If your visitors do not exercise regularly, help them organize short trips they can take while you exercise. Sightseeing trips are ideal. If relatives or friends are nearby, perhaps they can entertain your visitors while you exercise. What is required is some ingenuity, rather than interruption of your training.

$\mathcal{S}$UMMARY

Psychosocial Factors to Consider

To plan a fitness program, you need to know certain things about yourself. These include your locus of control, the degree to which you feel socially isolated, and your level of self-esteem (in particular, your bodily self-esteem).

Locus of control is your perception of the amount of control you exert over events in your life. If you believe you have a great deal of control, you have an internal locus of control. If you believe you have little control, you have an external locus of control.

People who are socially isolated are susceptible to illness and disease. Fitness programs can be organized to respond to social needs as well as to physical ones.

What you think of yourself and your body has significant influence on your health and wellness. Body cathexis is the esteem in which you hold your body and bodily functions. Fitness programs can improve self-esteem while they improve more traditional fitness components.

Strategies for Achieving Your Fitness Goals

Among the more effective strategies for achieving your fitness goals are goal-setting and behavior-change techniques. When you are determining fitness goals, be realistic about what is possible and periodically assess your progress toward meeting your goals. Behavior-change techniques that can be used to help you achieve your fitness goals include developing social support, contracting with yourself and others, reminder systems, gradual programming, tailoring, chaining, and the covert techniques of rehearsal, modeling, and reinforcement.

Maintaining Your Fitness Program

Strategies to use to maintain your fitness program include material and social reinforcement, joining a group, boasting, self-monitoring, and making your program fun.

Exercising under Difficult Circumstances

Periodically there will be obstacles to maintaining your fitness program. Among these are traveling, being confined to a limited space, being injured, being busy, and having visitors. In spite of these and other obstacles, adjustments can prevent interruption of your program. All that is required is a little ingenuity and determination to continue exercising.

Lab Activity 3.1

Locus of Control Assessment

INSTRUCTIONS: *Circle the answers that best describe your beliefs.*

1. a. Grades are a function of the amount of work students do.

   b. Grades depend on the kindness of the instructor.

2. a. Promotions are earned by hard work.

   b. Promotions are a result of being in the right place at the right time.

3. a. Meeting someone to love is a matter of luck.

   b. Meeting someone to love depends on going out often in order to meet many people.

4. a. Living a long life is a function of heredity.

   b. Living a long life is a function of adopting healthy habits.

5. a. Being overweight is determined by the number of fat cells you were born with or developed early in life.

   b. Being overweight depends on what and how much food you eat.

6. a. People who exercise regularly set up their schedules to do so.

   b. Some people just don't have the time for regular exercise.

7. a. Winning at poker depends on betting correctly.

   b. Winning at poker is a matter of being lucky.

8. a. Staying married depends on working at the marriage.

   b. Marital breakup is a matter of being unlucky in choosing the wrong marriage partner.

9. a. Citizens can have some influence on their governments.

   b. There is nothing a citizen can do to effect governmental function.

10. a. Being skilled at sports depends on being born well coordinated.

    b. Those skilled at sports work hard learning the skills.

11. a. People with close friends are lucky to have met people with whom to be intimate.

    b. Developing close friendships takes hard work.

12. a. Your future depends on whom you meet and on chance.

   b. Your future is up to you.

13. a. Most people are so sure of their opinions that their minds cannot be changed.

   b. A logical argument can convince most people.

14. a. People decide the direction of their lives.

   b. For the most part, we have little control over our futures.

15. a. People who do not like you just do not understand you.

   b. You can be liked by anyone you choose to like you.

16. a. You can make your life a happy one.

   b. Happiness is a matter of fate.

17. a. You evaluate feedback and make decisions based on it.

   b. You tend to be easily influenced by others.

18. a. If voters studied nominee's records, they could elect honest politicians.

   b. Politics and politicians are corrupt by nature.

19. a. Parents, teachers, and bosses have a great deal to say about your happiness and self-satisfaction.

   b. Whether you are happy depends on you.

10. a. Air pollution can be controlled if citizens get angry about it.

   b. Air pollution is an inevitable result of technological progress.

To determine your locus of control, give yourself one point for each listed response:

ITEM	RESPONSE	ITEM	RESPONSE	ITEM	RESPONSE
1	a	8	a	15	b
2	a	9	a	16	a
3	b	10	b	17	a
4	b	11	b	18	a
5	b	12	b	19	b
6	a	13	b	20	a
7	a	14	a		

Scores of 10 or above indicate you believe you are generally in control of events that affect your life, an internal locus of control. Scores below 10 indicate you believe you generally do not have control of events that affect your life, an external locus of control.

Name _____

Date _____

Lab Activity 3.2

Alienation Assessment

INSTRUCTIONS: *For each statement, place a letter in the blank space provided:*

A = strongly agree   D = disagree
B = agree   E = strongly disagree
C = uncertain

_____ **1.** Sometimes I feel all alone in the world.

_____ **2.** I do not get invited out by my friends as often as I would like.

_____ **3.** Most people today seldom seem lonely.

_____ **4.** Real friends are as easy as ever to find.

_____ **5.** One can always find friends if one is friendly.

_____ **6.** The world in which we live is basically a friendly place.

_____ **7.** There are few dependable ties between people anymore.

_____ **8.** People are just naturally friendly and helpful.

_____ **9.** I do not get to visit friends as often as I would like.

You have just completed a scale measuring a concept called *social isolation*, which is the lack of significant others (friends, relatives, and so forth) in whom to confide. To score this scale, record the number of points indicated for each of your responses:

Question 1:	A = 4	B = 3	C = 2	D = 1	E = 0
Question 2:	A = 4	B = 3	C = 2	D = 1	E = 0
Question 3:	A = 0	B = 1	C = 2	D = 3	E = 4
Question 4:	A = 0	B = 1	C = 2	D = 3	E = 4
Question 5:	A = 0	B = 1	C = 2	D = 3	E = 4
Question 6:	A = 0	B = 1	C = 2	D = 3	E = 4
Question 7:	A = 4	B = 3	C = 2	D = 1	E = 0
Question 8:	A = 0	B = 1	C = 2	D = 3	E = 4
Question 9:	A = 4	B = 3	C = 2	D = 1	E = 0

The average score for male undergraduates is 11.76 and for female undergraduates is 14.85. If you scored below the average, perhaps you should consider physical fitness activities that involve other people. In that way, you will be responding to your need for developing a social network while at the same time becoming physically fit.

Source: From Dean, Dwight G. "Alienation: Its Meaning and Measurement," *American Sociological Review* 26 (1961): 753–758. Used by permission.

Lab Activity 3.3

Body Self-Esteem Assessment

INSTRUCTIONS: *Using the scale, place the number alongside each body part or body function that represents your feelings about that part of yourself.*

✦ **Scale**

1. Have strong feelings and wish a change could somehow be made
2. Do not like, but I can put up with
3. Have no particular feelings one way or the other
4. Am satisfied with
5. Would not change, consider myself fortunate

✦ **Body Part or Function**

_____ hair	_____ appetite	_____ shoulder width
_____ hands	_____ fingers	_____ energy level
_____ nose	_____ waist	_____ shape of head
_____ wrists	_____ ears	_____ body build
_____ back	_____ weight	_____ ankles
_____ chin	_____ profile	_____ height
_____ neck	_____ chest	_____ eyes
_____ arms	_____ lips	_____ skin texture
_____ hips	_____ teeth	_____ forehead
_____ legs	_____ voice	_____ health
_____ feet	_____ posture	_____ face
_____ knees	_____ facial complexion	

✦ **Scoring**

Now sum up the point values you assigned and divide the sum by 33. Your score should fall between 1 and 5. If your score is below 2.5, you do not hold your body in high esteem. If your score is above 2.5, you do think well of your body. In particular, look at those items you assigned a 1 or a 2. Those are the parts of your body or bodily functions which you think are most in need of improvement. Concentrate on making those parts or functions better and you will think better of your body.

4

PRINCIPLES OF EXERCISE

Chapter Objectives

By the end of this chapter, you should be able to:

1. Identify the key components of a complete fitness program.

2. Apply the progressive resistance exercise (PRE) principle to your specific workout program.

3. Design formal warm-up and cool-down sessions for your exercise program.

4. Identify your target heart rate range, and determine whether your exercise program is intense enough to elevate and maintain your heart rate within that range.

5. Evaluate various exercise programs in terms of their effectiveness in developing aerobic fitness, muscular strength, muscular endurance, and flexibility, and in lowering body fat and improving lean body mass.

FOR THE PAST year, I have seen Maya in the university gymnasium almost every time I work out. It doesn't seem to matter what time I choose to exercise, she is also there exercising. Finally, I couldn't resist asking her about her exercise habits and was not surprised to learn that she trains 7 times weekly for two to three hours each session in a combination of formal aerobic classes, weight training, jogging, and stationary cycling. Nor was I surprised to hear that she has recovered from a number of overuse injuries, is tired most of the time, and suffers from aching muscles and sore knees.

Although Maya is doing a lot of things correctly, it is obvious that she is overdoing the training and does not thoroughly understand the basic principles of exercise such as the PRE principle, cross training, altering light and heavy workouts, and other key concepts that protect the body from injury and ensure safe progression to higher levels of fitness.

You may know someone like Maya. The situation is a common one that can be avoided through the application of the exercise principles discussed in this chapter.

Once the decision to begin a fitness program has been made, you are ready to master the principles that will help you achieve a higher level of aerobic (cardiorespiratory) fitness; increase muscular strength, muscular endurance, and flexibility; and help you lose or maintain body weight and fat. It is important to keep in mind that participation in an exercise program or a sport is no guarantee that your fitness level will improve unless you apply the exercise principles discussed in this chapter to your routine.

THE IDEAL EXERCISE PROGRAM

The following principles can be applied to most exercise choices to develop the five key components of health-related fitness: (1) cardiorespiratory endurance, (2) body composition (fat, muscle, and bone), (3) flexibility, (4) muscular strength, and (5) muscular endurance. Programs that improve these components also provide the health benefits discussed in chapter 1. Since motor skill-related areas such as agility, explosive power, balance, coordination, and speed are important to competitive athletes but have very little to do with health-related fitness, these components are not addressed in this chapter.

Cardiovascular Respiratory Function

Cardiovascular respiratory function, or aerobic fitness, is the most important health-related fitness component, and it should be the foundation of your complete program. It is necessary for you to choose at least one aerobic exercise activity that requires 20 to 30 minutes of continuous, uninterrupted exercise.

Preconditioning period A period of several weeks taken to prepare the body slowly for maximum effort testing or engagement in a vigorous activity or sport.

Progressive resistance exercise (PRE) The theory of gradually increasing the amount of resistance to be overcome and/or the number of repetitions each workout.

Stroke volume The amount of blood ejected per beat.

Cardiac output The volume of blood pumped by the heart per minute.

Walking (4 miles per hour [mph] or faster), jogging, running, cycling, lap swimming, aerobic dance, aerobic exercise classes, and conditioning classes are excellent aerobic choices. If you choose the sports approach to aerobic fitness, you may want to consider racketball or squash (singles with a player of similar skill), tennis or handball (singles), soccer, rugby, lacrosse, or full-court basketball. These exercise and sports activities can help prevent heart disease and other disorders and can also contribute heavily to fat and weight loss or maintenance.

Body Composition

Aerobic exercise burns more calories than do other exercises. Activities such as walking, jogging, cycling, and lap swimming allow you to exercise for longer periods of time (20 to 60+ minutes) than do activities requiring a higher intensity such as sprinting and full-court basketball. The key to fat loss through exercise is volume, not intensity. The longer you can continue to exercise, the more calories you burn and the more your fat cells shrink. To reduce body fat, lower your weight, and improve appearance, you need only three ingredients: (1) a reduced caloric intake to put yourself into a negative daily calorie balance; (2) daily aerobic exercise to burn calories and tone the body; and (3) flexibility, strength, and endurance training to add muscle mass and eliminate skin sagging. These areas are discussed in detail in chapter 9.

Flexibility, Muscular Strength, and Muscular Endurance

Improved flexibility may help reduce the incidence of both home and exercise-related injuries and allow you to perform various activities more efficiently and effectively.

Strength training will increase the strength and the size of your muscles. The additional muscle mass also elevates metabolic rate (calories burned at rest over a 24-hour period) and assists you in losing and maintaining body weight and fat. By improving the ratio of muscle mass to body fat, you are also able to exercise longer and more intensely and efficiently.

Improved muscular endurance also enables you to exercise for longer periods of time and is critical to participants in sports requiring short, all-out efforts such as sprinting, football, field hockey, and soccer. Depending on the design of your weight-training program (see chapter 6), you will develop muscular endurance and strength simultaneously.

FITNESS CONCEPTS

Study this section carefully until you can apply each concept discussed here to your specific exercise choice.

Begin with a Preconditioning Program

It requires a minimum of six to eight weeks to improve your aerobic fitness. Attempts to move quickly from one fitness level to another should be avoided in the early stages of your program. *Too much too soon* can produce muscle soreness, increase the chances of soft tissue injury (see chapter 12), and cause you to quit long before results are noticeable.

The first two to three weeks of your new program should be considered a **preconditioning period** during which you progress very slowly and enjoy each workout session. Although preconditioning will help reduce residual muscle soreness, you can expect some delayed soreness following an exercise session that involves unconditioned muscles. The time between the exercise session and the highest soreness level is somewhat dependent on your age—the older you are, the longer it takes to experience the soreness. Even with use of a preconditioning period, maximum-effort fitness tests may result in severe muscle soreness the following day.

Apply the Progressive Resistance (PRE) Principle

The **PRE principle** is simple to understand and has fascinating implications when it is correctly applied. If you gradually overload one of the body's systems (muscular, circulatory, or respiratory), it will develop additional capacity. When you repeatedly perform more strenuous exercise, the body repairs itself through elaborate cellular changes to prepare for more challenging, difficult exercise demands. Application of the PRE principle produces dramatic changes in the heart and also in the circulatory system. Regular exercise places stress on the heart, causing it to become larger and stronger and improving **stroke volume** (by pumping more blood each beat). A trained heart muscle with improved **cardiac output** pumps considerably more blood per beat and per minute, allowing the heart to slow down, beat fewer times per minute, and rest longer between beats. As the heart muscle adapts to the stress of exercise, the arteries that supply it also enlarge.

Diversity Issues

Income Level Affects Physical Activity Level

The majority of people in the United States are now aware that exercise is a crucial component to maintaining health. They also realize that physical inactivity is a serious threat to the health of the nation. Yet, some groups in our society, such as individuals in the lower-income groups, engage in exercise considerably less often than others.

The association between income level and physical inactivity makes maintaining physical health difficult for the lower-income population. Twelve percent of people aged 18 and older and 66 percent of youth aged 10 to 17 engage in vigorous physical activity that promotes the development and maintenance of cardiorespiratory fitness 3 or more days per week for 20 minutes or more per occasion. Yet only 7 percent of lower-income people are as physically active. In fact, 32 percent of people with family incomes lower than $20,000 per year do not engage in any leisure-time physical activity.

A number of factors contribute to the exercise habits of lower-income families. A higher school dropout rate in this group immediately eliminates both the required and the voluntary school exercise programs. For inner city residents, opportunities are virtually eliminated simply because there is no affordable place to exercise. For those who do not drop out, after-school hours are often needed to work and help supplement family income. Regardless of whether low-income families live in urban or rural settings, experts realize that it is difficult to influence these individuals to practice good health habits such as regular exercise and proper nutrition when they are fighting for their economic lives.

Making school and recreational facilities available at hours when low-income youth are less likely to be working is one way to improve the situation. One such successful approach to increasing the exercise habits of inner-city youth and encouraging a productive use of time during so-called high crime hours is the midnight basketball program in Chicago. Similar programs that open and supervise school and recreational facilities for as many evening and weekend hours as budgets permit are needed in both rural and urban settings. ✦

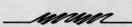

Myth and Fact Sheet

Myth	Fact
1. Aerobic development can be achieved in half the time by doubling the workout intensity.	1. Short, high-intensity workouts will improve anaerobic, not aerobic, fitness. There are no shortcuts to aerobic development.
2. More of a good thing results in added health benefits.	2. Health fitness levels for life can be achieved by following the concepts described in this text. Going too far beyond the FIT limits increases the risk of injury. Those persons who exercise beyond the health fitness level are usually seeking conditioning for athletic competition rather than health.
3. You should stretch before you begin your exercise program.	3. It is important to avoid stretching cold muscles. Light jogging or walking that results in some sweating will prepare you for your stretching session.
4. The use of a rubber suit during exercise aids weight loss.	4. In hot, humid weather, a rubber suit traps heat, prevents cooling by evaporation, raises body temperature, increases fluid loss, and contributes to heat-related injuries and illnesses such as muscle cramps, heat exhaustion, and heat stroke. Since not even one extra calorie is burned from use of such clothing, additional weight and fat loss do not occur. In winter months, perspiration may be trapped and frozen to the skin, thus causing frostbite.
5. A hat should be used when exercising.	5. Although extremely popular in tennis, baseball, and some other activities, the value of a hat depends on the type you choose. Hats help keep sun off the face, reduce glare, and allow you to see better. A hat with an open top (visor) should be used in hot, humid weather since considerable heat loss and cooling occurs through the head. In cold weather, a full hat is recommended to prevent heat loss.

Although everyone starts at a different conditioning level, let us examine what happens to your body when you begin an exercise program. You start the program at a certain functioning, or conditioning, level (level A in Figure 4.1). During and immediately after your first workout, this conditioning level temporarily declines to point B. You are now actually in worse shape, in terms of physical capacity to exercise, than you were before the workout. During the recovery phase, however, tissue will rebuild beyond your original level of conditioning to point C. You are now able to perform more work than you could before you began your exercise program with no more effort. You are also in better physical condition 24 hours later than you were before you completed your first workout. Repetition of this simple process will lead to continued improvement of conditioning levels, as indicated in Figure 4.1 by A–2, A–3, and A–4, providing you follow certain basic guidelines:

- Exercise must be sufficiently strenuous to cause an initial decrease in the conditioning level; the depth of the valley (A to B) and the corresponding increase (B to C) in Figure 4.1 is in proportion to the intensity and duration of your workout.

- Sufficient time must be allowed for recovery; improvement will not occur and conditioning will suffer if your second workout is performed before the recovery phase is complete (48 hours for strength training and 18 to 24 hours for aerobic and other workouts). Failure

Figure 4.1 ✦ Concept of Work Hypertrophy. (A) preexercising functioning level; (B) functioning level following exercise; (C) elevated functioning level following recovery; (A-2) elevated functioning level at the proper point to reconvene exercise; (A-3 and A-4) elevated functioning levels following additional workout and rest periods.

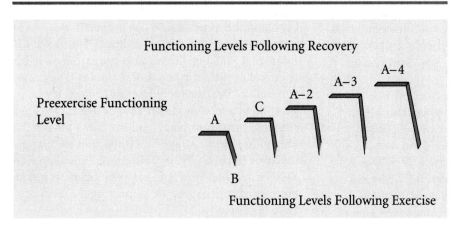

to follow this principle of recuperation can lead to overuse injuries and reduce the benefits of your workout.

- The next workout must occur within 24 to 48 hours; a greater time lapse will cause your conditioning level to decline.

If you apply this concept to any training program, improved conditioning is guaranteed. Even strength training (see chapter 6) uses this approach to acquire muscle mass and increase strength and endurance.

The resistance principle also applies to the skeletal system. Gradual stress to the bones stimulates the accumulation of calcium and other minerals. In the adult years, **osteoporosis** occurs. This process happens to astronauts freed from the stress of resisting gravity. It is also very common in postmenopausal women. When you walk, jog, run, or perform other aerobic exercise, the force of your feet hitting the ground sends an important signal to your body to maintain bone density. At this point, more of the calcium consumed in your diet reaches the orthopedic system. Other key factors that are also important in the prevention and treatment of osteoporosis are discussed in chapters 8 and 14.

Exercise Four Times a Week for 30 Minutes at Your Target Heart Rate (THR)

Although results can be attained without lengthy workouts, there are no shortcuts. Ten-second con-

tractions, massage, mechanical devices, steam baths, three-minute slimnastic programs, and other such approaches vary from slightly effective to worthless.

To receive the health-related benefits of exercise, you must apply the FIT principle:

Frequency	3 to 4 times weekly
Intensity	at or above your target heart rate
Time	20 to 30 minutes of continuous exercise

Frequency of exercise is the key to the success of your program. Exercising three to five times per week rather than one hard workout per week will greatly increase the chances of meeting your training objectives. Frequency is also strongly related to weight and fat loss, cardiovascular development, and preventive disease. One 30-minute session will not transform you into a lean, mean, muscle machine, but 3 to 4 sessions weekly for 6 to 12 months will do wonders. Regularity is also a critical factor in changing the way your body handles fats (cholesterol and triglycerides).

Intensity (work per unit of time) is the aspect of your training that determines whether you are receiving any cardiorespiratory (heart-lung) benefits. Researchers have developed simple formulas to determine how much your heart rate must increase during

Osteoporosis An abnormal decalcification of bones causing loss of bone density.

Fitness Heroes

Columbia University boasts a wealth of fitness heroes. Through an Olympic mentor fitness program, Columbia has created an atmosphere in which Olympic stars of the past help create Olympic stars of the future.

Former Olympic medalists and competitors joined together to create this program. They offer their time and expertise to future Olympic hopefuls—helping them reach for their Olympic dreams, as well as helping the United States achieve Olympic success. Among the Olympic mentors are 1984 basketball gold medalist Lynette Woodard, 1984 gold-medal cyclist Connie Carpenter-Finney, 1984 gymnast and gold medal winner Mitche Gaylord, 1976 swimmer and gold medalist John Naber, and Olympic diver Jenny Kine. These athletes are fine examples of fitness success, and they represent the true meaning of *fitness hero*. ✦

exercise and how long you need to keep it elevated (20 to 30 minutes) to improve cardiovascular fitness. In the early stages of your newly started program, you will need to work up to 20 to 30 minutes of continuous activity slowly, in four to six weeks, rather than attempt to maintain such a high intensity in early workout sessions. To locate your THR, complete Lab Activity 4.1: Finding Your Target Heart Rate at the end of this chapter.

Time (the duration of your workout) is the final one-third of the complete cardiorespiratory exercise session. Exercise duration is affected by intensity. Obviously, you cannot sprint at near-maximum

---

Afterburn The period of time following exercise when resting metabolism remains elevated.

Neuromuscular specificity Training a specific muscle group.

Metabolic specificity Training a specific energy system (citric acid cycle or glycolysis cycle).

Warmup The preparation of the body for vigorous activity through stretching, calisthenics, running, and specific sport movements designed to raise core temperature.

---

effort for 20 minutes. If aerobic conditioning is your goal, the session should maintain your target heart rate for 20 to 30 minutes. If the purpose of your program is cosmetic—to lose weight and fat and to improve your appearance—duration is the key. In general, the longer you exercise, the more calories you burn and the more fat you use as fuel. If weight loss is your primary objective, it is important to keep in mind that walking three miles burns only slightly fewer calories than running three miles. The longer you walk or run, the more calories you use. It may be good advice to slow down your walking, pedaling, running, rope jumping, and so on and exercise longer. To exercise longer, it is important to stay near the lower portion of your THR range. Providing your THR is reached, you are not only burning a high number of calories, you are improving the cardiovascular system as well.

Running or walking three miles on each of two successive days also burns more calories than one six-mile run. This is because of the extra 60 to 150 calories burned because of metabolic rate increases (calories burned while the body is at rest) following the exercise period. In other words, two short exercise sessions burn more calories than one long session since metabolic rate will become, and remain, elevated for several hours after each session. This extra calorie usage after exercise ceases is called **afterburn**. If you walk or run too far in one day and are unable to exercise the next day, you will eliminate one afterburn period and forfeit 60 to 150 calories. Late afternoon, when metabolic rates begin to slow in most people, may be one of the best times to exercise. You then burn calories while exercising and activate a faster metabolic rate for two to four hours at a time in the day when metabolic rate normally slows down.

Apply the Principle of Specificity

The effect of training is unique to an activity or sport. Football or field hockey players who have just completed seasons, for example, will find that they are not capable of meeting the physical demands of wrestling or basketball. The scientific basis for this is that training occurs, in part, within the muscles themselves, and that training is specific to the energy system being used. Thus complete training transfer, regardless of the closeness of the activities, is not possible. Training a particular muscle group is referred to as **neuromuscular specificity** whereas training one of the energy systems is called **metabolic specificity**. If your main training objective is to improve aerobic fitness, you must include activities such as jogging, running, cycling, aerobic dance, and distance swimming. Although gains in cardiorespiratory fitness will occur from each of these activities, a specific activity that closely simulates the movement of the sport for which you are training provides the most transfer. In other words, swimming is the preferred training method to improve distance swimming, running is the preferred training method for 10-K races, and so on.

Alternate Light and Heavy Workouts

The body responds best to training programs that alternate light and heavy workouts. This approach reduces the risk of injury, provides several emotionally relaxing workouts each week, and allows the body time to recover. In other words, it helps you receive maximum benefits from a fitness program. Consider: (1) never training extremely hard on consecutive

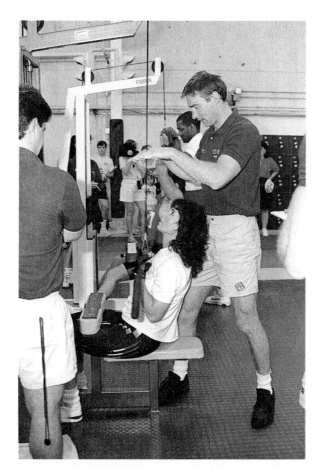

Alternating light and heavy workouts reduces the risk of injury and gives the muscles time to recover. (Photo Courtesy of the Aspen Hill Club.)

days, (2) training hard no more than three times a week, (3) scheduling one extra-hard, all-out workout once a week, and (4) knowing your body and allowing it to direct you (if pain continues or worsens or if you get heavy-legged, stop regardless of whether it is a light- or heavy-workout day). The PRE principle is applied by increasing the volume and/or intensity on the heavy-workout days.

Warm Up Properly before Each Workout

A **warmup** is almost universally used at the beginning of an exercise or activity session to improve performance and prevent injury. The theory behind the warmup is that muscular contractions are dependent on temperature. Since increased muscle temperature improves work capacity and a warmup increases muscle temperature, it is assumed that one is necessary. The amount of knee fluid is also increased with a warmup; oxygen intake is improved; and the amount of oxygen needed for exercise is reduced. Nerve messages also travel faster at higher temperatures.

Suggestions that can be drawn from the findings of well-controlled studies on the warmup include:

1. A warmup period of 10 to 15 minutes prior to the actual workout or exercise session. A longer period is needed in a cold environment to allow the body to reach the desired temperature prior to activity.

2. The main purpose of a warmup is to elevate core temperature by one to two degrees before engaging in explosive muscular movements; you will generally reach this point at the same time your warmup routine causes sweating.

3. Only a few minutes should elapse from completion of the warmup until the start of activity.

4. Warmup will not cause early fatigue and hinder performance.

Warmup methods fall into four categories:

1. **Formal** The skill or act that will be used in competition or in your workout, such as running before a 100-meter dash, jogging before a 3-mile run, or shooting a basketball and jumping before a basketball game.

2. **Informal** The general warmup involving calisthenics or other activity unrelated to the workout routine to follow.

3. **Passive** Applying heat to various body parts.

4. **Overload** Simulating the activity for which the warmup is being used by increasing the load or resistance, such as swinging two bats before hitting a baseball.

Each of these methods has been shown by some researchers to be helpful and by other researchers to be of little value. Formal warmup appears superior to informal procedures. When body temperature is elevated and sweating occurs, your muscles are ready for a brief stretching or flexibility session (see chapter 7).

How long you decide to engage in warmup activities is also important. The temperature of your muscles will rise in about 5 minutes and continue to rise further for 25 to 30 minutes. If you stop exercising and become inactive, your muscle temperature will decline significantly, and you may need an additional warmup period. The best advice is to use a 10- to 15-minute warmup period that ends in an all-out effort and causes you to perspire. You should plan to complete your warmup period about 5 minutes before an exercise session or competition begins. Find the magic combination for you and your activity and stay with it.

Cool Down Properly at the End of Each Workout

The justification for a **cooldown** period following a vigorous workout is quite simple. Blood returns to the heart through a system of vessels called *veins.* The blood is pushed along by heart contractions and the veins' milking action is assisted by muscle contractions during exercise. Veins contract or squeeze and

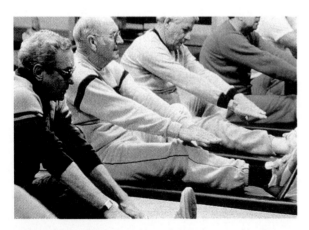

Warming up muscles improves performance and prevents injuries. (Photo Courtesy of the American Heart Association.)

move the blood forward against gravity while valves prevent the blood from backing up. If you stop exercising suddenly, this milking action will stop and blood return will drop quickly and may cause blood pooling (blood remaining in the same area) in the legs, leading to shock or deep breathing, which may in turn lower carbon dioxide levels and produce muscle cramps.

It is at this point also that blood pressure can drop precipitously and cause trouble. The body compensates for the unexpected drop in pressure by secreting as much as 100 times the normal amount of **norepinephrine**. This high level of norepinephrine can cause cardiac problems for some individuals during the recovery phase of vigorous exercise such as a marathon or a triathlon.

Postexercise peril occurs in some individuals immediately after exercise, particularly among those who fail to use a cooldown period. The least desirable postexercise behavior is standing. Lying down flat is acceptable; the preferred activity, however, is walking or jogging (light exercise).

You should also cool down following a long aerobic exercise session. A general routine might consist of walking or jogging a quarter-mile to a mile at a pace of three to four minutes per quarter mile, each quarter-mile slower than the previous one. The ideal cooldown routine should take place in the same environment as the workout (except in extremely hot or cold weather), last at least five minutes, and be followed by a brief stretching period.

Dress Appropriately for Ease of Movement and Heat Regulation

What you wear depends on your exercise program and the weather. The general rule is to have good shoes and to wear as little clothing as the weather permits.

Shoes To avoid injuries, quality shoes are essential for most aerobic activities. The primary criteria are fit, comfort, and quality. Most activities require a specialized shoe, and although they often look identical, the construction styles affect individuals differently. Specialty stores are more likely to provide sound advice about the best shoe for your aerobic goals. Since fit is so important, wear the same style socks you use for exercising when you are selecting a shoe.

Clothes For indoor and warm-weather outdoor exercise, wear the least clothing possible. The cooling process requires air to pass over the skin and evaporate; clothing must allow this process to take place.

Some individuals mistakenly feel they will lose weight by wearing multiple layers of clothes to increase fluid loss. It is the total calories expended, however, not the total sweat count, that determines weight and fat loss.

When you are exercising outside during the winter, do not either overdress or underdress. Like summer clothing, winter attire must allow the skin to breathe. Windbreakers and other nylon garments are therefore not recommended. Combining a T-shirt with a wool sweater, a hat, and gloves is usually sufficient for protection down to temperatures below 32 degrees F (0 degrees C). Under extremely cold conditions, however, frostbite is a real danger, particularly to exposed skin. The skin can be protected, but only to a degree, with creams and jellies. Men, for example, must protect the penis and testicles from frostbite; nylon shorts are of little value, and frostbite can occur without warning.

Take Special Precaution When You Are Exercising Outdoors

Weather conditions are not your only concern when you exercise outside. *Pollution*, particularly lack of clear air, is indeed a danger worth paying attention to. Although the benefits of exercise overshadow the dangers of unclear air, workouts during smog alerts and in high traffic areas should be avoided. *Motor vehicles* and even *bicycles* can present life-threatening situations to runners and others who exercise outside. Cars and bicycles should be given the right-of-way no matter what you or the law indicates. It is also advisable to run or walk toward traffic and to use reflective gear at night. Do not be aggressive since you are no match for a 3000+ lb vehicle. *Dogs* tend to have considerable bark and little bite, but the exceptions can produce disaster. Since dogs are extremely territorial, it is wise to avoid crossing property lines. For the occasional dog that comes after you, the best action is to stop, face the dog, and assume a passive posture before slowly backing away. As you vacate the property, the animal generally becomes less aggressive. *Two-legged animals* are far more dangerous than any of the four-legged varieties. Women in particular must be alert to dangerous situations and take care to exercise with others, avoid outside exercise at night, ignore taunts, and remain alert at all times.

Choose Soft Surfaces Whenever Possible

Although exercise involves some risk of injury (see chapter 12), choice of surface can reduce the risk. Generally speaking, the harder the surface, the greater the injury potential. A surface that is too soft or uneven also increases the risk of certain types of exercise injuries. A soft, uneven surface, such as a beach, can cause ankle and knee injuries. Dirt and gravel paths and trails covered with wood chips are best for walking and running, but the isolated nature of most trails increases the chances of assault. Public park, vitae courses usually provide relatively safe, soft places to exercise. Exercising on concrete floors, sidewalks, hard tennis courts, and gymnasium floors should be avoided whenever possible. Daily activity on such surfaces is almost certain to produce injury.

Use Cross Training in the Aerobic Component of Your Program

Repetitive motion syndrome can produce both injury and loss of interest in exercise. Daily step classes or a five-mile run, for example, both involve the same motion, movement, muscles, and joints over and over and are almost certain to result in injury over long periods of time. More and more individuals use **cross training** and avoid these dangers by varying their exercise choices weekly. Runners may choose to ride a stationary cycle or swim once or twice a week. Aerobic dance participants may alternate with cycling, walking, swimming, or racket sports. Such an approach provides a more complete workout and eliminates exercise boredom and burnout.

Use a Maintenance Approach after Reaching Your Desired Level of Fitness

It is possible to alter your exercise program to maintain the level of conditioning you have acquired.

Cooldown The use of 3 to 10 minutes of very light exercise movements at the end of a vigorous workout designed to cool the body slowly to near-normal core temperature.

Norepinephrine An end product of some of the secretions of the adrenal gland; influences nervous system activity, constricts blood vessels, and increases blood pressure.

Postexercise peril Illness, dizziness, nausea, and sudden death following vigorous exercise, particularly when a cooldown period is not used.

Cross training The practice of alternating exercise choices throughout the week to avoid overuse injuries from repetitive movements.

Considerable strength, for example, can be maintained by completing one or two hard weight-training workouts weekly. Maintaining your cardiorespiratory endurance may require two to three workouts weekly. During times when you are unable to exercise daily, you may choose to alter your routine by increasing the intensity and duration of the workouts you complete.

Monitor Your Progress Carefully

Records can be a source of motivation in addition to aiding in the prevention of injury. Keeping records of resting heart rate, the number of miles walked or run, laps swum, weight lifted, and number of workouts completed can provide the needed incentive to continue an exercise program.

Recordkeeping also helps you apply the PRE principle to guarantee continued improvement. It is difficult to improve and work harder today when you are not aware of the intensity and duration of your previous workouts. See Lab Activity 4.2: Evaluating Your Exercise Program.

If an overuse injury occurs, a perusal of records can aid in determining its cause and help you in setting a course toward recovery. Unfortunately, records can also lead to compulsive behavior known as negative addiction. To the addicted, records are made to be broken, more is better, and the record rather than the fitness benefits becomes the goal. Such individuals experience frequent injury intermixed with emotional stress in attempting to maintain or break records.

The daily log in Table 4.1 can help you apply many of the exercise concepts discussed in this chapter. The log information should include the number of minutes spent in aerobic activity, distance covered, and rest intervals between repetitions, if applicable. Your log should also contain weather conditions, water temperature, heart rate, how you felt, particular problems that indicate the possibility of future injury, number and type of activities completed, and (for weight training) the weight and number of repetitions for each exercise.

Aerobics Activity performed in the presence of oxygen, using fat as the major source of fuel.

Anaerobics High-intensity activity, such as sprinting, that is performed in the absence of oxygen, using glucose as the major source of fuel.

Oxygen debt The difference between the exact amount of oxygen needed for an exercise task and the amount actually taken in.

MAKING THE RIGHT EXERCISE CHOICES

The ideal, complete exercise program should have four components: aerobics, muscular strength, muscular endurance, and flexibility. The aerobic component will provide the health-related benefits in addition to controlling and maintaining body weight and fat. A sound weight-training program will improve muscle tone, strength, and endurance; prevent the loss of lean muscle mass; add muscle mass; and help control body weight and fat by increasing metabolism. Stretching exercises will help maintain and improve your range of motion and prevent joint stiffness.

Aerobic Choices

It is important to select a program that is effective in developing the cardiorespiratory system, and is compatible with your training objectives, amount of time available, and interests. Table 4.2 on page 66 compares aerobic exercise choices based on the characteristics of the ideal program. Study this table carefully before making your selection. It is also a good idea to sample different approaches to help you find activities you enjoy to use in cross training later.

If you are interested in the sports approach to aerobic fitness, study Table 4.3 on page 67 before making your selections. As you are now aware, the term **aerobic** means *with oxygen* and describes extended vigorous exercise that stimulates heart and lung activity enough to produce a training effect. This occurs when your target heart rate is reached and maintained at that level for 20 minutes or more. Many sports are more **anaerobic** than aerobic and fail to improve heart-lung endurance or provide the health benefits you desire. Anaerobic means *without oxygen* and describes short, all-out exercise efforts such as the 100-, 200-, or 400-meter dash and sports such as football and baseball. Anaerobic metabolism is the immediate energy source of all muscle work at the beginning of any type of exercise. This energy source, called adenosine triphosphate (ATP), is formed in the muscles primarily through the metabolization of carbohydrates. Every muscle needs ATP to perform its work. The process is anaerobic because

Table 4.1 ✦ Daily Exercise Log

Date _____   Time of day _____

Distance covered or total exercise time _____

Weather conditions _____

Terrain (flat, hills, soft, hard, and so forth) _____

Intensity: Heart rate _____

            Repetitions _____

            Rest interval _____

            Distance covered _____   Pace _____

Duration: _____

Positive impressions of workout:

Unusual feelings or problems during workout:

Overall rating on a scale of 1 to 10 _____
(10 = Excellent, 1= Dreadful)

ATP is metabolized without the need for oxygen. For short sprints and all-out efforts, the heart and lungs cannot deliver atmospheric oxygen to the muscles fast enough; anaerobic energy sources therefore must provide the fuel. The very instant that the amount of oxygen breathed in is not enough to supply active muscles, **oxygen debt** occurs and you begin to breathe heavily. After you stop exercising, oxygen debt is repaid and normal breathing returns. Unfortunately, anaerobic activities cannot be sustained for long periods of time, burn fewer calories, and fail to provide some important health benefits. It is difficult to improve your aerobic fitness through mere participation in a sport, and we recommend that you supplement such participation with a minimum of two aerobic workouts weekly.

Table 4.2 ✦ Evaluation of Exercise Programs

CHARACTERISTICS OF THE IDEAL PROGRAM	AEROBIC EXERCISE AND DANCE	ANAEROBICS	CALISTHENICS	CYCLING	ROPE JUMPING	RUNNING PROGRAMS	SPORTS[a]	WALKING	SWIMMING (LAPS)	WEIGHT TRAINING
Easily adaptable to individual's exercise tolerance	P	Y	Y	Y	Y	Y	P	Y	Y	Y
Applies the progressive resistance principle	Y	Y	Y	Y	Y	Y	P	Y	Y	Y
Provides for self-evaluation	Y	Y	P	Y	Y	Y	P	Y	Y	Y
Practical for use throughout life	Y	N	N	Y	Y	Y	P	Y	Y	Y
Scientifically developed	Y	Y	P	Y	Y	Y	U	Y	Y	Y
Involves minimum time	Y	P	N	Y	Y	Y	N	Y	Y	Y
Involves little or no equipment	P	Y	Y	N	Y	Y	N	Y	Y	N
Performed easily at home	N	N	Y	Y	Y	Y	N	Y	Y	N
Widely publicized	Y	N	N	Y	Y	Y	Y	Y	Y	Y
Accepted and valued	Y	P	N	Y	Y	Y	P	Y	Y	Y
Challenging	Y	Y	N	Y	Y	Y	Y	Y	Y	Y
Firms body	Y	Y	Y	Y	Y	P	P	Y	Y	Y
Develops flexibility[b]	Y	N	Y	N	Y	Y	Y	N	P	N
Develops muscular endurance	Y	Y	Y	Y		Y	Y	Y	Y	Y
Develops cardiovascular endurance: Prevents heart disease	Y	N	Y	Y	Y	Y	Y	P	Y	P
Develops strength	P	P	Y	P	P	Y	Y	P	P	Y
High caloric expenditure: Weight loss	Y	P	P	Y	Y	P	Y	Y	Y	N

Note: Y = yes, P = partially, N = no provision, U = unknown (referring to meeting ideal characteristics).

[a]The value of the sports approach depends on the activity and the level of competition.

[b]Flexibility can be improved only if the complete range of movement is performed in each exercise, applying static pressure at the extreme range of motion before returning to starting position.

Source: Adapted from John Unitas and George B. Dintiman, *Improving Health and Fitness in the Athlete* (Englewood Cliffs, NJ: Prentice-Hall, 1979), p. 180.

Table 4.3 ◆ Ratings of Sports

Sport	Type	Cardiovascular	Caloric Expenditure	Legs	Abdomen	Arms/ Shoulder	Age Range Recommended
Archery	Anaerobic	L	L	L	L	L	Ages 10 and up
Backpacking	50% Aerobic	M-H	H	H	M	L	All ages
Badminton	40% Aerobic	M-H	H	H	L	M	Ages 7 and up
Baseball/softball	Anaerobic	L	L	M	L	L	All ages
Basketball	25% Aerobic	M	H	H	L	L	Ages 7 to 40
Bicycling (competitive)	Aerobic	H	H	H	L	M	All ages
Bowling	Anaerobic	L	L	L	L	L	All ages
Dance (aerobic)	Aerobic	M-H	M-H	M	M	M	All ages
Canoeing/rowing							
Recreational	Anaerobic	L	M	L	L	M	Ages 12 and up
Competitive	Aerobic	H	H	M	M	H	Ages 12 to 40
Fencing	Anaerobic	L-M	M	M	L	M	Ages 12 and up
Field hockey	40% Aerobic	M-H	M-H	H	L	M	Ages 7 and up
Golf (motor cart)	Anaerobic	L	L	L	L	L	All ages
Walking	Aerobic	L	M	M	L	L	All ages
Handball/racketball/ squash (singles)	40% Aerobic	M-H	H	H	L	H	Under 45
Hiking	Aerobic	L-M	M	H	L	L	All ages
Hunting	Aerobic	L-M	M	M	L	L	All ages
Ice/roller skating							
Speed	Anaerobic	L-M	M	H	L	L	Under 45
Figure	Aerobic	L-M	H	H	M	M	All ages
Lacrosse	40% Aerobic	M-H	H	H	M	M	Under 45
Orienteering	50% Aerobic	M-H	H	H	M	L	All ages
Rugby	60% Aerobic	H	H	H	L	H	Under 45
Skiing (cross-country)	Aerobic	H	H	H	H	H	Under 45
Skin and scuba diving	Aerobic	M	M	M	M	L	All ages
Soccer	50% Aerobic	H	H	H	L	H	Under 45
Surfing	Anaerobic	L	M	H	M	L	Ages 7 and up
Tennis (singles)	40% Aerobic	M	M	H	L	L	All ages
Touch football	Anaerobic	L	L-M	H	L	L	Under 45
Volleyball	Anaerobic	L	L	M-H	L	M	All ages
Water skiing	Anaerobic	L-M	M	H	L	M	All ages
Weight training	Anaerobic	L	L	H	H	H	All ages
Wrestling	30% Aerobic	M	H	H	H	H	Under 45
Jogging	Aerobic	M-H	H	H	L	L	Ages 7 and up
Swimming	Aerobic	M	H	M	L	H	Ages 7 and up
Walking	Aerobic	L-M	M	H	L	L	All ages

H = high; M = medium; L = low

Behavioral Change and Motivational Strategies

There are many things that might interfere with your application of sound exercise principles. Some of these barriers (roadblocks) and strategies for overcoming them are:

Roadblock	Behavioral Change Strategy
Exercise just isn't fun anymore, and you no longer look forward to your afternoon workout session. Even if you do get into the workout, there is no motivation to put forth much effort.	You may be experiencing some of the emotional and physical effects of over-training or exercising too often. To renew your interest: 1. Change aerobic activities every other day as a cross-training technique. If you are jogging or using STEP daily, for example, substitute cycling, lap swimming, aerobic dance, or a sports activity two to three times weekly. 2. Change the time you exercise. Try early mornings, noon, or just before bedtime to see if time will improve your mood. 3. Apply the light-heavy concept discussed in this chapter and avoid two consecutive workouts of the same level of difficulty. 4. Add one or two fun workouts weekly, and exercise with a group of friends.
Muscle soreness the following morning is making your day unpleasant since sitting, standing, and moving around on the job is somewhat painful.	A number of factors may be causing the problem. You may be exercising untrained muscles; training much too hard; not consuming enough fluids before, during, and after your workout; or stretching improperly or not at all. Try some of these remedies for at least one week: 1. Hydrate 15 to 30 minutes before your workout by drinking three or four eight-ounce glasses of water. 2. Record the amount of water and other fluids you consume daily, making certain to drink at least eight glasses of water. 3. Alternate light and heavy workout days. 4. Warm up for a longer period of time than you normally do, then stretch carefully for at least 10 minutes. 5. At the end your workout, cool down properly, and end with a mild five-minute stretching session.
Although you have been exercising daily for a month, little weight and fat loss seems to be taking place.	To lose body fat and weight, you need to change your exercise emphasis and reduce your caloric intake. Don't give up. Be certain you: 1. Monitor both your exercise sessions and your food intake by keeping accurate records of total exercise volume and the daily calories consumed. 2. Increase the duration of your workout and exercise every day. If you are walking, try to walk continuously for at least one hour. Reduce the intensity of your workout and continue exercising longer each workout. 3. Schedule your workout about two hours before mealtime or two hours after your evening meal to help control hunger and the temptation to overeat or snack.
List other roadblocks that you are experiencing that seem to be reducing the effectiveness of your program and limiting your success.	Now list behavior change strategies that can help you overcome the roadblocks you listed. If you need to, refer to chapter 3 for behavior change and motivational strategies.
1. _____	1. _____
2. _____	2. _____
3. _____	3. _____

Choosing Muscular Strength and Endurance Programs

Chapter 6 describes numerous choices for increasing your muscular strength and endurance effectively. Your choice of workout routine depends on your training objectives, which also help you decide between free weights and the other types of exercise equipment. Chapter 6 gives you enough details to help you make the correct decision.

Selecting an Appropriate Flexibility Training Program

Although a simple, static stretching routine is the wisest choice for effectively improving your flexibility, specific exercise choices depend on your objectives, including that of the particular activity for which you are training. The detailed information in chapter 7 will help you make the right decision. In less than ten minutes daily, you can maintain and even improve range of motion in your major joints.

Summary

The Ideal Exercise Program

A complete exercise program should bring about improvement in five key health-related fitness areas: cardiorespiratory endurance, body composition, muscular strength, muscular endurance, and flexibility. Aerobic exercise is the most important component and should form the foundation of the ideal program. The principles of exercise must be applied specifically to your workout choice to guarantee continued improvement.

Fitness Concepts

A preconditioning period may be necessary before beginning a new exercise program, particularly for people who have previously been inactive. This three- to four-week period will prepare you for more vigorous workouts and allow you to reach and maintain your THR for 20 to 30 minutes safely.

The PRE principle can easily be adapted to aerobic, muscular strength and endurance, and flexibility training to ensure steady progress and improvement in these areas. To train for a specific sport or activity, you must apply the principle of specificity by using movements and exercises that closely simulate those performed in the sport. The use of a warmup and cooldown period, the application of FIT to your aerobic workout, alternating light and heavy workout days, dressing appropriately for the weather, monitoring your progress with recordkeeping, and cross training will improve the benefits of each workout, keep you emotionally and physically healthy, and eliminate boredom and overtraining.

Making the Right Exercise Choices

It is important to select aerobic activities you enjoy that are also effective and that meet your training objectives. The sports approach to aerobic fitness requires special care in selecting activities, such as soccer, rugby, field hockey, and racketball (singles), that are primarily aerobic in nature. Anaerobic activity choices will provide very little in the way of health-related benefits. Two to three additional workouts weekly in an aerobic activity are also recommended.

Lab Activity 4.1

Finding Your Target Heart Rate (THR)

INSTRUCTIONS: *There are several acceptable methods for determining your THR. To use this method, carefully complete each step:*

✦ **Step 1:** Find your predicted maximum heart rate (PMHR)—the total number of times your heart can potentially beat in one minute.

Men: PMHR 205 minus half your age

Women: PMHR 220 minus your age

Example: A 22-year-old male has a PMHR of 194 (205 minus 11). A woman of the same age has a PMHR of 198 (220 minus 22).

✦ **Step 2:** Take 60 percent of your PMHR, the lower level of your THR. Now take 90 percent of your PMHR to find the upper level.

Men: 194 times .60 equals 116 (lower level);
194 times .90 equals 175 (upper level)
THR range: 116 to 175

Women: 198 times .60 equals 119 (lower level);
198 times .90 equals 178 (upper level)
THR range: 119 to 178.

If your heart rate during exercise is within this range, an aerobic or cardiovascular training effect is taking place. It is just as important to avoid exceeding the upper level of your THR. Working above 90 percent of your maximum heart rate is not recommended unless you are a highly conditioned aerobic athlete.

Lab Activity 4.2

Evaluating Your Exercise Program

INSTRUCTIONS: *You can easily evaluate the effectiveness of your aerobic exercise program by taking your heart rate immediately after you complete the final seconds of your workout. Follow the steps below to determine whether you need to increase or decrease the intensity of your exercise session.*

✦ **Step 1:** Find your resting heart rate by locating your radial pulse. To do this, place the index and middle fingers of your right hand in the wrist groove just below your thumb. Count the number of beats for 15 seconds and multiple by 4 to find the beats per minute. A faster approach is to obtain the number of beats in exactly 6 seconds before adding a 0 to determine the number of beats per minute. This may be a more accurate method of estimating the rate while you were exercising. In general, the lower heart rate, the higher the aerobic fitness level. As you improve your cardiovascular fitness, your resting heart rate will decrease. The carotid pulse, located just under the jaw, can be used for those unable to feel a strong pulse at the wrist. Pressing too hard on the carotid pulse may slow heart rate and cause dizziness.

✦ **Step 2:** Complete your normal workout. Just prior to entering the cooldown phase, after a minimum of 20 minutes of continuous activity, stop and take your radial or carotid pulse and record the number of beats per minute.

✦ **Step 3:** Refer to Lab Activity 4.1 to see if this figure (number of beats per minute) falls within your THR range. If it is below the lower limit, you must run, walk, swim, or cycle faster or take shorter breaks between points in tennis, racquetball, handball, basketball, and so forth. If it is above the upper limit, you need to exercise at a slower pace and rest more.

Exercise activity _____

Exercise heart rate (number of beats per minute) _____

THR range _____ to _____

Recommended change _____

5

$\mathcal{E}$XPLORING
$\mathcal{C}$ARDIORESPIRATORY $\mathcal{F}$ITNESS

$\mathcal{C}$hapter Objectives

By the end of this chapter, you should be able to:

1. Give alternate names for cardiorespiratory endurance.

2. Express benefits to be derived from participating in a cardiorespiratory conditioning program.

3. Describe maximal oxygen uptake (VO_2) and show different ways of expressing it.

4. Assess your VO_2 and determine cardiorespiratory fitness.

5. Explain guidelines for safely beginning and progressing in an aerobic fitness program.

6. Develop your own cardiorespiratory conditioning program.

$\mathcal{R}$ECENTLY TWO WOMEN were shopping in a department store. Ms. Green, a professional, 40-year-old, single female, was purchasing exercise clothing and accidentally bumped into Mrs. Taylor, a 45-year-old, lower-income woman, who was purchasing clothing for her grandchildren. As the two women struck up a conversation, Ms. Green explained that she had just enrolled in the new Jane Fonda Step Aerobics class at the local health club. She asked Mrs. Taylor if she had considered joining the class because step aerobics is very popular and is a great form of exercise. Mrs. Taylor responded, "Well, you know, I'm so busy cleaning houses that I just don't have the time or the energy to join an exercise class!"

Unfortunately, the cardiorespiratory exercise boom has not reached all segments of the U.S. population for various reasons. Many obstacles, such as increased time demands, may make exercise seem impossible. As your time management skills improve, however, finding time to exercise will not be as difficult as it may seem. Also, many people mistakenly believe, as Mrs. Taylor does, that participating in an exercise class will make them more fatigued. In reality, the opposite is true. Improved cardiorespiratory fitness often increases your energy level. Many other benefits are to be derived from participating in an aerobic conditioning program.

Cardiorespiratory endurance is referred to by many names, including aerobic power, **maximal oxygen consumption** (VO_2), physical fitness, and **aerobic metabolism**. **Cardiorespiratory endurance** is the ability of the heart, blood vessels, and the lungs to deliver oxygen to the exercising muscles in amounts sufficient to meet the demands of the workload. **Endurance** is the ability to perform prolonged bouts of work without experiencing fatigue or exhaustion. As your cardiorespiratory endurance level increases, so does your ability to engage in sustained physical activity. By the end of several months of cardiorespiratory activities, you will be able to exercise for long periods of time without experiencing prolonged fatigue.

As your body adapts to an aerobic conditioning program, you will also feel better and have a much higher energy level. A high level of cardiorespiratory fitness actually increases the daily energy level as well as your level of productivity. A high level of cardiorespiratory endurance is also beneficial in helping to postpone or delay several chronic diseases, such as heart disease and high blood pressure. Recent research has even shown that people with high levels of cardiorespiratory endurance are less susceptible to

developing cancer. Since heart disease, high blood pressure, and cancer are among the leading causes of death in the United States, it is especially important to maintain a healthy cardiorespiratory system.

Let us examine the physiological benefits (see Table 5.1) to be derived from participating in a cardiorespiratory endurance conditioning program. While the list presented in Table 5.1 may seem overwhelming at first glance, all these physiological changes can be reduced to one primary benefit—increased aerobic power. What effect do all these changes have on level of performance? First, all the changes that occur to the heart, blood, blood vessels, and lungs, which comprise the **cardiorespiratory system**, are all geared to increase the amount of blood that is delivered to the muscles. Also these benefits make exercise feel easier at workloads below maximum. They increase your ability to perform at maximal exercise intensity. The changes that occur in the muscles, bones, and joints are all designed to increase your ability to extract oxygen from the bloodstream and use it to produce energy for exercise. Exercise duration is increased as well as exercise intensity. In short, the total amount of work that you are able to do increases as a result of cardiorespiratory adaptations from an aerobic conditioning program.

In the remainder of this chapter, we explore aerobic exercise choices and discuss the differences in VO_2 for various sports. We will also discuss guidelines for beginning and safely progressing in an aerobic conditioning program and conclude with some sample starter programs for aerobic activities. You will then have the opportunity to design your own aerobic exercise program.

Maximal oxygen consumption (VO_2) The optimal capacity of the heart to pump blood, of the lungs to fill with larger volumes of air, and of the muscle cells to use the oxygen and remove waste products that are produced during the process of aerobic metabolism.

Aerobic metabolism The process of breaking down energy nutrients such as carbohydrates and fats in the presence of oxygen in order to yield energy in the form of ATP.

Cardiorespiratory endurance The ability of the heart, blood vessels, and lungs to deliver oxygen to the exercising muscles in amounts sufficient to meet the demands of the workload.

Endurance The ability to work a long time without experiencing fatigue or exhaustion.

Cardiorespiratory system Joint functioning of the respiratory system (the lungs and airway passages) and the circulatory system (the heart and blood vessels).

Glycogen The stored form of carbohydrate in the muscles and liver.

Adenosine triphosphate (ATP) The basic substrate used by the muscle to provide energy for muscle contractions.

OVERVIEW AND ANALYSIS OF AEROBIC EXERCISE CHOICES

Only aerobic activities will increase your level of cardiorespiratory endurance. Fortunately, there are numerous aerobic choices available, including walking, jogging/running, swimming, bicycling, aerobic dancing and step aerobics, water aerobics, rope skipping, cross-country skiing, racket sports, and stepping.

Nearly all aerobic sports will lead to the same benefits with respect to increased aerobic power so it makes little difference whether you choose to walk, jog, or ride a bike. When you choose a conditioning program, however, it is important for you to realize that the larger the amount of muscle mass used in an activity, the greater will be your level of endurance,

Table 5.1 ✦ Physiological Benefits of Increased Cardiorespiratory Endurance after Participating in an Aerobic Training Program

HEART, BLOOD VESSELS, AND LUNGS	MUSCLES, BONES, JOINTS
Lower resting heart rate	Increased bone strength and density
Lower submaximal exercise heart rate	Increased thickness of cartilage, tendons, and ligaments
Increased maximal cardiac output	Increased oxygen consumed by muscles
Increased stroke volume	Increased number of mitochondria
Decreased recovery time	Increased size of mitochondria
Increased strength of heart muscle	Increased concentration of oxidative enzymes
Increased blood flow to muscles during exercise	Increased size of slow-twitch muscle fibers
Decreased resting blood pressure in hypertensives	Increased muscle glycogen stores
Increased number of capillaries in muscles	Increased ATP and phosphocreatine stores
Increased total blood volume	Increased ability to burn fat for energy
Increased hemoglobin (carries oxygen to muscles)	Decreased body fat percentage
Increased vital capacity (lung capacity)	Increased muscular endurance
Decreased blood lipids	Increased flexibility
Increased high-density lipoprotein (HDL) cholesterol	
Decreased low-density lipoprotein (LDL) cholesterol	
Decreased triglycerides (fats)	

especially during the initial phase of a conditioning program. For example, if you walk 45 minutes, you will probably not become fatigued as quickly as if you play tennis for 45 minutes. That is because the muscles that grip the tennis racket tire more quickly since you place a high energy demand on a very small muscle mass. Whereas your leg muscles, as used in walking, are a much larger group, they are more accustomed to this activity and will not fatigue as quickly. For this reason, you will find that your endurance is greater when you engage in activities such as swimming, walking, and jogging/running than is the case with activities that rely primarily on the arms. Remember that in the initial phase of a conditioning program, you can expect to fatigue sooner when small muscle groups are used.

Regardless of how exciting a new aerobic conditioning program may be, eventually boredom might creep in. Hence we recommend that you participate in a variety of aerobic activities in order to maintain cardiorespiratory fitness. The greater the diversity in your program, the greater the likelihood that you will maintain a lifetime of physical fitness. Also, whenever it is possible, exercise with a partner or with a group of people. The benefits of exercising with other people are discussed elsewhere in this book, but a major benefit is that exercising with a partner or a group increases the likelihood you will stay with your conditioning program.

MAXIMAL OXYGEN CONSUMPTION (VO₂)

Cardiorespiratory endurance is synonymous with VO₂, or maximal oxygen uptake. When a person is tested either in a laboratory or in the field, the highest level of oxygen uptake achieved is called the VO₂, which actually represents the volume of oxygen consumed by the muscles. The VO₂ is regarded as the single best indicator of cardiorespiratory endurance or aerobic fitness.

A high VO₂ indicates an increased ability of the heart to pump blood, of the lungs to fill with larger volumes of air, and of the muscle cells to use the oxygen and remove waste products that are produced during the process of aerobic metabolism. The two primary factors influencing maximal aerobic power are (1) the ability of the cardiorespiratory system to deliver oxygen to the muscles and (2) the ability of the muscles to extract oxygen from the blood.

Oxygen is used in the process of aerobic metabolism. When you exercise for prolonged periods of time, vast quantities of energy are needed by the muscles. Foodstuffs stored in the muscles, such as fats and **glycogen** (the stored form of carbohydrate in the muscles) are broken down continuously in order to provide **adenosine triphosphate (ATP)**, which is used by the muscles to provide energy for contrac-

Fitness Heroes

Arthur Ashe is often referred to as the eternal example of a sportsman and was the first eminent African-American male tennis player. As a child, he lived in Richmond, Virginia, with his father and brother (his mother died when he was six years old). His family lived in a house located near four tennis courts. Because his father forbade him to play football, Arthur spent all of his free time on the tennis court. This was very unusual because few African-American children played the game.

In 1955, at age 12, Arthur was not allowed to play in a Richmond city tennis tournament because of his color. Nonetheless, he persevered and became a tennis prodigy. His cool demeanor made him one of the most dangerous opponents in tennis. He won a scholarship to UCLA. He won the U.S. Open in 1968 and the Australian Open in 1970. The crowning event in his professional tennis career was defeating Jimmy Connors in the Wimbledon finals in 1975.

In 1979, at age 36, Arthur had a heart attack, forcing him to retire from tennis. It was virtually unheard of for such a highly conditioned athlete to have a heart attack at such a young age. However, his family history was considered to be the primary risk factor. Consistent with his fighting spirit, Arthur became chairman of the national campaign for the American Heart Association within one year of his heart attack. He also started the Arthur Ashe Tennis Center to teach sports to children in inner cities.

After his heart attack, Arthur had two bypass surgeries. He contracted the human immunodeficiency virus from a blood transfusion after the second operation in 1983. He died of AIDS-related complications on February 6, 1993.

Arthur Ashe is a fitness hero because of his distinguished career on and off the tennis court. Despite many obstacles, he persevered and proved that he was a true hero. ✦

longer able to supply adequate amounts of oxygen to the muscles, and for a short period of time, glycogen is broken down anaerobically (in the absence of oxygen). You can only exercise for a brief period of time when energy is provided through **anaerobic metabolism**. Fat is the major energy source used for sustained physical activity, and it cannot be burned through anaerobic processes. Hence the higher your level of aerobic fitness, the more fat you can burn during an exercise session.

Oxygen uptake is influenced by factors such as age, sex, genetic background, and physical training. Typically, as you get older, your maximal level of aerobic power declines. After age 30, sedentary individuals experience a decrease in VO_2 of about one percent per year. The rate of decline is much slower among active individuals. Also, men tend to have a higher level of aerobic power than women of similar ages. This is primarily due to the larger body size of men and to a greater amount of lean muscle tissue. Some people are born with a genetic predisposition to be elite endurance athletes. They inherit larger, stronger hearts, greater lung capacity, better blood supply in their muscles, larger quantities of red blood cells, and higher percentages of slow-twitch muscle fibers, which are found in greater percentages in the muscles used in aerobic exercise. These muscle fibers contain energy foodstuffs and enzymes that enhance aerobic metabolism and promote exercise of longer durations. As shown in Table 5.1, aerobic training also leads to many of these same changes. Thus even if you are not born an elite marathon runner, you can become a pretty good one by engaging in a prolonged aerobic conditioning program.

The VO_2, or aerobic power, of an individual is expressed in volume (in liters) per unit of time (in minutes). Scores in the range of three to four l/min are common for the average healthy individual who exercises three to four times per week. Highly trained endurance athletes, however, may have a VO_2 ranging from five to six l/min. Usually, the greater the amount of muscle mass used in a sport, the higher the maximal oxygen uptake obtained through training. Thus people who engage in activities such as running, cross-country skiing, and cycling often have the highest measured VO_2.

There are several ways of expressing the maximal oxygen uptake. When expressed in units of l/min (**absolute** expression), it is often difficult to compare the actual fitness level of one individual to another. The reason is that the larger the body size, the higher the oxygen uptake, regardless of the level of fitness. Expressing VO_2 **relative** to a person's body weight

tions. The greater the quantity of ATP available, the greater your work capacity is.

As long as adequate amounts of oxygen are delivered to the muscles, the process of breaking down glycogen proceeds aerobically (in the presence of oxygen). When you reach VO_2, however, you are no allows individuals of different sizes to be compared. Hence, a smaller individual may have a lower VO$_2$ when it is expressed in units of l/min but when expressed in units of milliliters oxygen per kilogram of body weight per minute (ml $\times$ kg^{-1} $\times$ min^{-1}), the smaller person may actually have a much higher level of cardiorespiratory fitness.

Let us use an example to illustrate this point. Antony weighs 165 lbs and has a maximal oxygen uptake of 4.2 l/min. Miranda weighs 130 pounds and also has a maximal oxygen uptake of 4.2 l/min. Who is more fit? Antony's maximal oxygen uptake expressed in relative units is determined by:

$$\frac{4200\ (1000\ ml = 1l)}{75\ kg\ (1\ kg = 2.2\ lb)} = 56\ ml/kg\ of\ body\ weight$$

Miranda's oxygen uptake expressed in relative units is determined by:

$$\frac{4200\ (1000\ ml = 1l)}{59.1\ kg\ (1\ kg = 2.2\ lb)} = 71.1\ ml/kg\ of\ body\ weight$$

Were you surprised? What a big difference between their levels of fitness when you express the oxygen consumption relative to their body weight. Apparently, Miranda has a much higher level of fitness even though she has a much smaller body size than does Antony. Normally, active college-aged females have average maximal oxygen uptake values of 38 to 42 ml/kg $\times$ min^{-1}, compared to a value of 44 to 50 ml/kg $\times$ min^{-1} for college-aged males.

The most accurate method of measuring maximal oxygen uptake is through direct gas analysis in a laboratory setting. This procedure involves the use of computerized equipment such as a treadmill or a bicycle ergometer, and a mouthpiece, which is cumbersome to the individual. This procedure is quite sophisticated and the equipment is expensive. Thus, indirect methods of assessing the VO$_2$ in healthy individuals are often used.

Anaerobic metabolism The process of breaking down carbohydrates (glucose or glycogen) in the absence of oxygen in order to yield energy in the form of ATP.

Absolute VO$_2$ Expressing the volume of oxygen consumption in the units of liters of oxygen consumed per minute (l/min).

Relative VO$_2$ Expressing the volume of oxygen consumption in the units of milliliters of oxygen per kilogram of body weight per minute (ml/kg $\times$ min^{-1}).

Diversity Issues

Gender Differences

More U.S. women are exercising in the 1990s than ever before. The aerobic dance and exercise movement, the tennis and golf boom, and the thousands of new fitness centers attest to the number of women in the United States who are reaping the benefits of exercise.

Thanks to the Title IX section of the Educational Amendments Act of 1972 forbidding discrimination on the basis of sex in educational programs for activities in schools receiving federal funds, old attitudes and misconceptions about women and exercise are dissipating. Unfortunately, some still think that exercise makes women less feminine and that weight training makes them too masculine.

Women are equally as skilled as men and capable of performing well in any type of exercise. In fact, in some fitness areas, women are superior to men. Women have greater buoyancy than men because of a higher portion of fatty tissue, which is advantageous in swimming, as it means they require less energy to stay afloat. They are more flexible than men, as is evidenced in their ability to perform dance and aerobic routines. Even sedentary women can be as flexible as active men, and remain so throughout life. Women have a definite edge in the areas of grace and beauty of movement, which is important in competitive gymnastics and dance. Women have as great a physical skill-learning rate and capacity as men, and only in the areas of strength and endurance do women have some catching up to do. In fact, women's finishing times in marathons are coming closer to men's times every year.

Although women's bodies do not respond to training at the same rate as men's, they have a tremendous capacity for improving their muscular strength, muscular endurance, flexibility, body composition, and aerobic fitness levels. ✦

There are several field tests used to measure aerobic power indirectly. The most commonly used field tests include the 1-mile walking test, the 1.5-mile run, the 12-min run test, the 3-mile walking test, the 12-min swimming test, and the YMCA bicycle test. If

Table 5.2 ✦ Cardiorespiratory Fitness Classification for Women and Men According to Maximal Oxygen Uptake in ml/kg per min and METS

Sex	Age	(VO₂)	FITNESS CLASSIFICATION			
			Fair	Average	Good	Excellent
Women	< 30	ml/kg/min	24–30	31–37	38–48	> 49
		METS	7–8	9–10	10–14	> 14
	30's	ml/kg/min	20–27	28–33	34–44	> 45
		METS	5–8	8–9	10–13	> 13
	40's	ml/kg/min	17–23	24–30	31–41	> 42
		METS	5–6	7–8	9–12	> 12
Men	< 30	ml/kg/min	25–33	34–42	43–52	> 53
		METS	7–9	9–12	12–15	> 15
	30's	ml/kg/min	23–30	31–38	39–48	> 49
		METS	6–8	8–11	11–14	> 14
	40's	ml/kg/min	20–26	27–35	36–44	> 45
		METS	5–7	8–10	10–12	> 13

you have been involved in a physical conditioning program, you may elect to complete the 1.5-mile run test. If you are just beginning your aerobic exercise program, however, you should assess your maximal oxygen uptake by completing Lab Activity 5.1: Assessing Your Level of Aerobic Fitness by the Three-Mile Walking Test at the end of this chapter.

The 3-mile walk test is an excellent means of assessing cardiorespiratory endurance with a low risk of injury for someone who is just beginning an exercise program. Once you complete Lab Activity 5.1, use Table 5.2 to determine your fitness classification based on sex and age. If you are in the poor or fair fitness category, begin with the sample walking program presented later in this chapter. If you are in the good or excellent fitness category, begin with the sample jogging/running program also presented later in this chapter.

ℋOW TO SAFELY BEGIN AND PROGRESS IN AN AEROBIC FITNESS PROGRAM

We recommend following seven guidelines in order to minimize risk of injury when you begin an aerobic fitness program.

1. **Total work concept** The total amount of work you do each week is important when you are attempting to increase cardiorespiratory fitness and change body composition. Total work is usually calculated in units of calories (kcal) per week. Total work is assessed by quantifying the frequency, intensity, and duration of your exercise sessions. For instance, if you burn 300 kcal per 30-minute exercise session, four times per week, your total energy expenditure is 1200 calories per week. The next week, however, you might exercise three times per week for 45 minutes at the same exercise intensity and burn 400 calories per session. Your total work would still be 1200 calories. Thus if your schedule fluctuates constantly, you might still maintain your exercise schedule and meet your energy expenditure goals by manipulating exercise intensity, frequency, or duration. By the way, there are 3500 kcal in one lb of fat.

2. **Shin splints** Exercisers who engage in hard-impact, high-intensity exercise for extended periods of time are at risk of developing shin splints. This condition is an inflammation of the muscle-tendon junction on the outer front side of the lower leg. Shin splints are believed to be caused by overuse, improper shoes, poor exercise technique, hard surfaces, and back defects. To avoid shin splints, use a variety of activities, especially water aerobics, and avoid chronic exercise on hard surfaces so that you will not overstress the lower extremities.

3. **Stitch-in-the-side phenomenon** Adequate breathing while running is essential for maintaining suf-

ficient oxygen to exercising muscles. Diaphragmatic breathing (from the chest muscles) often results in the pain associated with the stitch-in-the-side phenomenon. The cause of this condition is unknown, but it is believed to be associated with an inability of the diaphragm muscle to use oxygen. If you use the abdominal muscles while breathing, the *stitch-in-the-side* phenomenon is less likely to occur. Expand your abdomen rather than your chest. Breathing should be rhythmic and closely associated with your stride. Most exercise physiologists recommend that you take a deep breath every two to four strides.

4. **Blisters** These can be very painful and are often debilitating. Friction develops at the point of contact between your foot and the running surface and initially causes hot spots. If this friction is not minimized, fluid will eventually develop between the layers of skin at the point of contact and swelling will occur, leading to a blister. To prevent blisters from developing, wear two pairs of cotton socks, especially when you are doing hard-impact exercises for long periods of time. Also, if you place a Bandaid® at the point of contact before the exercise session, the skin is protected, and blisters are less likely to develop. If a blister ruptures, you should treat it as an open wound and keep it sterile.

5. **Muscle soreness. Delayed-onset muscle soreness** (DOMS) often occurs within 12 to 24 hours after a high-intensity exercise session. During the initial phases of an exercise program, DOMS is most likely to occur. Most physiologists believe the cause is related to minute tears in the muscle fibers and connective tissue. After one or two days, the pain eventually subsides. You may take aspirin or another pain killer, such as acetaminophen, to relieve the pain. Gentle stretching after the workout, mild-intensity exercise, and light massage may also help decrease the pain.

6. **Heat illness symptoms** Most heat problems arise because of inadequate fluid intake and/or improper heat dissipation. As you begin exercising, your body temperature increases greatly because of the increased rate of metabolism. Normally, the body temperature is regulated by sweating. As the sweat evaporates from your body, it is cooled, and its inner temperature decreases. When you do not drink enough fluids before and during exercise, especially in hot, humid or hot, dry weather, however, the sweating

mechanism becomes less effective and your inner-body temperature remains elevated. Also, when you do not wear proper exercise clothing, the sweating mechanism becomes ineffective, and the core temperature remains elevated.

As your core temperature rises, symptoms such as muscle cramps, excessive fatigue, nausea, dizziness, light-headedness, headaches, diminished coordination, and cotton mouth, or dry lips, may develop. You may have any combination of these symptoms when heat illness occurs. As **heat exhaustion** develops, your rate of sweating increases, and you develop cold, clammy skin. As it intensifies, you may lose consciousness, and suddenly sweating will cease. If the skin becomes hot and dry and your pulse becomes rapid and strong, you may have suffered **heat stroke**.

If any of these symptoms occur while you are exercising, stop immediately, and begin removing layers of clothing. Also, drink as much fluid as you can tolerate, and elevate your feet. Begin cooling your body by using cold, wet towels; place ice on the body in more severe cases; and get out of the sun. Heat illness is extremely dangerous, and you should see a physician if it occurs.

7. **Rest, ice, compression, and elevation (RICE)** Avoidance of injury is crucial as you begin your conditioning program. RICE is the acronym for the recommended steps to follow in the immediate treatment of an injury. We recommend isolating the injured extremity instead of trying to walk it off in order to avoid creating a more serious condition. Place ice on the injured part for 20 to 30 minutes repeatedly for one to three days, depending on the severity of the injury. This will help decrease pain and minimize swelling. Compressing the injury with an Ace® bandage and elevating the injured part above the level of the heart and head also help reduce swelling. Protect your body at all times by warming up before, and

---

Delayed onset muscle soreness (DOMS) Muscle soreness that typically occurs 12 to 24 hours after a high-intensity exercise session.

Heat exhaustion (heat prostration) Collapse due to loss of fluid and salts caused by oversweating.

Heat stroke Severe, sustained rise in fever due to the failure of the body-heat-regulating mechanism after a prolonged period of elevated temperature.

Myth and Fact Sheet

Myth	Fact
1. Smoking is not harmful as long as you exercise.	1. Smoking limits your level of performance because it increases the airway resistance and decreases the amount of oxygen available to muscles. It also increases your heart rate by as much as 12 to 20 beats per minute, so your exercise endurance is compromised. Even after training, smokers do not improve as much as nonsmokers.
2. You should exercise every day in order to increase your level of cardiorespiratory fitness.	2. When you begin an exercise program, you should *not* exercise every day because you will increase the risk of getting injured. It is best to exercise on alternate days to allow adequate time for recovery. After you reach your maximal level of aerobic fitness, it is safe to exercise daily because your risk of injury will be lower after a long period of training.
3. You should wear a rubberized suit while exercising to increase the number of calories you burn during a workout.	3. You should *never* wear any type of rubber exercise clothing because of the increased amount of heat that is trapped in the body. Rubberized clothes will not allow the sweat to evaporate from the surface of the body, and if sweat does not evaporate, your inner body temperature does not decrease. This leads to heat exhaustion and even heat stroke. Always wear loose-fitting, cotton clothing to aid the sweating mechanism.
4. Jogging or rope skipping will cause a woman's breasts to stretch or sag.	4. No researchers have found this to be true. Giving birth to children and getting older often contribute to stretching and sagging breasts, but not exercise. Some women complain of tenderness or soreness in the breasts, especially when they fail to wear a suitable bra. A well-fitted bra will often eliminate any such discomfort during exercise.

cooling down after, each exercise session. Also remember that pain is your body's mechanism for letting you know that something is wrong so do not ignore it or try to *push through it*. Stop and investigate the problem in order to minimize the risk of developing a more serious situation.

SAMPLE STARTER PROGRAMS

Sample Walking Program

In recent years, walking has become one of the most popular of all aerobic activities. One reason for its popularity is that it does not require any specialized skills and is both safe and painless when the guidelines we discuss in this chapter are followed. You can walk almost anywhere, at any time, and at little cost. Many people choose walking over activities like jogging because it puts less stress on the hips, knees,

and ankles and results in a reduced risk of orthopedic injuries. Also, exercisers have found walking to be an excellent means of reducing body weight and lowering body fat percentage.

Many people feel that because they have been walking all their lives, they do not need instructions on how to begin a walking program. Any successful walking program depends, however, on your understanding of a few basic guidelines and principles. The basic principles of beginning an exercise program were covered earlier so we will limit our discussion here to special considerations for the beginning and for the advanced walker.

Duration During the initial phase of a walking program, you should walk 10 to 15 minutes at a pace that is comfortable to you. After one or two weeks, you can advance to 30-minute sessions. Continue walking for 30 minutes per session for at least four weeks in order to decrease your risk of injury and to minimize fatigue. After approximately six weeks, you can increase the exercise period to 45 minutes. The more advanced walkers typically progress to 60-minute walking sessions.

Intensity The first step in regulating exercise intensity is to *forget* the familiar saying "no pain—no gain." Calculate your target heart rate (THR); begin your walking program at 50 to 60 percent of that rate. Once you advance to 30-minute walking sessions, you can increase your exercise intensity to 60 to 65 percent of your THR. As you advance to 45- to 60-minute exercise sessions, remember to stay within your THR.

It is best to use your THR as a measure of intensity rather than using a particular walking speed. That will give you the best measure of the cardiorespiratory benefits of your workout. During the initial phase of your walking program, check your exercise heart rate every 5 minutes. Use a 10-second pulse count while walking, multiplying the result by six to determine your heart rate per minute. At the end of your exercise session, if you have walked at a comfortable pace, your heart rate should drop below 100 beats per minute following a 10-minute cool down period.

A great way of monitoring exercise intensity while walking without actually counting your pulse is to use the talk test. Any time you are walking with a partner, if your breathing rate is so fast that you cannot carry on a conversation with that person, you are probably walking too fast. Beginning to feel winded is an instant indication that you should slow down the pace.

If you are walking alone, a simple test to monitor exercise intensity is to take one inward breath with every three strides and one outward breath with the following three strides. If you are inhaling and exhaling at every two strides, you are probably exercising above your THR and should slow down. Remember: Exercise intensity is inversely related to exercise duration. If your exercise heart rate is too high, you will tire more quickly and exercise for shorter periods of time, and you will also increase your risk of getting injured. Exercise should be fun and relaxing; it is not meant to cause pain.

Frequency At the beginning of your exercise program, you should walk every other day up to a maximum of three to four days per week. After the first six weeks you can increase your frequency to four to five days per week. Limit your exercise frequency to a maximum of five days per week in order to allow a few days for recovery, thereby minimizing your risk of injury.

Calorie Cost When you begin your walking program, choose some premeasured distance, whether on a track, a cross-country trail, or a treadmill. This will enable you to calculate the number of calories burned as an estimate of the total amount of work you have completed. Table 5.3 shows one method of

Table 5.3 ✦ Energy Costs of Walking (kcal/min)

Body weight (lb)	Miles per hour/METs						
	2.0/2.5	2.5/2.9	3.0/3.3	3.5/3.7	4.0/4.9	4.5/6.2	5.0/7.9
110	2.1	2.4	2.8	3.1	4.1	5.2	6.6
120	2.3	2.6	3.0	3.4	4.4	5.6	7.2
130	2.5	2.9	3.2	3.6	4.8	6.1	7.8
140	2.7	3.1	3.5	3.9	5.2	6.6	8.4
150	2.8	3.3	3.7	4.2	5.6	7.0	9.0
160	3.0	3.5	4.0	4.5	5.9	7.5	9.6
170	3.2	3.7	4.2	4.8	6.3	8.0	10.2
180	3.4	4.0	4.5	5.0	6.7	8.4	10.8
190	3.6	4.2	4.7	5.3	7.0	8.9	11.4
200	3.8	4.4	5.0	5.6	7.4	9.4	12.0
210	4.0	4.6	5.2	5.9	7.8	9.9	12.6
220	4.2	4.8	5.5	6.2	8.2	10.3	13.2

Source: From *Fitness Leader's Handbook* (p. 149) B.D. Franks and E.T. Howley, Champaign, IL: Human Kinetics Publishers. Copyright 1989 by B. Don Franks, Edward T. Howley, and Susan Metros. Reprinted by permission.

Table 5.4 ✦ Days Required to Lose 5 to 25 Pounds by Walking* and Lowering Daily Caloric Intake

MINUTES OF WALKING	+	REDUCTION OF CALORIES PER DAY (IN KCAL)	DAYS TO LOSE 5 LB	DAYS TO LOSE 10 LB	DAYS TO LOSE 15 LB	DAYS TO LOSE 20 LB	DAYS TO LOSE 25 LB
30		400	27	54	81	108	135
30		600	20	40	60	80	100
30		800	16	32	48	64	80
30		1000	13	26	39	52	65
45		400	23	46	69	92	115
45		600	18	36	54	72	90
45		800	14	28	42	56	70
45		1000	12	24	36	48	60
60		400	21	42	63	84	105
60		600	16	32	48	64	80
60		800	13	26	39	52	65
60		1000	11	22	33	44	55

*Walking briskly (3.5–4.0 mph), calculated at 5.2 kcal/minute.

Source: From Frank Konishi, *Exercise Equivalents of Foods: A Practical Guide for the Overweight.* Carbondale, IL: Southern Illinois University Press, 1973.

determining the energy cost of walking in units of kcal per minute. To use this table, find horizontally the approximate speed you walk in miles per hour (or METs). One MET is equal to the resting metabolic rate. If your walking speed is four METs, the intensity is four times greater than that of the resting metabolic rate.

Next locate your approximate body weight on the vertical column. The figure at the intersection represents an estimate of the kcal used per minute. Multiply this figure by the number of minutes you exercise to get the total number of kcal used.

For example, Jennifer weighs 140 lbs and walks at a speed of 3.5 mph for 45 minutes:

$$3.9 \text{ (kcal/min)} \times 45 \text{ (minutes)} = 176 \text{ calories}$$

Her total caloric expenditure based on this table is approximately 176 kcal per exercise session.

An additional benefit of participating in activities that increase your level of cardiorespiratory fitness is that they also influence your body composition. Table 5.4 expresses the number of days required to lose 5 to 25 lbs by walking and lowering your daily caloric intake. This table demonstrates the combined benefits of exercise and caloric reduction in maintaining your body weight and lowering your body fat percentage. As you can see, the longer you exercise and the greater your caloric reduction, the quicker you

lose weight. For instance, if Daniele walks 45 minutes a day and decreases her caloric intake by 400 kcal per day, it should take her approximately 23 days to lose five pounds. And if Karen walks 30 minutes per day and reduces her caloric intake by 400 kcal per day, it should take her approximately 27 days to lose five pounds. Thus the longer you exercise, the quicker the results in terms of changes in body composition.

Rate of Progression Do not get discouraged if you do not see immediate progress, especially if you have not been exercising on a regular basis. During the initial phases of a walking program, first slowly increase the distance that you walk at a slow pace for a few weeks, and then increase the speed that you walk. This will give your body time to adjust to your new training program and reduce your chances of injury. It is best to increase your exercise time by no more than 10 percent a week. Most people will use from 90 to 150 calories per session during a 30-minute walk covering 1.5 miles. When you reach this level you are ready to move on to a more advanced phase of walking.

Advanced walkers typically use 200 to 350 calories per session by manipulating their exercise intensity and duration. Once you reach an advanced level of walking you may choose to begin a walk/jog/run program. Many people enjoy just walking, however, reaping many fitness benefits with little risk of injury.

As you begin your walking program, try to:

1. Maintain good postural alignment to avoid tension in the neck, back, and shoulders.

2. Hold your head high to help maintain good posture.

3. Use full, deep, abdominal breathing to enhance relaxation and monitor your walking pace.

4. Hold your arms in a relaxed position with the elbows flexed at a 90-degree angle.

5. Form a slightly clenched, relaxed fist with your hands.

6. Swing your arms naturally back and forth to add power to each stride.

7. Begin each stride with a slight forward lean of the body at the ankles.

8. As the foot contacts the surface, make contact on the outer edge of the heel.

9. On impacting the surface, roll the foot smoothly forward with most of the body weight distributed along the outer edge of the foot, transferring the weight to the ball of the foot and on to the toes for the push off.

10. Walk at a pace of 3 to 3.5 mph for a comfortable workout.

11. Walk at a pace of 3.75 mph for a vigorous workout.

12. Walk faster than 4 mph if you are an advanced walker.

13. Walk on dirt trails or grass for a more comfortable workout than if you walk on concrete sidewalks.

14. Be cautious when walking on uneven surfaces such as grass or dirt because of the increased risk of ankle sprains.

15. Walk in shoes with a comfortable fit, a cushioned sole, and good arch support.

16. Wear loose-fitting clothing to allow freedom of movement and dissipation of heat.

17. In cold weather, wear several layers of clothing to slow down the rate of heat loss.

18. In cold weather, wear a cap to avoid heat loss through the scalp.

19. Wear cotton socks to avoid getting blisters and to absorb perspiration.

20. Warm up before, and cool down after, each walking session.

Sample Jogging/Running Program

Once you complete an advanced walking program, you may be ready for a jogging program. Some people find walking so enjoyable that it is their exercise of choice. If you are not excessively overweight and do not have any orthopedic problems, however, you may decide to increase your exercise intensity and begin jogging. If you have any congenital heart defects or metabolic and/or cardiorespiratory diseases, consult a physician before beginning a jogging program.

For purposes of changing body composition, increasing muscular endurance, and improving cardiorespiratory endurance, jogging is one of the most effective activities. The energy costs of running are greater than those of walking the same distance (see Table 5.5 on page 86). Thus if you have reached a moderate to high level of fitness and want to increase your caloric expenditure but are unable to increase the amount of time you exercise, you should increase the exercise intensity by jogging instead of walking.

Complete the most advanced level of a walking program before you begin a jogging program. This will allow adequate time for the development of your cardiorespiratory system and the strengthening of your ligaments and tendons to reduce the risk of injury. There are many options in beginning a jogging program dependent on your initial level of fitness and prior exercise experience. Here are a few guidelines for jogging.

Duration In the initial phase of a jogging program, exercise 15 to 30 minutes. During the session, alternate brief periods of slow jogging (approximately five to six mph) with intervals of walking. Gradually increase the amount of time spent jogging and decrease walking time until you reach a level of fitness in which you can jog continuously for 30 minutes within your THR. As you reach an advanced level of running, exercise sessions may last as long as 60 minutes. Most people jog two to three miles an exercise session during the first 10 weeks of a jogging/running program. When you can jog three miles comfortably within 27 to 30 minutes, you are probably ready to advance to a running program. More advanced runners can cover five miles per session within 35 to 40 minutes.

Intensity An important factor in a jogging/running program is to monitor your exercise heart rate. During the initial phase of your program, stay in the 60 to 75 percent training heart rate zone. As you reach a higher level of fitness, you may increase exer-

Table 5.5 ✦ Energy Costs of Jogging and Running (kcal/min)

Body Weight (lb)	MILES PER HOUR/METS							
	3.0/5.6	4.0/7.1	5.0/8.7	6.0/10.2	7.0/11.7	8.0/13.3	9.0/14.8	10.0/16.3
110	4.7	5.9	7.2	8.5	9.8	11.1	12.3	13.6
120	5.1	6.4	7.9	9.3	10.6	12.1	13.4	14.8
130	5.5	7.0	8.6	10.1	11.5	13.1	14.6	16.1
140	5.9	7.5	9.2	10.8	12.4	14.1	15.7	17.3
150	6.4	8.1	9.9	11.6	13.3	15.1	16.8	18.5
160	6.8	8.6	10.5	12.4	14.2	16.1	17.9	19.8
170	7.2	9.1	11.2	13.1	15.1	17.1	19.1	21.0
180	7.6	9.7	11.8	13.9	15.9	18.1	20.2	22.2
190	8.1	10.2	12.5	14.7	16.8	19.1	21.3	23.5
200	8.5	10.8	13.2	15.4	17.1	20.1	22.4	24.7
210	8.9	11.3	13.8	16.2	18.6	21.1	23.5	25.9
220	9.3	11.8	14.5	17.0	19.5	22.2	24.7	27.2

Source: From *Fitness Leader's Handbook* (p. 150) B.D. Franks and E.T. Howley, Champaign, IL: Human Kinetics Publishers. Copyright 1989 by B. Don Franks, Edward T. Howley, and Susan Metros. Reprinted by permission.

cise intensity to 70 to 85 percent. Remember, however, that as your exercise intensity increases, you tend to exercise less because of an earlier onset of fatigue. Keep the training heart rate in the moderate range in order to receive the double benefits of improving cardiorespiratory fitness and to increase the percentage of fat calories used. You will see changes in body fat percentage more quickly by exercising at a moderate intensity (60 to 75 percent training heart rate zone).

Frequency The optimal frequency for jogging is every other day. If you want to exercise every day, use walking as a form of exercise on alternate days in order to decrease the amount of stress on your hips and the joints of the legs and feet. Even exercisers who participate in road races seldom exercise seven days per week. They recognize the need to allow a rest period between workouts. If you want to increase total work done on a weekly basis, it is better to increase exercise duration gradually and to maintain a moderate exercise intensity with a frequency of four to five times per week instead of jogging seven days per week.

Calorie Cost Table 5.5 shows one method of estimating the energy costs of jogging and running, expressed in units of kcal per minute. Let us consider the differences between walking and running for the same time periods.

If Joseph weighs 150 lbs and jogs at 7 mph for 45 min, he will burn 13.3 kcal per min. To find his total energy expenditure:

$$13.3 \text{ (kcal/min)} \times 45 \text{ (min)} = 599 \text{ kcal}$$

If Daniel weighs 150 lbs and walks at 3 mph for 45 min, he will burn 6.4 kcal per min. To find his total energy expenditure:

$$6.4 \text{ (kcal/min)} \times 45 \text{ (min)} = 288 \text{ kcal}$$

Both of these young men, with similar body weights and exercise durations, but with different exercise intensities, had vastly different caloric expenditures. Joseph burned more than twice as many calories as Daniel did. And since Joseph was moving at a faster pace, he covered more distance and had a higher caloric expenditure.

Another explanation for the difference in their energy expenditures is that the caloric cost of walking one mile and running one mile are not the same. Walking at speeds slower than 3.5 mph requires approximately half the energy cost of running at speeds greater than 6 mph. That is because more energy is required to lift the body from the ground when you are running than is necessary when you are moving the body forward on a horizontal plane as you do when you are walking. If a person walks at speeds of 5 mph, the energy cost of walking and running is similar. That is because your exercise heart rate will probably be nearly as high walking at 5 mph as it is when you are running at 6 mph. Thus the caloric cost is similar for walking at fast speeds and

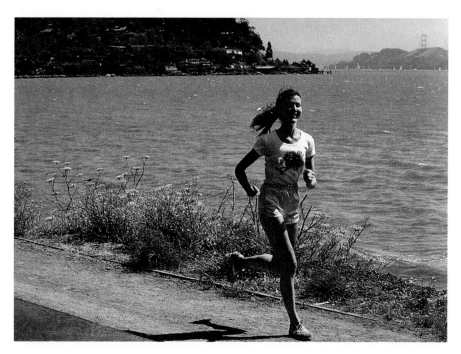

Jogging is one of the most effective activities for increasing muscular endurance, changing body composition, and improving cardiorespiratory endurance. (Photo Courtesy of the National Cancer Institute.)

jogging at relatively slow speeds. Remember that walking at slow speeds burns half the calories as does jogging the same distance at faster speeds, but walking at fast speeds can burn the same number of calories as jogging.

Table 5.6 shows the estimated number of days required to lose 5 to 25 pounds by jogging and lowering your daily caloric intake. To illustrate the difference between walking and jogging by using this chart, recall the example of Daniele who walked 45

Table 5.6 ✦ Days Required to Lose 5 to 25 Pounds by Jogging* and Lowering Daily Caloric Intake

Minutes of Jogging	+	Reduction of Calories per Day (in kcal)	Days to Lose 5 lb	Days to Lose 10 lb	Days to Lose 15 lb	Days to Lose 20 lb	Days to Lose 25 lb
30		400	21	42	63	84	105
30		600	17	34	51	68	85
30		800	14	28	42	56	70
30		1000	12	24	36	48	60
45		400	18	36	54	72	90
45		600	14	28	42	56	70
45		800	12	24	36	48	60
45		1000	10	20	30	40	50
60		400	15	30	45	60	75
60		600	12	24	36	48	60
60		800	11	22	33	44	55
60		1000	9	18	27	36	45

*Jogging: Alternate jogging and walking, calculated at 10.0 kcal/min.
Source: From Frank Konishi, *Exercise Equivalents of Foods: A Practical Guide for the Overweight.* Carbondale, IL: Southern Illinois University Press, 1973.

minutes and reduced her caloric intake by 400 calories per day. It took Daniele 23 days to lose 5 pounds. Now let us assume that Joseph jogs for 45 minutes a day and reduces his caloric intake by 400 calories per day. It will only take him 18 days to lose 5 pounds because of the increased energy expenditure for jogging as compared to walking. Naturally, the greater your exercise duration, the higher the intensity, and the greater the reduction in caloric intake, the quicker you will see changes in your body composition.

Rate of Progression During the initial phase of a jogging program, you should combine walking and jogging. If you maintain a constant walking interval of 60 seconds, you can increase the jogging intervals until you are doing more jogging than walking. Always be careful to use exercise heart rate as your guide for determining the jogging/walking intervals. As your fitness level increases, you should be able to jog for longer periods of time while remaining within your target training zone. Most people use 350 to 750 kcal per session in a jogging/running program.

Concentrate on slow steady progress. As long as you are constantly increasing the total amount of calories used from your weekly workouts, remaining within your THR zone, and having no problems with injuries, you are probably working out at a suitable level.

After the first two months of a jogging program, you may notice that you do not seem to be improving as much as you expected. During this time, you might easily become discouraged and bored with your training program. That is when you might consider changing the intensity and duration of your workouts or training for a short road race. Alternatively, you can change your exercise route so that the environment becomes more exciting. Try running with a partner or listening to music while you jog. By changing the environment and increasing the amount of visual or auditory stimulation during the workout, you will find that time seems to pass more quickly, and you become less focused internally on your body and more focused on external factors. This shift in your attention away from your body may enable you to exercise for longer periods of time without becoming bored.

Sample Swimming Program

Swimming Swimming is an excellent aerobic activity. Patients in cardiac rehabilitation programs and in physical therapy often use a pool as their primary means of aerobic conditioning because of the decreased stress on hips, knees, and ankles that exer-

cising in water affords. In addition, the warmer water temperatures of a pool are therapeutic for arthritic patients. Furthermore, since body weight is supported, obese persons have fewer injuries while exercising in water. As a consequence, a growing number of people are choosing aquatic exercises as their primary mode of fitness. Since the cardiorespiratory benefits derived from water exercises are similar to those derived from jogging and cycling, consider including water exercises as a part of your training program.

Water Exercises Water aerobics are highly touted by exercise physiologists because they cause virtually no impact to the muscles and the skeletal system and are safe for people of all ages regardless of health status.

For years, water exercises were avoided because it was believed there was insufficient resistance in the pool to stimulate cardiorespiratory endurance. In reality, water is nearly 1000 times more dense than air and thus creates greater resistance. This increased resistance provides a higher workload for the muscles. We now know that the resistance of the water is sufficient to challenge even the most elite athlete, and an increase in cardiorespiratory fitness can easily be experienced by participating in water exercises.

An added benefit is that this cushioned medium promotes a virtually injury-free environment. The density of water gives almost any object placed in it a certain buoyancy. Your body will weigh less in water because of buoyancy, so less stress is placed on it when you exercise in water.

Obese people may especially enjoy exercising in water because it is much easier for them to dissipate heat. When you exercise, a great deal of heat is generated as a result of metabolism. This heat is often difficult for an obese person to release because of the thick layer of fatty tissue underneath the skin. Heat is much easier to dissipate in water than it is in air so the obese find exercising in it much more comfortable. One advantage water aerobics provides over jogging is that jogging does nothing to work the upper body, but water greatly increases strength and endurance in the upper body as well as the lower body. Here are guidelines to follow when you begin a water exercise program.

Duration Start at a comfortable level. This will vary depending on your initial level of fitness. If you are a swimmer but have been inactive for a long period of time, you may need to spend a few weeks walking across the width of the pool in chest-deep water until you can complete two 10-minute intervals at your exercise heart rate. Gradually alternate walking and

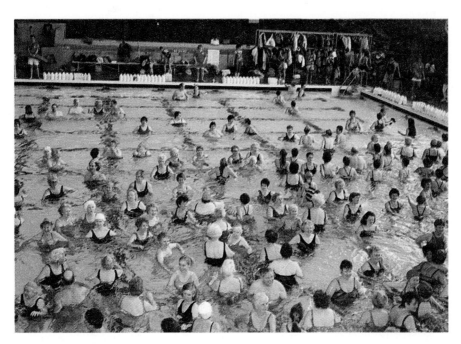

Water exercise places less stress on the body than many other exercises, and is a great way for people of all ages to improve their cardiorespiratory fitness. (Photo Courtesy of the United States Water Fitness Association.)

jogging across the pool until you can complete four 5-minute intervals of jogging at your training heart rate. As you progress, you can jog across the pool and swim back. Repeat this pattern until you jog/swim for about 20 to 30 minutes. As your level of fitness increases, spend more time swimming and less time jogging until you can swim continuously for 20 to 30 minutes. Advanced swimmers can swim 30 to 45 minutes each exercise session.

Intensity Research has shown that a person's maximal heart rate is approximately 10 beats lower in the water than it is on land. Thus when women calculate their training heart rate for water activities, use the formula 210 (rather than 220) minus your age to determine your maximal heart rate. From there, follow the standard formula for calculating your training heart rate that appeared in chapter 4. During the initial phase of your swimming program, begin at a pace that keeps your heart rate at 50 percent of your target training zone. Gradually increase exercise duration and intensity as level of fitness increases, but be careful to remain within your heart rate zone.

Frequency As with other forms of aerobic exercise, you should swim three to four days per week. If you have trouble tolerating chlorinated pools, you can alternate swimming with other forms of aerobic exercise. You can also wear swimming goggles to protect your eyes from irritation.

Calorie Cost It is difficult to estimate the energy costs associated with swimming because there are vast differences between individuals based on the efficiency of the stroke used. Table 5.7 on page 90 shows the estimated caloric cost per mile of swimming the front crawl for men and women according to skill level. The values are expressed in units of kcal per mile. You may be surprised to find that the lower the skill level, the higher the energy expenditure for both men and women. That is because unskilled swimmers often fight the water and waste a lot of energy during each stroke. As the level of skill rises, however, the swimmer becomes more efficient and the caloric cost decreases. This might lead you to believe that poorly skilled swimmers will burn a lot more calories per workout than highly skilled swimmers will. This is not true. Unskilled swimmers exercise for a shorter period of time because they tire earlier than skilled swimmers do and will probably spend more time resting than actually swimming. For this reason, poorly skilled swimmers should use a combination of water exercises with swimming to increase their caloric expenditure.

Table 5.7 ✦ Caloric Cost Per Mile (kcal/mile) of Swimming the Front Crawl for Men and Women, by Skill Level

SKILL LEVEL	WOMEN	MEN
Competitive	180	280
Skilled	260	360
Average	300	440
Unskilled	360	560
Poor	440	720

Source: From *Fitness Leader's Handbook* (p. 155) B.D. Franks and E.T. Howley, Champaign, IL: Human Kinetics Publishers. Copyright 1989 by B. Don Franks, Edward T. Howley, and Susan Metros. Reprinted by permission.

Table 5.8 shows the estimated number of days required to lose 5 to 25 pounds by swimming and lowering daily caloric intake. When this table is compared to Table 5.6, which shows the same estimates for weight loss by jogging, you can see that swimming is very similar to jogging in terms of caloric expenditure. For instance, if Alexandra swims for 30 minutes and decreases her caloric intake 800 kcal per day, it should take her 14 days to lose 5 pounds. If she jogs for 30 minutes and decreases her caloric intake 800 calories per day, it should take her the same 14 days to lose 5 pounds. But if she walks for 30 minutes at the same caloric reduction, it should take her 16 days to lose 5 pounds. Undoubtedly, swimming is as beneficial as jogging in terms of changing body composition.

Rate of Progression Unless you are a very good swimmer, you may become exhausted after swimming only one or two laps. Since continuous exercise is essential for improving cardiorespiratory fitness, in this case begin with a walk/jog/swim program. As your level of aerobic conditioning increases and your swimming skills improve, you should be able to spend more time swimming and less time walking/jogging. It is not essential that you spend the entire workout actually swimming. You can easily achieve your exercise heart rate through other water exercises. As you begin your water aerobics program, follow these guidelines:

1. Always exercise in a supervised environment. It is possible to get muscle cramps in water, especially if you swim too soon after eating a meal. If you are exercising in chest-deep water, you could be in danger.

2. Exercise in water two to three inches above the waist. The depth of the water determines the amount of resistance experienced. When the water is too shallow, more stress is placed on the

Table 5.8 ✦ Days Required to Lose 5 to 25 Pounds by Swimming* and Lowering Daily Caloric Intake

MINUTES OF SWIMMING	+	REDUCTION OF CALORIES PER DAY (IN KCAL)	DAYS TO LOSE 5 LB	DAYS TO LOSE 10 LB	DAYS TO LOSE 15 LB	DAYS TO LOSE 20 LB	DAYS TO LOSE 25 LB
30		400	23	46	69	92	115
30		600	18	36	52	72	90
30		800	14	28	42	56	70
30		1000	12	24	36	48	60
45		400	19	38	57	76	95
45		600	15	30	45	60	75
45		800	13	26	39	52	65
45		1000	11	22	33	44	55
60		400	16	32	48	64	80
60		600	14	28	42	56	70
60		800	11	22	33	44	55
60		1000	10	20	30	40	50

*Swimming at about 30 yards/min, calculated at 8.5 kcal/min.

Source: From Frank Konishi, *Exercise Equivalents of Foods: A Practical Guide for the Overweight.* Carbondale, IL: Southern Illinois University Press, 1973.

lower extremities. Conversely, when the water level is too high, buoyancy increases and less resistance results, making the exercises less effective.

3. Avoid excessive twisting in the water in order to minimize the risk of injury.

4. If the surface of the pool is rough, wear cotton socks to avoid scratching the soles of your feet.

5. Stand with your knees slightly bent, and avoid locking your joints.

6. Keep your arms in the water to generate more resistance. This helps raise the heart rate into the target training zone.

7. Cup your hand during water activities to increase the amount of resistance.

8. Ankle weights may be used to increase the intensity of lower body workouts.

9. To improve your balance in the water, use a stride stance (one foot forward, the other behind) in the pool.

10. You may opt to use hand paddles, fins, pull buoys, and/or wrist weights to increase resistance.

11. When you are doing lower body exercises, keep your pelvis tilted upward to help support the lower back.

12. Include warmup exercises before, and cooldown exercises after, your water workout.

Sample Bicycling Program

Bicycling, or cycling, has become an increasingly popular aerobic activity especially for those who have joint problems or those who are overweight. For them, cycling is ideal because their weight is supported. Consequently they can often exercise for longer periods of time. Today, stationary bikes are as popular as 10-speed and mountain bikes are. Cycling has a high energy expenditure per minute and can result in tremendous increases in cardiorespiratory endurance and muscular strength and endurance.

Duration Each cycling session should last approximately 30 to 45 minutes. When you can cycle several miles within a 30-minute period, you have reached a high level of cardiorespiratory fitness.

Intensity As long as you are at the beginning of your cycling program, you may have to exercise below your THR in order to cycle 1 to 2 miles. After a few weeks of cycling this distance, however, you should be able to exercise at 60 percent of your heart rate zone. As you progress to cycling 3 to 5 miles, you may increase your exercise intensity to as high as 70 to 75 percent. Be careful to limit the intensity so that you can maintain your endurance. Once you reach a maximal level of fitness and can cycle 10 to 15 miles, you may increase your exercise intensity to 80 percent of your heart rate zone. A word of caution to those using stationary bikes: Periodically check your resistance setting because the work load tends to shift when you ride for long periods of time.

Frequency As with other forms of cardiorespiratory exercise, you should cycle three to five times per week. Bike on alternate days to allow adequate rest. During the first phase of a cycling program, bike a maximum of three days per week. Since cycling is not a familiar exercise to many people, they may experience more muscle soreness initially than they would with other activities such as walking.

Calorie Cost The type of bike you ride will effect the calories you expend. A person riding a 10-speed bike can cover the same distance as a person riding a mountain bike and probably burn fewer calories, depending on which gear the bike is in. Thus estimates of the calorie cost are approximations and may be less accurate than the estimates for activities such as walking and jogging.

Table 5.9 on page 92 shows estimates for the calorie cost for cycling 10 to 60 minutes for distances of 1 to 15 miles on a flat surface. To use the table, find the time closest to the number of minutes you cycle on the horizontal line. Then find the approximate

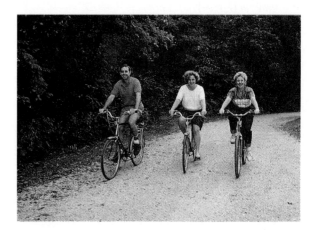

A regular bicycling program can result in tremendous increases in cardiorespiratory endurance. (Photo Courtesy of the National Cancer Institute.)

Table 5.9 ✦ Determining Calorie Cost for Bicycling

DISTANCE (IN MILES)	TIME (IN MIN)										
	10	15	20	25	30	35	40	45	50	55	60
1.00	.032										
1.50	.042	.032									
2.00	.062	.039	.032								
3.00		.062	.042	.036	.032						
4.00			.062	.044	.039	.035	.032				
5.00			.097	.062	.045	.041	.037	.035	.032		
6.00				.088	.062	.047	.042	.039	.036	.034	.032
7.00					.081	.062	.049	.043	.040	.038	.036
8.00						.078	.062	.050	.044	.041	.039
9.00							.076	.062	.051	.045	.042
10.00							.097	.074	.062	.051	.045
11.00								.093	.073	.062	.052
12.00									.088	.072	.062
13.00										.084	.071
14.00											.081
15.00											.097

Source: From Ivan Kusinitz and Morton Fine, *Your Guide to Getting Fit*, 2d ed. Mountain View, CA: Mayfield Publishing Company, 1991.

distance in miles you cover on the vertical column. The number at the intersection represents an approximate calorie cost.

For example, Anita weighs 185 lbs and cycles 1.5 miles in 16 minutes. To find out her caloric expenditure:

185 (lbs) × .032 (kcal/lb) = 5.92 × 16 min = 95 kcal burned

Table 5.10 shows the number of days required to lose 5 to 25 pounds by cycling and lowering daily caloric intake. If we assume that Christine rode her bike for 60 minutes and reduced her caloric intake by 400 calories per day, it would take her 19 days to lose 5 pounds. By comparing this table to Table 5.6 you can see that the energy expenditure for cycling is very similar to that for jogging. Thus cycling is an excellent activity for both increasing cardiorespiratory endurance and changing body composition.

Progressive Cycling Program Begin a cycling program by riding one or two miles at a comfortable pace until your level of fitness increases to the point that you can train at the low end of your THR. Depending on your level of fitness, you may ride 1 to 2 miles per session for several weeks. Soon you should be able to ride approximately 3 to 5 miles. Continue at this level for several weeks. Gradually add mileage until you are able to cycle 10 to 15 miles each session. Depending on your rate of progression, you may be in a cycling program for six months or more before you can cycle continuously for 10 to 15 miles. Those who are very fit may need to ride faster than 13 to 15 miles per hour in order to reach their THR zone.

Rate of Progression As was mentioned earlier, it is crucial to start at a comfortable pace in order to avoid injuries and extreme muscle soreness. It is better to increase the distance that you cycle instead of increasing your speed until you reach a high level of fitness. Following this advice will allow your body to adapt to this form of aerobic exercise. Do not be embarrassed to take rest periods during the early phases of your cycling program, and if you ride a 10-speed bike, switch gears periodically to lessen the resistance and make the ride a little easier. The key to a successful cycling program is to increase your total work gradually. Follow these guidelines when beginning your cycling program:

Table 5.10 ✦ Days Required to Lose 5 to 25 Pounds by Bicycling* and Lowering Daily Caloric Intake

MINUTES OF BICYCLING	+	REDUCTION OF CALORIES PER DAY (IN KCAL)	DAYS TO LOSE 5 LB	DAYS TO LOSE 10 LB	DAYS TO LOSE 15 LB	DAYS TO LOSE 20 LB	DAYS TO LOSE 25 LB
30		400	25	50	75	100	125
30		600	19	38	57	76	95
30		800	17	34	51	68	85
30		1000	13	26	39	52	65
45		400	22	44	66	88	110
45		600	17	34	51	68	85
45		800	14	28	42	56	70
45		1000	12	24	36	48	60
60		400	19	38	57	76	95
60		600	15	30	45	60	75
60		800	13	26	39	52	65
60		1000	11	22	33	44	55

*Bicycling calculated at 6.5 kcal/min at approximately 7 mph.

Source: From Frank Konishi, *Exercise Equivalents of Foods: A Practical Guide for the Overweight.* Carbondale, IL: Southern Illinois University Press, 1973.

1. Adhere to all traffic rules and wear appropriate safety gear when you are cycling outdoors.

2. Adjust the seat height so that your knee has a slight bend when your foot is at the bottom of a pedal swing. This position gives you maximum power without creating stress on your spine.

3. Saddle soreness occurs because of either chafing caused by friction on the skin of the buttocks or increased pressure on the genital area and the buttocks that causes pain and numbness. To avoid or minimize saddle soreness, use corn starch or talcum powder. You may also consider purchasing a larger seat for the bicycle.

4. Wear cycling shorts padded by soft chamois sewn in the seat to increase the cushioning and reduce friction.

Sample Rope-Skipping Program

On days when you cannot do outdoor aerobic activities or when you want to try a different form of aerobic conditioning, rope skipping is an excellent alternative. One factor that deters many exercisers from using rope skipping as their primary form of exercise is the amount of skill involved in turning and jumping. Since exercise needs to be continuous in order for you to achieve maximal cardiorespiratory benefits, you need to become proficient in jumping and turning. With practice, however, even a novice can become a good rope skipper.

It is important to purchase a rope of the correct length. The rope should be long enough to reach from armpit to armpit while it is passing under both feet. When the rope is too short, you are forced to jump in a humped position, and poor posture while exercising at high intensities causes increased strain on the back muscles. In addition, buy a good pair of exercise shoes because of the stress to the balls of your feet.

Duration Most beginners use an interval program consisting of brief periods of jumping followed by periods of rest. Unless you are already involved in a physical conditioning program, start with a beginning-level walking program to improve your level of fitness and strengthen your joints, tendons, and ligaments before you begin rope skipping. Since rope skipping can cause fatigue in the arms, stretch before and after each exercise session. Initially, the amount of time actually spent jumping may be small. As you continue exercising and your coordination improves, you will be able to increase the amount of time you spend jumping.

Intensity During the initial phase of a rope-skipping program, you may actually exercise at an intensity below your training heart rate zone. Do not push too hard too soon. Rope skipping requires constant im-

Behavioral Change and Motivational Strategies

There are many things that might interfere with your ability to improve your cardiorespiratory fitness. Here are some barriers (roadblocks) and strategies for overcoming them.

Roadblock	Behavioral Change Strategy
Your schedule fluctuates from week to week because you travel for your job. It is difficult to establish a regular time for exercise, and you find that your exercise frequency decreases during the weeks that you travel.	Several strategies included in chapter 3 apply to your situation. First, you need to consider *tailoring* a program to suit your needs. Since your schedule constantly changes, you should consider including a variety of cardiorespiratory activities in order to increase your fitness level. While you are traveling, you could use exercise equipment in the fitness center of your hotel. You could also jog, providing you are in a safe environment. Use the exposure to a new surrounding to increase your likelihood of exercising rather than as an excuse not to exercise. You could also manipulate your total work so that during the weeks when your exercise frequency decreases, you can extend the duration of exercise sessions and/or increase exercise intensity. Another principle from chapter 3 also applies here. Use *reminder systems* to help you remember the appropriate exercise intensity, frequency, and duration for the upcoming week based on your traveling schedule.
You are at the end of your second year of college and are horrified to find that you have gained 25 pounds in two years! You have never been involved in an aerobic conditioning program and find it difficult to get started.	Begin by *contracting*. Once you establish exercise goals, develop a contract and have it witnessed by someone (see Figure 3.1 on page 42). Your chances of adhering to your exercise program will also be much greater initially if you use *social support*. Try to find an exercise partner who will motivate you to stick with the program. Finally, we recommend that you use *gradual programming*. Since you have not been a regular exerciser, it may be difficult to jump right into a program and maintain it. Do not get discouraged if you are not 100 percent adherent initially. You will find that, as the weeks pass and you begin to experience benefits from exercising, your level of motivation will increase and it will become easier to get off the couch and exercise.
Your friends have decided to join a health club. You were never good at sports and have gained 15 pounds since graduation from college. Your level of fitness really is not great, but you don't want to be left out of the group.	Remember first that increasing your level of cardiorespiratory fitness can be fun. Select activities that you enjoy doing that require little skill. Many aerobic exercises require very little skill, so don't be discouraged if you are not ready for strenuous exercise at the club. You will find that, as your level of cardiorespiratory fitness increases, you will have greater stamina. Your coordination will also improve and you may find yourself trying sports that were beyond you when you first joined. Begin with a walk/jog program. Find a friend who has a fitness level similar to yours, and begin exercising together. By using these methods, you will feel more confident and not as self-conscious about exercising at the club.
List other roadblocks preventing you from participating in a cardiorespiratory endurance program or factors hindering your progress in your current program.	Now cite behavior change strategies that can help you overcome these roadblocks.

1. _____   1. _____

2. _____   2. _____

3. _____   3. _____

pact on the bones in the feet and can cause trauma to them. As your level of fitness increases, you will be able to exercise at 65 to 75 percent of your heart rate zone. Avoid very high exercise intensities while rope skipping because of the stress to your hips, knees, ankles, and feet.

Frequency As with other forms of aerobic exercise, rope skip no more than three days per week on alternate days. Because a lot of stress is placed on the lower parts of the body, you may choose to alternate rope skipping with other forms of exercise to reduce the risk of injury. Water exercises are an especially good alternative because of the lack of stress on the joints.

Calorie Cost Table 5.11 shows the gross energy cost of rope skipping in units of kcal/min. By way of example, Natasha weighs 110 lbs and skips slowly for 20 minutes. Her estimated caloric expenditure is calculated as:

$$7.5 \text{ kcal/min} \times 20 \text{ min} = 150 \text{ kcal}$$

If Joyce also weighs 110 pounds and skips at a fast pace for 20 minutes her caloric expenditure would be:

$$9.2 \text{ kcal/min} \times 20 \text{ min} = 184 \text{ kcal}$$

Hence these two women, who have the same body weight, would have different energy expenditures based on the speed of turning the rope.

Table 5.11 ✦ Gross Energy Cost of Rope Skipping (kcal/min)

BODY WEIGHT (LBS)	SLOW SKIPPING	FAST SKIPPING
110	7.5	9.2
120	8.2	10.0
130	8.9	10.9
140	9.5	11.7
150	10.2	12.5
160	10.9	13.4
170	11.6	14.2
180	12.3	15.0
190	13.0	15.9
200	13.6	16.7
210	14.3	17.5
220	15.0	18.4

Source: From *Fitness Leader's Handbook* (p. 154) B.D. Franks and E.T. Howley, Champaign, IL: Human Kinetics Publishers. Copyright 1989 by B. Don Franks, Edward T. Howley, and Susan Metros. Reprinted by permission.

Rate of Progression Most beginners skip rope at 60 turns per minute. This is usually a comfortable pace that allows time for the beginner to develop coordination between turning and jumping. As you advance, you should be able to increase the number of turns to 70 to 100 per minute. Rope skipping can become boring so, as your skill level increases, you may use tactics such as jumping on one foot or changing the direction of the rope to introduce variety into your program. If you have trouble with coordination, try jumping while you listen to music.

SUMMARY

Many physiological benefits can be derived from participating in an aerobic fitness program, including a lower resting heart rate, a stronger heart, and a greater blood supply to exercising muscles. All these benefits will increase aerobic power and make exercise feel easier at workloads below maximum.

Overview and Analysis of Aerobic Exercise Choices

Only aerobic exercises will increase your cardiorespiratory endurance. There are many options for aerobic activities of which a number are not dependent on your having a high skill level. During the initial phase of your program, participate in activities that rely on large muscle groups to increase your endurance and minimize your risk of injury.

Maximal Oxygen Consumption

Cardiorespiratory endurance is synonymous with maximal oxygen consumption. The maximal oxygen uptake is influenced primarily by (1) the ability of the cardiorespiratory system to deliver oxygen to the muscles and (2) the ability of the muscles to extract oxygen from the blood. When comparing the fitness level of individuals, it is best to express the maximal oxygen uptake in units of ml/kg $\times$ min^{-1}. Although the maximal oxygen uptake is best measured by gas analysis, field tests are often used to decrease the expense while still providing an accurate indication of aerobic fitness.

How to Safely Begin and Progress in an Aerobic Fitness Program

It is important to manipulate the exercise intensity, duration, and frequency to both (1) maintain the targeted amount of total work and (2) adjust to the schedule. If you have a busy week planned, you can easily manipulate these factors and still maintain your caloric expenditure. Avoid shin splints by wearing good running shoes, exercising on soft surfaces, and using a variety of aerobic exercise choices. Use the abdominal breathing technique to reduce the pain associated with the stitch-in-the-side phenomenon. Wear two pairs of cotton socks and place a Bandaid® on hot spots to reduce blisters. When muscle soreness occurs, use light massage, static stretching, and light-intensity exercise to decrease pain and stiffness. Always maintain your level of hydration, and wear adequate clothing to avoid heat illness. Use RICE as the immediate form of therapy for injuries.

Sample Starter Programs

Walking is one of the most popular aerobic activities because it does not require any specialized skills. When you start a walking program, begin walking 10 to 15 minutes per session at a comfortable pace at 50 to 60 percent of your THR three to four times per week. Gradually increase your rate of progression until you reach a distance of five miles. At this point you may consider beginning a jogging program.

Complete the advanced walking program before beginning a jogging/running program. Gradually increase the amount of time spent jogging until you can jog continuously for 30 to 45 minutes. The aver-

age distance covered by more advanced runners is five miles per session within 35 to 40 minutes. During the initial phase, remain in the 65 to 75 percent training heart rate zone. The optimal frequency is three to four days per week. Overuse can quickly result in injuries. To prevent injury, increase your distance before you increase your speed.

Swimming and water aerobics have increased in popularity because of the high rate of musculoskeletal injuries associated with other aerobic activities. The resistance in water is sufficient to elicit increased cardiorespiratory endurance while providing a virtually injury-free environment. If you are not a strong swimmer, begin with a walking program, and spend more time doing water exercises. As both your level of fitness and your swimming ability increase, you may make your total workout program one of swimming. The exercise heart rate is lower in water, so be careful to adjust for that.

Cycling is a great aerobic activity because your body weight is supported. Begin cycling a distance of one or two miles, even if you are exercising below your THR zone. Increase your intensity and duration until you can cycle three to five miles at 70 to 75 percent intensity. The type of bike used will effect caloric expenditure; thus the caloric cost of cycling is difficult to estimate.

Rope skipping is too often avoided by aerobic exercisers because of the skill needed and of the high amount of impact involved. Begin with brief periods of jumping followed by periods of rest. Complete a beginning walking program first in order to increase your level of fitness and decrease your risk of injury. Begin at 65 to 75 percent of your training heart rate and exercise three days per week on alternate days. You may choose to participate concurrently in alternative aerobic activities, such as swimming, to experience a more rapid increase in cardiorespiratory fitness with little risk of injury.

Lab Activity 5.1

Assessing Your Level of Aerobic Fitness by the Three-Mile Walking Test

INSTRUCTIONS: *The objective of this walking test is to cover three miles in the fastest time possible without running. It can be performed on a track or on any distance that has been accurately measured. (If you are a jogger/runner, you may choose to substitute the 1.5-mile run test.)*

◆ Step 1: Pretest Screening

1. If you are over 35 years of age, seek the advice of your physician before taking this test.

2. Do not eat or drink anything except water for at least three hours before taking the test.

3. Avoid using any type of tobacco, including cigarettes and chewing tobacco, for at least three hours before taking the test.

4. Avoid heavy physical activity on the day of the test.

5. If you are on medication, report it to your instructor before you begin the test.

6. Wear loose-fitting clothes, such as shorts and a T-shirt, and running shoes.

◆ Step 2: Administration of the Test

1. Divide participants into two groups.

2. Each participant in the first group should choose a partner from the other group.

3. Those taking the test first complete a thorough warmup session and slowly walk one lap around the track.

4. The partner maintains a scorecard that records time in minutes and seconds and keeps track of the number of laps walked.

5. The instructor explains the procedures again and instructs the first group to begin.

6. As the walker completes each lap, the partner lets the walker know how many laps remain and encourages the partner to maintain a steady pace.

7. The instructor calls out the time in minutes and seconds periodically.

8. The partner writes the final time on the scorecard.

9. After all walkers in the first group have finished, the second group takes the test while the first group acts as partners.

✦ Step 3: Interpreting the Results

1. The following table contains five fitness classifications based on age and sex.

2. To use the table, find on the horizontal line the approximate length of time it took for you to walk three miles in your age category. Then locate on the vertical column your fitness category, according to sex.

3. For example, if you are an 18-year-old male and it took 36 minutes and 12 seconds for you to walk three miles, you are in the *good* fitness category.

4. Review Table 5.2 on page 80 to obtain an estimate of your maximal aerobic power based on your performance in this test.

Three-Mile Walking Test (No Running) Time (Minutes)

Fitness category		AGE (YEARS)			
		13–19	20–29	30–39	40–49
1. Very poor	(men)	> 45:00*	> 46:00	> 49:00	> 52:00
	(women)	> 47:00	> 48:00	> 51:00	> 54:00
2. Poor	(men)	41:01–45:00	42:01–46:00	44:31–49:00	47:01–52:00
	(women)	43:01–47:00	44:01–48:00	46:31–51:00	49:01–54:00
3. Fair	(men)	37:31–41:00	38:31–42:00	40:01–44:30	42:01–47:00
	(women)	39:31–43:00	40:31–44:00	42:01–46:30	44:01–49:00
4. Good	(men)	33:00–37:30	34:00–38:30	35:00–40:00	36:30–42:00
	(women)	35:00–39:30	36:00–40:30	37:30–42:00	39:00–44:00
5. Excellent	(men)	< 33:00	< 34:00	< 35:00	< 36:30
	(women)	< 35:00	< 36:00	< 37:30	< 39:00

*< Means *less than*, > means *more than*.

✦ Step 4: Cardiorespiratory Endurance Record

Name _____   Date _____

Age _____   Sex _____   Body Weight _____ lbs

Walking Time _____   Fitness Category _____

Maximal VO$_2$ (ml/kg × min^{-1}) _____

Lab Activity 5.2

Assessing Your Level of Aerobic Fitness by the One-Mile Walking Test

INSTRUCTIONS: *This test is designed for older adults or for those who are just beginning an aerobic conditioning program. The time of the walk and the postexercise heart rate value are used to predict the subject's maximal oxygen consumption.*

✦ **Step 1: Pretest Screening**

1. If you are over age 35, seek the advice of your physician before taking this test.

2. Do not eat or drink anything except water for at least three hours before taking the test.

3. Avoid using any type of tobacco, including cigarettes and chewing tobacco, for at least three hours before taking this test.

4. Avoid heavy physical activity on the day of the test.

5. If you are on medication, report it to your instructor before you begin this test.

6. Wear loose-fitting clothes, such as shorts and a T-shirt, and running shoes.

✦ **Step 2: Administration of the Test**

1. Divide participants into two groups.

2. Each participant in the first group should choose a partner from the other group.

3. Those taking the test first complete a thorough warmup session and slowly walk one lap around the track.

4. The partner maintains a scorecard that records time in minutes and seconds and keeps track of the number of laps walked.

5. The instructor explains the procedures (such as the fact that the faster the participants walk, the higher their level of cardiorespiratory fitness will be) and instructs the first group to begin.

6. The students are to walk the mile as fast as possible, and only walking is allowed.

7. As the walker completes each lap, the partner lets the walker know how many laps remain and encourages the partner to maintain a steady pace.

8. The instructor calls out the time in minutes and seconds periodically.

9. The partner writes the final time on the scorecard.

10. The partner immediately takes the walker's 10-second heart rate. Instruct the walker that the heart rate count should be completed within 15 seconds after the end of the mile walk. Any further time delay will result in an overestimation of the maximal oxygen consumption.

11. After all walkers in the first group have finished, the second group of walkers takes the test while the first group acts as partners.

✦ Step 3: Interpreting the Results

1. The tables on pages 101 and 102 contain the estimated maximal oxygen uptake $(ml/kg \times min^{-1})$ for women and men 20 to 39 years old based on the one-mile walk test.

2. To use the tables, find the section that pertains to your age and sex. On the horizontal line across the top, find the amount of time (to the nearest minute) it took to walk a mile. In the vertical column, find the point of intersection for your walking time and your postexercise heart rate (listed in the far left column). The number where the postexercise heart rate and the one-mile time intersect is your maximal oxygen consumption expressed in $ml/kg \times min^{-1}$. For example, a 34-year-old woman who walked the mile in 17 minutes and had a postexercise heart rate of 170 would have an estimated oxygen consumption of 27.6 $ml/kg \times min^{-1}$. According to Table 5.2 on page 80, she would be in the *fair/good* fitness category.

3. Review Table 5.2 to obtain an estimate of your maximal aerobic power based on your performance in this walk test.

✦ Step 4: Cardiorespiratory Endurance Record

Name _____   Date _____

Age _____   Sex _____   Body Weight _____ lbs

Walking Time _____   Fitness Category _____

Maximal VO_2 $(ml/kg \times min^{-1})$ _____

Estimated Maximal Oxygen Uptake (ml/kg $\times$ min^{-1}) for Women, 20 to 39 Years Old

Heart rate	Min/mile										
	10	11	12	13	14	15	16	17	18	19	20
Women (20–29)											
120	62.1	58.9	55.6	52.3	49.1	45.8	42.5	39.3	36.0	32.7	29.5
130	60.6	57.3	54.0	50.8	47.5	44.2	41.0	37.7	34.4	31.2	27.9
140	59.0	55.7	52.5	49.2	45.9	42.7	39.4	36.1	32.9	29.6	26.3
150	57.4	54.2	50.9	47.6	44.4	41.1	37.8	34.6	31.3	28.0	24.8
160	55.9	52.6	49.3	46.1	42.8	39.5	36.3	33.0	29.7	26.5	23.2
170	54.3	51.0	47.8	44.5	41.2	38.0	34.7	31.4	28.2	24.9	21.6
180	52.7	49.5	46.2	42.9	39.7	36.4	33.1	29.9	26.6	23.3	20.1
190	51.2	47.9	44.6	41.4	38.1	34.8	31.6	28.3	25.0	21.8	18.5
200	49.6	46.3	43.1	39.8	36.5	33.3	30.0	26.7	23.5	20.2	16.9
Women (30–39)											
120	58.2	55.0	51.7	48.4	45.2	41.9	38.7	35.4	32.1	28.9	25.6
130	56.7	53.4	50.1	46.9	43.6	40.4	37.1	33.8	30.6	27.3	24.0
140	55.1	51.8	48.6	45.3	42.1	38.8	35.5	32.3	29.0	25.7	22.5
150	53.5	50.3	47.0	43.8	40.5	37.2	34.0	30.7	27.4	24.2	20.9
160	52.0	48.7	45.4	42.2	38.9	35.7	32.4	29.1	25.9	22.6	19.3
170	50.4	47.1	43.9	40.6	37.4	34.1	30.8	27.6	24.3	21.0	17.8
180	48.8	45.6	42.3	39.1	35.8	32.5	29.3	26.0	22.7	19.5	16.2
190	47.3	44.0	40.8	37.5	34.2	31.0	27.7	24.4	21.2	17.9	14.6

Calculations assume a body weight of 125 lbs for women. For each 15 pounds beyond 125 lbs, subtract 1 ml from the estimated maximal oxygen uptake given in the table.

Source: From *Fitness Leader's Handbook* (pp. 90–91) B.D. Franks and E.T. Howley, Champaign, IL: Human Kinetics Publishers. Copyright 1989 by B. Don Franks, Edward T. Howley, and Susan Metros. Reprinted by permission.

Estimated Maximal Oxygen Uptake (ml/kg $\times$ min^{-1}) for Men, 20 to 39 Years Old

Heart rate	MIN/MILE										
	10	11	12	13	14	15	16	17	18	19	20
Men (20–29)											
120	65.0	61.7	58.4	55.2	51.9	48.6	45.4	42.1	38.9	35.6	32.3
130	63.4	60.1	56.9	53.6	50.3	47.1	43.8	40.6	37.3	34.0	30.8
140	61.8	58.6	55.3	52.0	48.8	45.5	42.2	39.0	35.7	32.5	29.2
150	60.3	57.0	53.7	50.5	47.2	43.9	40.7	37.4	34.2	30.9	27.6
160	58.7	55.4	52.2	48.9	45.6	42.4	39.1	35.9	32.6	29.3	26.1
170	57.1	53.9	50.6	47.3	44.1	40.8	37.6	34.3	31.0	27.8	24.5
180	55.6	52.3	49.0	45.8	42.5	39.3	36.0	32.7	29.5	26.2	22.9
190	54.0	50.7	47.5	44.2	41.0	37.7	34.4	31.2	27.9	24.6	21.4
200	52.4	49.2	45.9	42.7	39.4	36.1	32.9	29.6	26.3	23.1	19.8
Men (30–39)											
120	61.1	57.8	54.6	51.3	48.0	44.8	41.5	38.2	35.0	31.7	28.4
130	59.5	56.3	53.0	49.7	46.5	43.2	39.9	36.7	33.4	30.1	26.9
140	58.0	54.7	51.4	48.2	44.9	41.6	38.4	35.1	31.8	28.6	25.3
150	56.4	53.1	49.9	46.6	43.3	40.1	36.8	33.5	30.3	27.0	23.8
160	54.8	51.6	48.3	45.0	41.8	38.5	35.2	32.0	28.7	25.5	22.2
170	53.3	50.0	46.7	43.5	40.2	36.9	33.7	30.4	27.1	23.9	20.6
180	51.7	48.4	45.2	41.9	38.6	35.4	32.1	28.8	25.6	22.3	19.1
190	50.1	46.9	43.6	40.3	37.1	33.8	30.5	27.3	24.0	20.8	17.5

Calculations assume a body weight of 170 pounds for men. For each 15 pounds beyond 170 pounds, subtract 1 ml from the estimated maximal oxygen uptake given in the table.

Source: From *Fitness Leader's Handbook* (pp. 90–91) B.D. Franks and E.T. Howley, Champaign, IL: Human Kinetics Publishers. Copyright 1989 by B. Don Franks, Edward T. Howley, and Susan Metros. Reprinted by permission.

6

IMPROVING MUSCULAR STRENGTH AND ENDURANCE

Chapter Objectives

By the end of this chapter, you should be able to:

1. Identify the factors that directly or indirectly effect muscular strength and endurance.

2. Cite the advantages of acquiring and maintaining adequate muscular strength and endurance throughout life.

3. Design a personalized strength-development program using weights that applies sound training principles and meets your fitness objectives.

4. Design a personalized muscular-endurance training program without weights that applies sound training principles and meets your fitness objective.

5. Complete a strength and endurance routine using one of the acceptable methods described in this chapter.

6. Design a sound girth control program to flatten your stomach.

ESTHER HAS BEEN interested in trying some form of strength training for years to firm her muscles and improve her appearance. She is also interested in it because she has heard something about this type of training aiding weight and fat loss. Some of her friends who use the weight room at the gym seem to have improved their bodies and are looking good. Esther wants to get started too, but she has many questions and concerns. What type of program should she choose? How often should she workout? Should she use heavy or light weights? Will she add too much muscle and lose her femininity?

The answers to these and many more questions are provided in this chapter to help Esther and others begin sound strength-training programs designed to meet their personal objectives.

Although muscular strength and endurance are closely related, it is important to differentiate between the two. Muscular strength is the amount of force or weight a muscle or group of muscles can exert for one repetition. It is generally measured by a single maximal contraction. The amount of weight you can bench press overhead one time, for example, measures the strength of the triceps muscle. You can measure the strength of other muscle groups the same way with specific tests (see chapter 2). Muscular endurance is the capacity of a muscle group to complete an uninterrupted series of repetitions as often as possible with light weights. The total number of bench presses you can complete with one-half of your maximum weight on the barbell, for example, measures the endurance of the triceps and pectoralis muscles. Depending on the desired outcome, you can manipulate the training variables (choice of equipment and exercises, amount of resistance or weight, number of repetitions and sets, length of rest interval) to make your program strength- or endurance-oriented or a balance of both.

This chapter addresses the key factors involved in training for the development of strength and endurance, including importance, influencing factors, training principles and suggestions, specific exercises, equipment, girth control, and other related concerns to help design a program to meet your specific needs.

THE IMPORTANCE OF STRENGTH AND ENDURANCE

The improvement of muscular strength and endurance will affect almost every phase of your life. Some of the benefits, such as the loss of body fat and improved self-concept, have been overlooked in the past because of overemphasis on adding muscle mass and improving performance. A closer look at the true value of strength and endurance training makes it clear that a sound program can help to improve both physical and mental health. Complete Lab Activity 6.1: Do You Need to Start a Strength-Training Program? to determine whether you need to begin a strength-training program.

The Management of Body Weight and Fat

Although strength training is generally associated with muscle weight gain and not with body weight and fat loss, it is a critical part of a total weight-control program. Unfortunately, although metabolism slows with age, the amount of calories (cal) we consume does not. As a result, body weight and fat increase and the amount of lean muscle mass decreases. From 25 to 50 years of age, **basal metabolism** slows by as much as 15 percent in some sedentary individuals. The typical 60-year-old, for example, burns about 350 fewer daily calories at rest than he or she burned at age 25. This is equivalent to one pound of fat (3500 cal = 1 lb of fat) every ten days, 3 lb per month, 36 lb per year. As you can see, even small decreases in metabolism produce large increases in body weight and fat. A 5 percent slowing of metabolic rate, for example, can add 6 to 9 lbs of body fat in just one year depending on your weight and size at the time (see chapter 9 for a more detailed discussion of basal metabolism).

This slowing of resting metabolism is a direct result of the loss of lean muscle mass through inactivity, something that happens to everyone who is, or becomes, inactive regardless of age. Although it requires energy (cal) to maintain muscle tissue at rest, fat or adipose tissue is almost metabolically inert and requires very few calories to maintain. A comparison of two individuals identical in weight, one with ten pounds more muscle than the other, clearly shows that the resting metabolism is significantly higher in the more muscled individual. According to some experts, resting metabolism increases by approximately 30 to 50 cal daily for every pound of muscle weight added. In other words, you burn enough extra calories at rest to lose three to five lbs a year for every pound of muscle mass you add.

Regular strength and endurance training and aerobic exercise can prevent much of this undesirable change in metabolic rate. In fact, a well-conceived weight-training program that emphasizes muscle-weight gain will actually increase basal metabolism regardless of age. For both women and men, aerobic exercise followed by a half-hour strength-training session three to four times weekly, coupled with sound nutrition, is an ideal approach to weight control throughout life.

Improved Appearance, Body Image, and Self-Concept

Muscular strength and endurance training can improve your physical appearance. By reducing your caloric intake, losing body fat and weight, improving muscle tone, and adding muscle weight, you will look better.

When weight loss occurs too rapidly, particularly without exercise, skin gives the appearance of not fitting the body very well. Sagging skin on the back of the arms, for example, is often an indication of either too rapid, or too large an amount of, weight loss. With reduced caloric intake, fat cells shrink but the skin does not keep pace to provide a tight fit. One way to improve appearance and help your skin fit better during and after weight loss is to include strength training as part of your total program. As fat cells shrink in the back of your arms, for example, strength training can enlarge the tricep muscle tissue to help avoid sagging skin.

Keep in mind that these changes will not occur overnight. Depending on age and current physical state, it may take 12 months or more of regular aerobic exercise, strength and endurance training, and dietary management of calories to decrease total body fat significantly, add 5 to 10 pounds of muscle weight, tone the entire body, give skin sufficient time to rebound to a tight fit, and adjust to the new body. These changes will alter the way you both perceive yourself and feel others perceive you. Practically everyone who stays with a program experiences improved body image and self-concept that positively affects their personal and professional lives. Patience is necessary, however; proper nutrition and exercise, rather than diets, are meant to be lifetime activities.

Increased Bone-Mineral Content

Recent studies suggest that regular strength training aids in optimal bone development by improving bone-mineral content. The use of strength training in addition to weight-bearing exercise, such as walking, jogging, racket sports, and aerobic dance, may help women reach menopause with more bone-mineral mass, an important factor in the prevention, and delay, of osteoporosis (see chapter 8).

Increased Strength and Endurance for Work and Daily Activities

Each of the training programs discussed in this chapter will effectively increase both muscular strength and endurance in the relatively short period of 8 to 12 weeks. If you are, for example, in the process of moving or helping a friend to move, you will notice an improvement in your ability to lift furniture and other heavy objects without undue fatigue. Additional strength and endurance will also

Basal metabolism The energy expended (calories burned), measured by oxygen consumption, during a resting state over a 24-hour period.

Diversity Issues

Strength and Endurance in Young People in the United States

Strength training, particularly in its most popular form of weight training, has traditionally been a man's activity at all age levels. Unfortunately, boys, girls, men, and women are equally in need of this key aspect of a complete fitness program. Studies continue to indicate that elementary school-aged children of both sexes are extremely weak in the upper body and in the abdominal area. A recent survey of 18,857 public school students at 187 schools revealed that 40 percent of boys aged 6 to 12 and 70 percent of girls in the same age group could not do more than one pull up, and 45 percent of boys aged 6 to 14 and 55 percent of girls in that age group could not hold their chins over a raised bar for more than 10 seconds. Special programs in our schools and universities, such as the Presidential Fitness Awards, have had little impact on the muscular strength and muscular endurance of the nation's youth. Overall, the performance of U.S. children in these areas has changed very little from surveys taken 10 to 20 years ago. Widespread use of strength training in our nation's schools could dramatically improve both upper body and abdominal strength and endurance in children, and could improve the future physical fitness of our nation.

This trend is unlikely to change unless the emphasis on muscular strength and endurance is increased in U.S. schools. Minimum standards should be developed with each individual required to meet and maintain the standards. Specific programs must then bring about improvement without totally disrupting the remaining phases of the physical education program. A major reason for neglect in the past is lack of strength-training facilities that accommodate entire physical education classes. Although free weights and special weight-training apparatus offer the most effective and quickest approach to improvement, they are certainly not the only methods or the most practical. The use of circuit training involving calisthenics stations or special strength-endurance obstacle courses are not only effective but extremely time efficient. Both could be used the first or last 10 minutes of each class period. With proper recordkeeping and planning, significant improvement would occur in both the strength and endurance of our nation's young people. ✦

help you perform daily personal and work activities more efficiently and provide you with the extra strength needed to cope with unexpected emergencies in life.

Improved Performance in Sports and Recreational Activities

Children and adults often lack strength and endurance in the upper body (arms and shoulders) and in the abdominal area. Many studies also show that most women are weak in the arms and shoulders because they think strength training will cause a loss of femininity, a totally unfounded fear. It is important to recognize that individualized, safe weight-training programs can be designed for both sexes at all ages and that these programs will improve muscular strength and endurance in the upper body, stomach, lower back, and other areas with little or no health risks or change in femininity. Increased upper-body and abdominal strength and endurance also helps to improve physical appearance and self-concept. Such a program helps children and young adults to engage in a wide variety of sports such as tumbling, gymnastics, baseball, basketball, field hockey, touch football, and soccer. You will also notice a difference when you perform an aerobic exercise or dance class, a conditioning class, or participate in your favorite recreational activity. The additional strength and endurance will delay fatigue and make free movement easier.

Muscle fibers Bundles of tissue composed of cells.

Myofibrils Thin protein filaments that interact and slide by one another during a muscular contraction.

Tendon A fibrous band into which some muscles narrow down for attachment to a bone.

Slow-twitch, oxidative muscle fiber Red muscle fiber used in aerobic activity that contracts and tires slowly.

Fast-twitch, glycolytic muscle fiber White muscle fiber used in anaerobic activity that contracts rapidly and explosively but tires quickly because it has a poor blood supply.

Fast-twitch, oxidative, glycolytic fiber An intermediate fiber that can be used in both anaerobic and aerobic activity.

Decreased Incidence of Sports and Work-Related Injuries

Improved strength in the musculature surrounding the joints helps prevent injuries to your muscles, tendons, and ligaments. With regular training, bones and connective tissue become stronger and more dense. These changes make you less vulnerable to muscle strain, sprains, contusions, and tears (see chapter 12 for more details). Even low back pain may be prevented by an improved balance of strength and flexibility in the abdominal and back extensor muscles.

Strength training is also an important part of recovery following certain injuries. Return to normal range of motion and strength following soft-tissue injuries occurs more rapidly and completely with rehabilitative strength training.

ℱACTORS EFFECTING MUSCULAR STRENGTH AND ENDURANCE

Muscle Structure

A cross section of various parts of a muscle are shown in Figure 6.1. Each muscle contains bundles of tissue composed of cells referred to as **muscle fibers**. A muscle fiber is composed of contractile units called **myofibril**s.

The entire muscle, consisting of the bundles and the muscle fibers, are covered and bound together by layers of connective tissue that blend together to form the **tendon**. When you contract your bicep, for example, the muscle shortens with the force moving through the tendon to the bones to bend the elbow.

Types of Muscle Fiber

The three types of muscle fibers contained in each muscle in the body can be classified by two factors: the speed with which they contract and their main energy system (see Figure 6.2 on page 108). **Slow-twitch, oxidative fiber** is used primarily in aerobic endurance activities such as jogging, marathon running, and cycling. These fibers contract slowly but are also slow to fatigue because of their tremendous vascular supply. **Fast-twitch, glycolytic fiber** is used primarily for explosive anaerobic movements such as sprinting, jumping, and throwing. These fibers contract explosively, tire rapidly, and are suitable for short-duration exercise. **Fast-twitch, oxidative, glycolytic fiber** has a speed of contraction that is faster than that of slow-twitch, oxidative fiber but slower than fast-twitch, gly-

Figure 6.1 ✦ The Structure of Muscle. The whole muscle (a) is composed of separate bundles of individual muscle fibers (b). Each fiber is composed of numerous myofibrils (c), each of which contains thin protein filaments (d) arranged so they can slide by one another to cause muscle shortening or lengthening. Various layers of connective tissue surround the muscle fibers, bundles, and whole muscles, which eventually bind together to form the tendon.

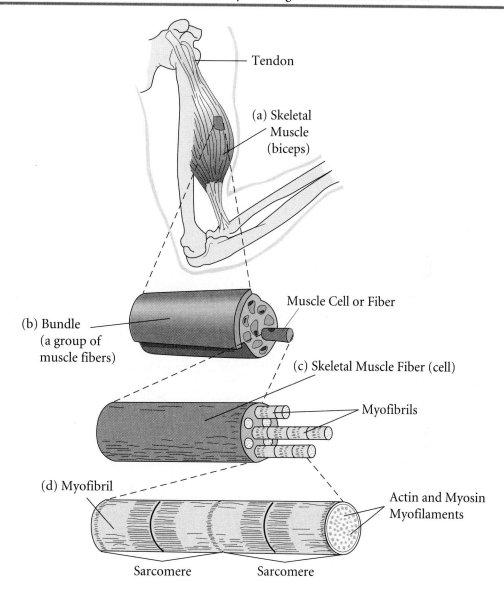

colytic fiber, and fatigue occurs much more slowly than that of the fast-twitch, glycolytic fiber.

How Muscles Become Larger and Stronger

The capability of a muscle or muscle group to generate force for one maximum repetition depends on such factors as size, type, number of muscle fibers activated, and the ability of the nervous system to activate these fibers. Although your strength potential is limited by genetics and the number and size of fast-twitch fibers, everyone can improve strength with proper training. As training progresses, muscle cells will increase in size (particularly the fast-twitch fibers), the myofibrils in each cell may increase in number, and the connective tissue around your muscle fibers and bundles of muscle may also thicken. These three factors will significantly increase the size of a muscle in 8 to 10 weeks. Although women generally do not progress at the same rate as men do, significant increases in cell size also occur after engaging in a sound weight-training program.

Fitness Heroes

Fred Hatfield was an orphan who learned early that he had only himself to rely on. He was a highly motivated student and athlete, but he seemed to have extra drive and a need for success. After college, Fred continued his studies and eventually earned his Ph.D. While in graduate school, Fred developed an interest in power lifting, and he participated in competitions throughout the world. With vigorous training and competition, his body changed from 165 pounds to over 225 pounds.

Dr. Fred Hatfield, affectionately referred to as *Dr. Squat,* is the founder and current President of the International Sports Society of America. He once held nine world records, including that for the greatest lift of all time—1008.5 pounds in the squat—a feat declared by some experts to be the single greatest athletic achievement of the twentieth century. No one in power lifting has achieved such success since. Fred not only made great personal strides in power lifting, but also has contributed to the success of others by encouraging young athletes with lectures, demonstrations, books, and leadership of the International Sports Society. ✦

You can improve your local muscular endurance by training both types of fast-twitch fiber by increasing the number of repetitions and by using lower weight. As training progresses, you will be capable of performing a greater number of repetitions for each exercise.

STRENGTH-TRAINING PRINCIPLES

The training principles discussed in this section will help you design a program to meet your specific needs. First, consult Table 6.1, and choose a primary training objective. This table allows you to approximate the weight and number of sets and repetitions needed to fit your training objectives. The table is based on:

1. Heavy weight and low repetitions (three to six) develop considerably more strength and muscle mass than endurance. Your starting weight for

Figure 6.2 ✦ Muscle Fiber Types   SO is the slow-twitch, oxidative fiber; FOG is the fast-twitch, oxidative, glycolytic fiber; and FG is the fast-twitch glycolytic fiber.

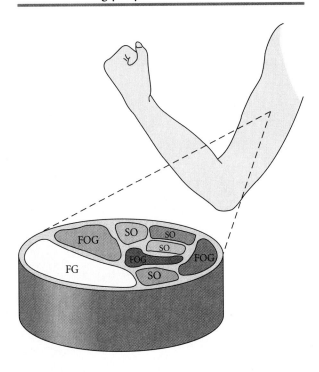

each exercise should be about 80 percent of your 1-RM (maximum amount of weight you can lift one time). If your maximum lift on the bench press is 100 lb, your starting weight is 80 lb (100 × .80).

2. The closer you work to the 1-RM, the greater the strength gains. Unfortunately, the chance of injury increases with weight so this approach is somewhat impractical.

3. Heavy weight, a moderate number of repetitions (six to eight), and multiple sets is more effective in adding muscle weight (mass).

4. Light weights and a high number of repetitions develops muscular endurance more than strength.

5. From a health standpoint, using 6-RM as the starting weight and progressing to nine repetitions is ideal for general bodily development and the improvement of muscular strength and endurance.

6. Regardless of your training objective, the final repetition in each set should result in complete muscle failure or the inability to perform even one more repetition.

Table 6.1 ✦ Strength and Endurance Training Objectives and Variable Control

DESIRED PHYSICAL OUTCOMES	VARIABLE CONTROL
Strength	Heavy weight (3-RM or 80% of 1-RM), low repetitions (3 to 9), slow negative phase, multiple sets (3 to 5), moderate rest between each set and exercise (90 seconds), use of maximum lift days.
Muscular endurance	Light weight (10-RM), high repetitions (10 to 15), slow negative phase, multiple sets (2 to 3), minimum rest between each set and exercise (2 min decreasing to 30 sec).
Strength and endurance/general body development/improved athletic performance	Moderate weight (6-RM), moderate repetitions (6 to 9), slow negative phase, multiple sets (2 to 3), moderate rest between each set and exercise (1 min)
Muscle mass or bulk	Heavy weight (3- to 5-RM), low repetitions, multiple sets (5 to 10), minimum rest between sets and exercises (1 min), use of a large number of different exercises for each muscle group and of periodization (2- to 3-week cycles that alter the resistance, repetitions, and sets from low through moderate to high).
Speed and explosive power	Moderate weight (5-RM), low repetitions (3 to 5), explosive contractions, slow negative phase, use of Olympic power lifts.
Rehabilitation from injury	Light weight and slow contractions performed without pain and to the full range of motion, 6 to 10 repetitions, 3 sets, and use of exercises that activate the supporting muscles of the joints (ankle, wrist, knee, and shoulder).

Types of Training

The three most commonly used strength and endurance training methods are isotonics, isokinetics, and isometrics, each with a number of variations and each requiring special equipment. During an isotonic contraction, such as the execution of an arm curl with free weights or universal or nautilus machines, the muscle shortens (**positive phase**) as the weight is brought toward the body and lengthens (**negative phase**) as it is returned to the starting position. Inertia helps move the weight during the positive phase, and the weight is slowly lowered under control during the negative phase. During an **isokinetic** arm curl with special equipment, the muscle also shortens and lengthens during the positive and negative phases; however, maximal resistance is provided throughout the full range of movement in both phases. Without the benefit of inertia or gravity to allow a weight to drop, the routine would be considerably more difficult. In an isometric contraction, the exercised muscle contracts but its overall length remains unchanged.

You are performing isotonic contractions when you use Free Weights, Universal, Nautilus, Cam II, Polaris, and other similar equipment. New Life Cycle equipment has found a way to eliminate cheating and take full advantage of the negative phase of contraction. During the negative phase of each repetition, the weight automatically increases by 25 percent. It is

Positive phase of muscular contraction The phase of a weight-training exercise when weight is brought toward the body and muscle shortening occurs.

Negative phase of muscular contraction The phase of a weight-training exercise when weight is returned to the starting position and muscle lengthening occurs.

Isokinetic contraction Muscular movement that involves both muscle shortening and lengthening during the positive and negative phase.

also nearly impossible to drop the weight and cheat as you return to the starting position in the negative phase or to use inertia to help during the positive phase.

The Mini-gym uses the isokinetic, or accommodating resistance, principle designed to overload the muscle group maximally through the entire range of motion. The harder you pull, the harder the Mini-Gym resists your pull. Since there is no negative phase, strength gains are not as rapid as they are with other equipment.

Hydra Fitness and Eagle Performance Systems combine the isotonic and isokinetic methods by automatically adjusting to the strength and speed of the individual.

Isometric exercises can be compared to weight-training movements in which the weight is so heavy that it cannot be moved. It involves a steady muscle contraction against immovable resistance for six to eight seconds. Strength gains appear to be specific to the angle and do not transfer into increased strength throughout the full range of motion.

Calisthenics is the oldest form of weight training. Using the body as resistance, it represents a safe, practical, and effective method of developing muscular strength and endurance. Since the resistance is low body weight and since a high number of repetitions must be used to bring about fatigue, the program is more effective for developing muscular endurance than it is for developing strength. Calisthenics is also an ideal, safe strength and endurance training method for preadolescent children.

Professional athletes and experts prefer isotonic movements with free weights for the development of muscular strength and endurance, muscle mass, and speed. Special equipment that allows either isotonic or isokinetic movement is excellent for rehabilitation from injury, focusing on specific body areas, and improving general body development. This equipment is relatively safe and can be performed without a spotter, or partner.

Amount of Resistance (Weight) to Use

The weight with which you can perform a specific number of repetitions is called the RM (repetitions maximum). The 9-RM, then, is the amount of weight that would bring you to almost complete muscle failure on the ninth repetition—you could not perform even one additional repetition. After you decide on the range of repetitions for your training objective, your starting weight is the RM for the lower repeti-

tion (for example, with a six to nine cycle, your starting weight is 6-RM).

Number of Repetitions to Complete

The number of consecutive times you perform each exercise is called **repetitions**. A high number (10 to 20) with lighter weights favors the development of endurance, whereas a low number (3 to 5) with heavier weights tends to favor strength development.

Number of Sets to Complete

One group of repetitions for a particular exercise is a **set**. Depending on your training objectives and the method of progression you select, three to five sets are recommended. Sets should be performed consecutively for each exercise before moving on to another muscle group. To avoid excess muscle soreness and stiffness, beginners should start with one set and gradually work up to three over a period of three to four weeks.

Amount of Rest between Sets

The time you take between each set is the **rest interval**. Muscle fibers will recover to within 50 percent of their capacity within 3 to 5 seconds and continue to near full recovery after about two minutes. In a program designed to increase strength only, the rest interval is less important and should approach one minute. For muscular endurance training, however, the rest interval should gradually decrease from two minutes to about 30 seconds over a six- to eight-week period. Unless you slowly decrease the rest interval between repetitions or increase the number of repetitions, you will not improve muscular endurance.

Amount of Rest between Workouts

For a total body workout, you will receive the best effect of training when you allow at least 48 hours of rest (alternate-day training) between each workout. With shorter rest periods, complete recovery is not taking place, and you are not receiving the full benefits of your workout. For split-body routines that emphasize the upper body one day and the lower body the next, it is possible to train for six consecutive days before taking a day of rest. If too much time (four or more days) passes before the next workout,

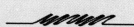

Myth and Fact Sheet

Myth	Fact
1. Strength training will make me inflexible.	1. Strength training will actually improve your flexibility providing you go through the full range of motion on each exercise and stretch properly before and after each workout.
2. Strength training makes females unfeminine and masculine.	2. With only three to four strength training sessions weekly, it is impossible to acquire large, bulky muscles. A program using a moderate number of repetitions and weight will only improve your feminine appearance.
3. Strength training will turn my fat to muscle.	3. Fat (adipose) and muscle are separate tissue types. You cannot convert one to the other. When you burn more calories than you eat, fat cells shrink. Strength training causes muscle tissue to increase in size and helps your skin fit you better after weight loss.
4. Sit ups are the best stomach flattening exercise.	4. Although exercises such as the curl are helpful in flattening the stomach, they are not as effective as decreasing your caloric intake. Reduced calories will shrink the fat cells in your stomach area; the girth control program described in this chapter will improve the muscular strength and endurance of your abdominal muscles. Both programs must be used to obtain a flat stomach.
5. If stomach exercises do not hurt, they will not work.	5. You can improve your abdominal strength and endurance without pain. In fact, it is good advice to back off when a burning sensation occurs to prevent muscle soreness and injury.
6. Without steroids, it is next to impossible to add muscle.	6. You can safely add one to two lbs of muscle a month (up to one-half lb per week) without steroids through weight training and sound nutrition.
7. Why should I start a strength training program? When I stop, my muscle will turn to fat.	7. As we indicated previously, fat cannot turn into muscle nor can muscle change into fat. When you stop exercising, muscles will get smaller and fat cells will get larger.

acquired strength and endurance gains begin to diminish.

Speed for Completing Exercises

For most training objectives, you should return the weight to the starting position (negative phase) twice as slowly as you completed the positive phase. If it took you one second to bench press the weight overhead, it should take two seconds to lower the weight. It is important to raise the weight slowly enough to eliminate the help of inertia in the positive phase and lower the weight under control to receive the full benefit of the negative phase. If you merely drop the weight in the negative phase of each exercise, your muscles are not being exercised during one-half of the workout and benefits are greatly reduced.

Repetitions The number of times a specific exercise is completed.

Set A group of repetitions for a particular exercise.

Rest interval Amount of time taken between sets.

Applying the Principle of Specificity

To gain strength and endurance in a particular muscle, muscle group, or movement in a sport or activity, you must specifically train the muscle or muscles in a similar movement. To improve sprinting speed by increasing your strength and endurance, for example, the muscles involved in sprinting must be identified and isotonic exercises chosen that strengthen those muscles in a movement similar to the sprinting action.

Applying the Overload Principle

Strength gains occur either by muscle fibers producing a stronger contraction or by recruiting a higher proportion of the available fibers for the contraction. The overload principle improves strength both ways, providing the demands on the muscle are systematically and progressively increased over time and the muscles are taxed beyond their accustomed levels. In other words, during each workout your muscles must perform a higher volume of work than they did in the previous workout. This is achieved by increasing the amount of resistance (weight) on each exercise or the number of repetitions and/or sets.

Applying the Progressive Resistance Exercise (PRE) Principle

As training progresses and you grow stronger, you must continuously increase the amount of resistance (weight) if continued improvement is to occur. One way to apply the PRE principle is to choose your starting weight and the lower limit of repetitions for each exercise. If you are using three sets of six to nine repetitions, for example, you would perform six repetitions for each exercise on your first workout. On the second, third, and fourth workouts, you would complete seven, eight, and nine repetitions, respectively. Then you would add 5 lb of weight to each upper-body exercise and 10 lb to each lower-body exercise and return to three sets of six repetitions.

Numerous other methods of progression in weight training have been shown to be effective. The *rest-pause* method involves completion of a single repetition at near maximal weight (1-RM) before resting one to two minutes, completing a second repetition, resting again, and so on until the muscle is fatigued and cannot perform one additional repetition. The *set system* involves use of multiple sets (3 to 10) of about five to six repetitions for each exercise.

The *burnout* method uses 75 percent of maximal weight for as many repetitions as possible. Without any rest interval, 10 lb are removed from the starting weight and another RM set is performed. The procedure is repeated until the muscle does not respond (burnout). Each designated muscle group is put through the same demanding process.

Supersets involve the use of a set of exercises for one group of muscles followed immediately by a set for their antagonist. For example, one set of arm curls (biceps) is followed by a set of bench presses (triceps). Each of the preceding methods has been effective in the development of muscular strength and endurance. To avoid boredom, add variation to your program, and help overcome plateaus (periods when improvement is slow or nonexistent). It is good to alternate your program among these methods every three to four weeks.

Engaging in Body Building

Body builders are generally more concerned with flex appeal (size, shape, definition, and proportion) than they are with muscle strength. They use dumbbells, barbells, and resistance-designed machines to carve out and define individual muscles. Beauty of physique is much more important to them than feats of strength. Competitors perform posing routines and are judged on symmetry (body parts having been equally developed top and bottom, left and right), muscle definition, and poise. Female competitors complete their competition by engaging in a brief freestyle routine to music, a cross between sport and cabaret.

When to Expect Results

You will see significant strength gains after about eight weeks of consecutive training. Be patient as it will take approximately 12 months to dramatically change the general appearance of your body and to add 12 to 14 lb of muscle mass.

Maintaining Strength and Endurance Gains

After you have acquired the level of muscular strength and endurance desired, one or two vigorous training sessions a week will maintain most of the improvement that has occurred.

Behavioral Change
and Motivational Strategies

A number of things may interfere with your strength-training progress. Some of these barriers (roadblocks) and strategies for overcoming them to keep you moving toward your training goals are:

Roadblock	Behavioral Change Strategy
You are aware of your need to engage in strength training but just cannot seem to stay interested enough to avoid skipping workouts.	The first month of any exercise program is the most difficult. Muscle soreness, discomfort, and a body that looks the same can discourage you at this stage. Try some of these techniques to overcome this critical period: 1. Set a realistic goal for each exercise such as only a 10-lb gain in the amount of weight you can move for three weeks. 2. Take a tape measure and record the size of your upper arm, upper leg, and abdominal area. 3. Avoid remeasuring yourself until you have added 10 lbs to most of the exercises in your program. You can be assured that you will meet this goal at your own pace and that, when you do, you will have acquired additional muscle mass. 4. Use a more realistic approach to determining your progress such as merely feeling various muscle groups and pinching fat to assure yourself of a new firmness, more muscle, and less fat.
After three to four months of training, you seem to have leveled off or reached a plateau. Improvement is occurring so slowly that you are becoming discouraged and feel you have already improved as much as possible.	What you are experiencing happens to everyone. Initial gains in strength and endurance are always much greater than those you achieve months later. Consider some behavioral changes to help overcome this leveling: 1. Incorporate one fun day into your weekly schedule, preferably on the day you are most likely to skip. Use lighter weights, rest longer between sets and exercises, and enjoy yourself. 2. Find a partner or group of people at about your level to work out with, and encourage one another to put a strong effort in your remaining two workouts weekly. 3. Incorporate a *maximum lift day* into your workout routine once every four weeks to demonstrate how you are progressing in each exercise. Use this session to reestablish your 1-RM and record the results.
List other roadblocks you are experiencing that seem to be reducing the effectiveness of your strength-training program. 1. _____ 2. _____ 3. _____	Now list the behavior change strategies that can help you overcome the roadblocks you listed. If you need to, refer back to chapter 3 for behavior change and motivational strategies. 1. _____ 2. _____ 3. _____

LIFTING TECHNIQUES

Warmup and Cooldown

To warm up properly, it is helpful to perform four to five minutes of walking or light jogging to raise body temperature and to follow it with a brief stretching period (see chapter 7). The first of three sets can be used as a light set with a high number of repetitions (15 to 20) and low weight (20-RM). A four- to five-minute stretching period at the close of your workout will help prevent muscle soreness and aid in improving your range of motion.

Full Range of Motion

Each exercise should move through the full range of motion without locking out the joint. The arm curl, for example, should result in the weight being moved as close to the chest as possible on the positive phase, before returning to the starting position without locking the elbow joint. When lifting heavy arm or leg weights, injuries are much more likely to occur to a joint that is fully extended at both the beginning and ending phases of an exercise.

Proper Breathing

One recommended breathing procedure is to inhale as the weight is lowered and to exhale as the weight is raised or pushed away from the body. You should attempt to blow the weight away from the body. This procedure will improve your efficiency and reduce the risk of holding your breath and blacking out during demanding exertion. Until the correct breathing is mastered, practice the technique with light weights.

Sequence of Exercises

Exercises should be arranged to prevent fatigue from limiting your lifting ability. One approach is to exercise the large muscle groups before exercising the smaller muscles. It is difficult to exhaust large muscle groups when the smaller muscles that serve as connections between the resistance and the large muscle groups have been prematurely fatigued. It is also important for the abdominal muscles, used in most exercises to stabilize the rib cage, to remain relatively unfatigued until the latter phases of the workout. A typical sequence that applies the concept of large to small is: (1) hips and lower back, (2) legs (quadriceps, hamstrings, and calves), (3) torso (back, shoulders, chest), (4) arms (triceps, biceps, and forearms), (5) abdominals, and (6) neck.

Form and Technique

It is important to follow the specific form tips identified for each exercise in Figure 6.3 carefully. In addition, you can apply these general techniques to most exercises and equipment:

1. The basic stance can be achieved by placing the feet slightly wider than shoulder-width apart with the toes parallel. The stronger leg is sometimes placed back in a heel-toe alignment depending on your preference.

2. Toes should be placed just under the bar in the starting phase of exercises in which the barbell is resting on the floor.

3. The back should remain erect (unless it contains the muscle group being exercised) with the head up and the eyes looking straight ahead.

4. The bar is grasped with the hands a shoulder-width apart using one of three grips:

   Overhand The bar is grasped until the thumb wraps around and meets the index finger. You may place the thumb next to the index finger without wrapping your hand around the bar if you prefer.

   Underhand The bar is grasped with the palms turned upward away from the body. The fingers and thumb are wrapped around the bar.

   Mixed Grip A combination of the overhand and underhand grip may be used with each hand assuming one of the grips.

5. Leaning backward to assist a repetition should be avoided.

6. Safety should be stressed at all times and should include workout partners to spot and protect you when you are using heavy free weights.

   - Avoid attempting to lift more weight than you can safely handle.
   - Secure collars and engage pins before attempting a lift.
   - Avoid holding your breath during the lift.
   - Return the barbell to the floor, rack, or starting position in a controlled manner.
   - Bend your knees when moving heavy weight from one place to another for storage.

Helpful hints for weight-training exercises are provided in Figure 6.3. These suggestions will help you prevent injury and improve the effectiveness of each exercise.

Figure 6.3 ✦ Barbell and Dumbbell Exercises
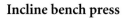

Bench press

Equipment: Barbell, bench rack, spotter

Movement: Using an overhand grip, slowly lower the bar to the chest, then press back to the starting position.

Hints: Bend knees at 90° and keep feet off the bench and the floor.

Muscle Groups: Shoulder extensors

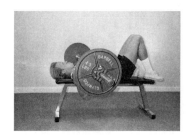
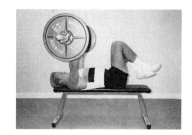

Incline bench press

Equipment: Incline bench, squat rack, spotter

Movement: Using an overhand grip, slowly raise and lower the bar to the chest (both feet flat on the floor).

Hints: Use a weight rack to support the weight above the bench. Avoid lifting the buttock or arching the back while lifting.

Muscle Groups: Upper pectoralis major, Anterior deltoid, Tricep

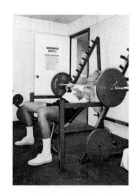
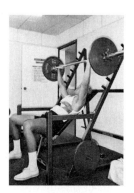

Power cleans

Equipment: Barbell

Movement: Using an overhand grip, pull the bar explosively to the highest point of your chest. Rotate hands under the bar and bend your knees. Straighten up to standing position. Bend the arms, legs, and hips to return the bar to the thighs, then slowly bend the knees and hips to lower to the floor.

Hints: Grasp the bar at shoulder width. Start with knees bent so hips are knee level. Keep head up and back straight.

Muscle Groups: Trapezius, Erector spinae, Gluteus, Quadriceps

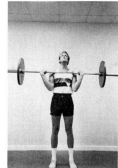
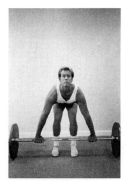
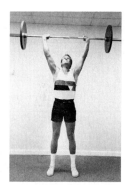

Deadlift

Equipment: Barbell

Movement: Using a mixed grip, bend knees so hips are close to knee level. Straighten knees and hips to standing position. Bend at knees and hips to return.

Hints: Keep the head up and back flat. Grasp bar at shoulder width.

Muscle Groups: Erector spinae, Gluteus, Quadriceps

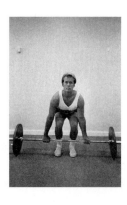
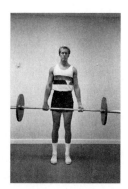

Figure 6.3 ✦ Barbell and Dumbbell Exercises *(continued)*

Bent arm flyes

Equipment: Dumbbells

Movement: Using an underhand grip, hold a dumbbell in each hand above the shoulders with the elbows slightly bent.

Hints: Keep elbows slightly bent at all times.

Muscle Groups: Pectoralis major

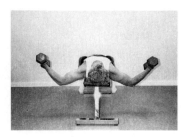
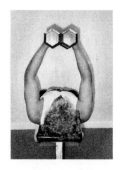

Barbell rowing

Equipment: Barbell

Movement: Using an overhand grip, hold the barbell directly below your shoulders. With elbows leading, pull the barbell to chest and hold momentarily. Then slowly return to the starting position.

Hints: Grasp bar slightly wider than shoulder width. Refrain from swinging or jerking the weights upward to the chest region.

Muscle Groups: Latissimus dorsi, Rear deltoid, Trapezius

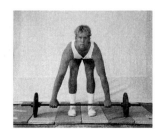
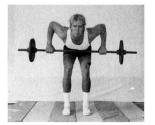

One dumbbell rowing

Equipment: Dumbbells

Movement: Using an underhand grip, kneel with one hand and one knee on exercise mat. Pull weight on support side upward to chest.

Hints: Hold dumbbell briefly at chest before returning.

Muscle Groups: Latissimus dorsi

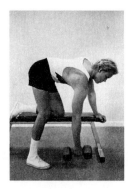
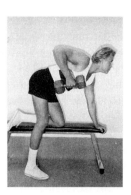

Shoulder shrug

Equipment: Barbell

Movement: Using an overhand grip, elevate both shoulders until they nearly touch the earlobes, then relax and return bar to the thighs.

Hints: Keep the extremities fully extended. Heavy weights (within limitations) will bring more rapid strength gains.

Muscle Groups: Shoulder girdle elevators

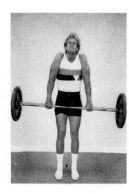

Figure 6.3 ✦ Barbell and Dumbbell Exercises *(continued)*

Military press

Equipment: Barbell

Movement: Using an overhand grip, slowly push bar overhead from chest until both arms are fully extended.

Hints: Keep neck and back erect, and knees extended and locked. Avoid jerky movements and leaning.

Muscle Groups: Abductors, Flexors, Arm extensors, Deltoids, Triceps

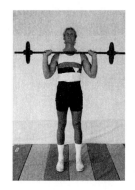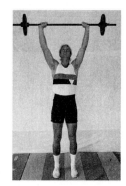

Upright rowing

Equipment: Barbell

Movement: Using an overhand grip, raise bar to the chin, and then return to thighs.

Hints: Grasp bar 6 to 8 inches apart. Keep elbows higher than the hands. Maintain an erect, stationary position.

Muscle Groups: Abductors, Arm flexors, Deltoids, Trapezius

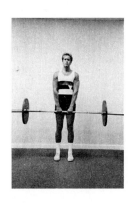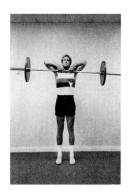

Bent-over lateral raise

Equipment: Dumbbells

Movement: Using an overhand grip, grasp dumbbell in each hand and draw arms to shoulder level. Slowly return to hanging position.

Hints: Keep knees and elbows slightly bent. Hold weights for 1–2 seconds before returning to hanging position.

Muscle Groups: Rear deltoid

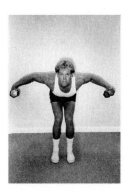

Two-arm curl

Equipment: Barbell

Movement: Using underhand grip, raise bar from thighs to chest level, and return.

Hints: Keep body erect and motionless throughout.

Muscle Groups: Upper arm flexors, Wrist flexors, Long finger flexors

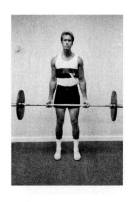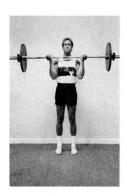

Figure 6.3 ✦ Barbell and Dumbbell Exercises *(continued)*

Reverse curl

Equipment: Barbell

Movement: Using overhand grip, raise bar from thighs to chest level, and return.

Hints: Use less weight than in two-arm curl.

Muscle Groups: Upper arm flexors, Hand extensors, Finger extensors

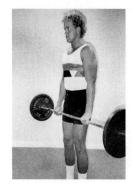 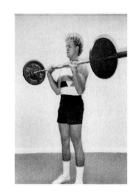

Seated dumbbell curl

Equipment: Dumbbells

Movement: Using an underhand grip, curl one or both dumbbells to the shoulder, then slowly return the weight to the sides of the body.

Hints: Keep the back straight throughout the entire movement.

Muscle Groups: Biceps

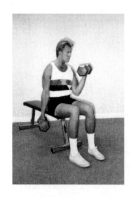

Close grip bench press

Equipment: Barbell, squat rack, spotter

Movement: Using an overhand grip, slowly lower the barbell to the chest and press back to the starting position.

Hints: Grasp center of bar (hands 2 to 4 inches apart). Bend knees at 90°; keep feet off the bench floor so as to avoid arching the back. Keep elbows in; extend arms fully.

Muscle Groups: Triceps, Anterior deltoid, Pectoralis major

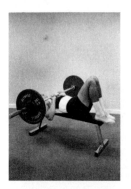 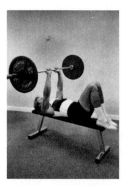

Standing or seated tricep

Equipment: Dumbbell

Movement: With both hands grasped around the inner side of one dumbbell overhead, lower the weight behind your head, then return.

Hints: Keep the elbows close together throughout the maneuver.

Muscle Groups: Triceps

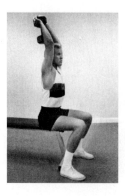 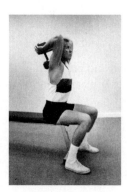

Figure 6.3 ✦ Barbell and Dumbbell Exercises *(continued)*

Barbell wrist curl

Equipment: Barbell

Movement: Using an underhand grip, let the bar hang down toward the floor and then curl toward you.

Hints: Grasp center of bar (hands 2 to 4 inches apart). Keep forearms in steady contact with the bench while moving the weight.

Muscle Groups: Forearm flexors

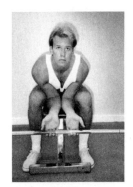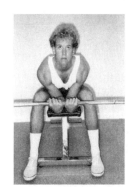

Reverse wrist curl

Equipment: Barbell

Movement: Using an overhand grip, and moving the wrists only, raise bar as high as possible, and return to the starting position.

Hints: Grasp barbell at shoulder width. Movement should only be at the wrist joint.

Muscle Groups: Forearm extensors

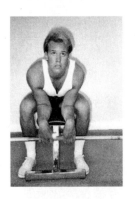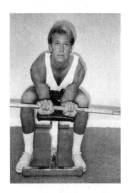

Front squat

Equipment: Barbell, squat rack, chair or bench, 2- to 3-inch board, spotters

Basic Movement: Using an overhand grip, flex legs to a 90° angle. Return to standing position.

Hints: Keep the heels up, and point the chin outward slightly. A chair or bench can be placed below the body (touch buttocks slightly to surface).

Muscle Groups: Thigh extensors, Lower leg extensors

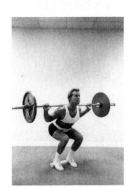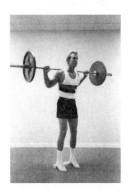

Lunge with dumbbells

Equipment: Dumbbells

Movement: Overhand grip; alternate stepping forward with each leg, bending the knee of the lead leg, and lowering your body until thigh of the front leg is level to the floor. Barely touch the knee of rear leg before returning to the starting position.

Hints: Keep your head up and upper body erect throughout the exercise. Avoid bending front knee more than 90°.

Muscle Groups: Quadriceps, Gluteus

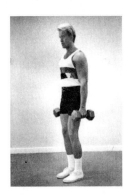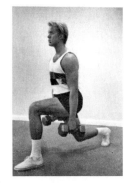

Figure 6.3 ✦ Barbell and Dumbbell Exercises *(continued)*

Heel raise

Equipment: Barbell, squat rack, spotters, 2- to 3-inch board

Movement: Using an overhand grip, the body is raised upward to maximum height of the toes.

Hints: Alter the position of the toes from straight ahead to pointed in and out. Keep the body erect.

Muscle Groups: Foot plantar flexors

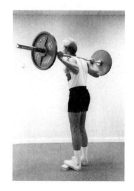 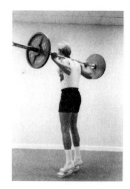

One dumbbell heel raise

Equipment: Dumbbell, 2- to 3-inch board

Movement: Using an overhand grip, shift entire body weight on the leg next to the dumbbell, and raise the foot off the floor behind. Raise the heel of the support foot upward as high as possible and hold momentarily.

Hints: A wall is useful for balance, but avoid using free hand for assistance.

Muscle Groups: Gastrocnemius, Soleus

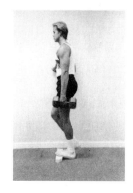 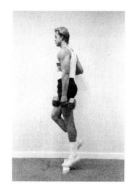

ℬARBELL AND DUMBBELL EXERCISES

Figure 6.3 shows specific exercises, describes the equipment needs, basic movement, and helpful hints and identifies the muscle groups involved. This information will help you choose exercises that train the important muscle groups in your sport or activity. Table 6.2 includes some of the many barbell and dumbbell exercises and their variations for a basic resistance program designed to improve your strength, local muscular endurance, and muscle size.

𝒢IRTH CONTROL

Almost everyone wants a flat tummy. In fact, a flat stomach is strongly associated with fitness and wellness in our society. A large belly can make people appear much older than they really are. It also can be a sign of poor health—evidence of accumulating fat that may lead to hypertension, stroke, heart disease, adult-onset diabetes, and other ailments. Some fat around the midsection is not necessarily unhealthy. Practically everyone acquires at least a small spare tire (fat on both sides of the hips) and some abdominal fat. Becoming obsessed with this somewhat natural change is a mistake. In fact, as you reach the third and fourth decades of life, maintaining the flat stomach you had in your teens may be impossible.

Most people attempt to solve the girth-control problem by using unnatural and worthless devices such as girdles, corsets, weighted belts, rubberized workout suits, and special exercise equipment that promises a flat stomach with just minutes of use daily. Although it is not an easy task, you can bring back some of the lost youth in your abdominal area by completing the program described in Lab Activity 6.2: Obtaining a Flat, Healthy Stomach at the end of this chapter.

Table 6.2 ✦ Basic and Alternate Weight-Training Programs: Programs for General Body Development

Exercises	Repetitions	Starting weight (RM)	Speed of contraction
Basic program			
Two-arm curl	6–10	8	Moderate
Military press	6–10	8	Moderate
Sit ups (bent-knee)	25–50	30	Rapid
Rowing (upright)	6–10	8	Moderate
Bench press	6–10	8	Moderate
Squat	6–10	8	Rapid
Heel raise	15–25	20	Rapid
Dead lift (bent-knee)	6–10	8	Rapid
Alternate I			
Reverse curl	6–10	8	Moderate
Triceps press	6–10	8	Moderate
Sit ups (bent-knee)	25–50	30	Rapid
Shoulder shrug	6–10	8	Moderate
Squat jump	15–25	20	Rapid
Knee flexor	6–10	8	Rapid
Knee extensor	6–10	8	Rapid
Pull overs (bent-arm)	6–10	8	Moderate
Alternate II			
Wrist curl	6–10	8	Moderate
Side bender	6–10	8	Moderate
Lateral raise	6–10	8	Moderate
Straddle lift	6–10	8	Rapid
Supine leg lift	6–10	8	Rapid
Hip flexor	6–10	8	Rapid
Leg abductor	6–10	8	Rapid
Forward raise	6–10	8	Moderate

SUMMARY

The Importance of Strength and Endurance

Strength and endurance training provides health-related benefits for people of all ages. Such training burns calories, adds muscle mass, prevents the slowing of metabolism with age, and is an important aspect of controlling body weight and body fat throughout life. Over a period of 6 to 12 months of this training, your general physical appearance, body image, and self-concept will improve. Strength training also aids in the development of the skeletal system and in improving bone mineral content. The added strength and endurance acquired also increases energy and productivity on the job and in recreational activities and reduces the incidence of sports- and work-related injuries. And finally, strength and endurance training plays a major role in the rehabilitation of soft-tissue injuries such as muscle strains, tears, contusions, and surgery.

Factors Affecting Muscular Strength and Endurance

A muscle is composed of fibers and myofibrils bound together by layers of connective tissue. There are three general types of fiber tissue: slow-twitch, oxidative (aerobic); fast-twitch, glycolytic (anaerobic); and fast-twitch, oxidative, glycolytic (aerobic and anaerobic). Strength training predominantly effects the fast-twitch fibers while endurance training effects the slow-twitch fibers. Your strength and endurance potential is governed by genetics and the number, size, and distribution of your fast- and slow-twitch fibers. Everyone can increase muscle size, strength, and endurance with training.

Strength-Training Principles

Three basic training methods are commonly used to develop strength and endurance: isotonics, isokinetics, and isometrics. On completion of an isotonic or isokinetic contraction, the muscle shortens during the positive phase as weight is brought toward the body and lengthens in the negative phase as the weight is returned to the starting position. No muscle shortening occurs when force is applied to an immovable object (isometric contraction). Isotonic and isokinetic workouts are more beneficial to sports performance than isometric workouts are.

Training variables can be altered to meet specific objectives. By manipulating the number of sets, repetitions, rest intervals, and speed of contraction, programs can be altered to focus on strength, muscular endurance, general body development, muscle mass, speed and explosive power, or rehabilitation from injury.

Lifting Techniques

Sound lifting techniques with free weights or special equipment require careful warmup and cooldown periods with stretching, the full range of motion on each repetition, proper breathing, use of a partner or spotter, and careful attention to ideal form in each exercise.

Barbell and Dumbbell Exercises

A variety of exercises can be chosen that focus on the major muscle groups of the body. One sound approach is first to identify the key muscles involved in the activity or those you want to train, then to select specific weight-training exercises that activate these muscles, preferably in a similar movement.

Girth Control

To obtain a flat stomach, it is necessary to restrict your daily calories enough to cause fat cells in the abdominal area to shrink in size and to engage in a series of high-repetition abdominal exercises daily. You cannot change fatty tissue to muscle tissue, and muscle tissue will not change to fatty tissue when exercise ceases. Abdominal exercises alone will only improve the strength and endurance of your stomach muscles; little or no change will take place in the size of the stomach unless calories are also restricted. The combination of these two methods can significantly reduce the size of your stomach and improve your abdominal strength and endurance.

Lab Activity 6.1

Do You Need to Start a Strength-Training Program?

INSTRUCTIONS: *Answer each question below before reading the interpretation section to find out how badly you are in need of a strength-training program.*

	Yes	No
1. Have you been on a diet within the past 6 to 12 months?	_____	_____
2. Have you ever lost, then regained, 8 to 10 lb in the same year?	_____	_____
3. Do you have difficulty controlling your body weight?	_____	_____
4. Do you have excess, sagging skin on the back of your upper arms, your thighs, back of your legs, stomach, or other body part?	_____	_____
5. Are you interested in changing your appearance by adding muscle and reducing the size of fat deposits?	_____	_____
6. Would a firmer, more muscular body help your body image, how you feel about yourself, and how you think others feel about you?	_____	_____
7. Would additional strength or muscular endurance improve your performance in any sports or recreational activities?	_____	_____
8. Would additional strength or local muscular endurance help you perform better on the job and at home?	_____	_____
9. Are there any specific muscle groups in your body that you would prefer to strengthen?	_____	_____
10. Have you sustained a soft-tissue injury within the past 12 months, such as an ankle sprain, a pulled muscle, or a contusion?	_____	_____

Interpretation: If you answered "yes" to two or more of the questions, a strength and endurance program may be needed.

Questions 1–3 are concerned with body weight and fat. Strength and endurance training can help your skin fit better, help you focus on your body, help you shrink fat cells, and add muscle mass.

Questions 4–6 are concerned with body image and your interest in improving your appearance through strength and endurance training.

Questions 7–9 are concerned with the need for additional strength and endurance to aid performance on the job, at home, and in recreational activities.

Question 10 is concerned with the prevention of job-, home-, and sports-related injuries.

Lab Activity 6.2

Obtaining a Flat, Healthy Stomach

INSTRUCTIONS: *Take a moment to measure and record the size of your waist. Now apply the pinch test or use skinfold calipers one inch to the right of your belly button and on the left side of your hip to locate the excess fat. If you can pinch more than an inch in these areas, consider following the program described in this lab activity.*

A girth-control program is designed to flatten your stomach and improve the strength and endurance of your abdominal muscles. It is based on two sound principles:

1. Consume fewer calories than you burn, and remain in a negative calorie balance daily for a few months. Keep in mind that fat or adipose tissue and muscle tissue are different tissue types; one cannot be transformed to the other no matter what you do. Reducing caloric intake to produce a fat loss of one to two pounds weekly (see chapter 9) will shrink the size of your fat cells in the abdominal area. It is important to engage in an aerobic exercise program three to four times weekly to help burn extra calories and to allow consumption of sufficient nutrients and calories to spare protein, thus reducing the amount of lean muscle-tissue loss that occurs when you diet without exercise.

2. Supplement your dietary management with aerobic exercise (see chapter 5) and the six abdominal exercises described in this lab activity. For each exercise, work toward 100 repetitions daily. Begin with the maximum number you can perform in one set and add 2 to 5 repetitions each day until you reach 100. Complete these exercises daily, and expect to train for three to four months before you notice significant results. Remember that these abdominal exercises only strengthen muscles that lie beneath the fat. Unless you reduce calories to shrink the fat cells, you will merely have firm abdominal muscles beneath the fat with little reduction in the size of your stomach.

   A. **Sit-ups** Lie flat on your back with knees slightly bent and both hands resting on your chest. Pull your chin to your chest and sit up slowly to approximately 60 degrees.

   B. **Crunches** Lie flat on your back with knees bent and pulled toward the chest. Raise your head and shoulders off the floor as you thrust your upper body toward your knees, then return to the starting position.

   C. **Twisting Crunches** Lie flat on your back with hands behind your head. Touch elbow to opposite knee while the other leg straightens; keep feet flexed.

D. **Alternate Knee Kicks** Lie flat on your back with hands under the buttocks. Bend one knee with the other leg straight and raised 6 inches off the floor. Straighten the bent knee, and bend the other leg as in walking or marching.

E. **Side Raise** Lie on your side with arm extended and head on bicep muscle. Hold both legs 6 inches off the floor with feet together. Raise top leg up, and return to leg-together position.

F. **Back Scissors** Lie on your stomach with hands at sides and palms down for support. Start with legs apart and feet off the floor; bring feet together, then move them apart.

7

ℱLEXIBILITY

Chapter Objectives

By the end of this chapter, you should be able to:

1. Identify the factors that directly or indirectly effect range of motion in various joints.

2. Cite the advantages of acquiring and maintaining lifelong adequate flexibility.

3. Describe the role of flexibility in the prevention of injuries.

4. Self-administer a series of tests that evaluates your flexibility.

5. Design a personalized flexibility-training program that applies sound training principles.

6. Complete a flexibility routine using one of the acceptable methods described in this chapter.

JOHN IS PROUD of the fact that he is muscular and athletic although he is troubled by his lack of flexibility. In the past, he thought limited flexibility was a normal part of developing muscles and becoming strong. He now realizes that his inflexibility is interfering with his ability to enjoy recreational activities and competitive sports and to perform daily tasks such as picking up an object, tying shoes, and even getting up out of a chair. Unfortunately, John does not know what to do to improve his range of motion and correct the problem.

Flexibility is the range of motion around a joint. Of the five components of health-related physical fitness, it is the aspect most neglected by the exercising population, by athletes, and by health-care professionals and practitioners. Like John, few individuals understand the importance of developing and maintaining acceptable levels of joint flexibility, yet the health, injury, and performance consequences of doing so are quite evident.

In this chapter, we will provide answers to all of John's questions and examine the many aspects of joint flexibility, such as the factors effecting range of motion, its importance, assessment techniques, sound training principles, and choice of specific stretching exercises to help evaluate range of motion and devise a program that meets your specific health and fitness needs.

FACTORS EFFECTING FLEXIBILITY

Since flexibility is specific to each joint, having good hip flexibility is no guarantee you will be flexible in the shoulders, back, neck, or ankles. Depending on your stretching routine and choice of exercises, you may become highly flexible in some joints and remain inflexible in others. A number of factors combine to determine the range of motion around each joint: heredity; gender; age; the elasticity of the muscles, ligaments, and tendons; previous injuries; lifestyle; adipose tissue (fat) in and around joints; and body type. Young children are more flexible than adults but seem to lose that flexibility more quickly than their more active counterparts of 20 years ago did; the tendency to become inflexible with age is closely associated with inactivity, which results in a loss of muscle elasticity, a tightening of tendons and ligaments, and an increase in fatty tissue in and around joints. Extra fat effects flexibility by increasing resistance to movement and creating premature contact between adjoining body surfaces. Sedentary living can lead to shortening of muscles and ligaments and can therefore restrict range of motion. Poor posture, long periods of sitting or standing, or immobilization of a limb can have a similar effect. Exercise that overdevelops one muscle group while neglecting opposing groups produces an imbalance that also restricts flexibility.

The formation of scar tissue following a muscle or connective-tissue injury (ligaments and tendons)

Muscle extensibility The ability of muscle tissue to stretch.

Vertebrae The 33 bones of the spinal column, some of which are normally fused together (sacral and the coccygeal vertebrae).

Sciatica Pain along the course of the great sciatic nerve (hip, thigh, leg, foot).

can decrease flexibility. Arthritis and calcium deposits can damage joints by causing inflammation, chronic pain, and restriction of movement.

Fortunately, everyone is capable of increasing range of motion in particular joints. Regular stretching routines cause permanent lengthening of ligaments and tendons. Muscle tissue undergoes only temporary lengthening following a warmup and stretching routine as **muscle extensibility** increases. Muscle temperature changes alone, attained through proper warmup, can increase flexibility by 20 percent.

THE IMPORTANCE OF FLEXIBILITY

A regular stretching routine will help increase range of motion, improve performance in some activities, help prevent soft-tissue injuries, aid muscle relaxation, and help you cool down at the end of a workout. It is a valuable part of a complete exercise program, and it provides some benefits to everyone.

Increased Range of Motion and Improved Performance

Since we have established the fact that range of motion is joint-specific, a well-rounded flexibility program must devote attention to all the body's major joints: neck, shoulder, back, hip, knees, wrist, and ankles. You can increase your range of motion in each of these major joints in six to eight weeks by following one of the recommended stretching techniques discussed in this chapter.

In sports such as gymnastics, diving, skiing, swimming, and hurdling and in other activities requiring a high level of flexibility, a stretching routine that focuses on the key joints can also help improve performance. Although there is little scientific evidence available, the association between flexibility and sports performance is almost universally accepted.

Injury Prevention

Regular stretching routines may help reduce the incidence of injury during exercise for athletes and others. Continuous exercise such as jogging, running, cycling, and aerobics tightens and shortens muscles, and tight muscles are more vulnerable to injury from the explosive movements common in sports. A brief warmup period followed by stretching will not only increase range of motion but will also provide some protection from common soft-tissue injuries such as strains, sprains, and tears. Striving to maintain a full, normal range of motion in each joint with adequate strength, endurance, and power throughout the range will reduce your chances of experiencing an exercise-induced injury.

Lower back pain Pain in the lower back occurs as frequently in our society as the common cold does. This twentieth-century plague affects an estimated 8 to 10 million people in the United States who lose over 200 million work days each year. Informal surveys of middle and senior high school athletes indicate that as many as 40 percent have experienced back problems severe enough to result in missed practice time. Although back pain affects all age groups, the elderly are the most vulnerable. The older you are, the more likely you are to have problems with your lower back. No one seems to be immune.

A brief description of your spinal column will help you understand why the back is so vulnerable to injury (see Figure 7.1 on page 130). The human body has 33 vertebrae that extend from the base of the skull to the tail bone. The **vertebrae** form a double *S*, reverse curve to ensure proper balance and weight-bearing. If the vertebrae were placed directly on top of one another, the back would be only five percent as strong as it is and one step would produce enough trauma and brain jolt to cause concussion. Shock absorbers, known as *discs,* are located between each vertebra. These capsules of gelatinous matter contain approximately 90 percent water in young people but only 70 percent in older individuals. With loss of water comes a loss of compressibility and increased vulnerability to injury often referred to as *slipped, ruptured,* or *herniated* disc. Ruptured disc material may bulge through the rear portion of the outer ring and pressure nerves, thereby producing pain in the lower back that may radiate down into the leg and toes (**sciatica**).

Not all sufferers of lower-back pain have bone or disc disorders. In fact, the problem for most individuals involves muscles, tendons, or ligaments. No one cause can be isolated that triggers an episode of back pain. Some of the more common factors include physical injury, hard sneezing or coughing, improper lifting or bending, standing or sitting for long hours, sitting slumped in overstuffed chairs or automobile seats, tension, anxiety, and depression, obesity, and disease (for example, arthritis and tumors). Some individuals merely have a genetically weak back involving one or more of the approximately 140 muscles that provide support to the back and control its movements. Typi-

cally, a muscle, ligament, or tendon strain or sprain causes nearby muscles to spasm to help support the back. It is estimated that 7 out of 10 problems are due to the improper alignment of the spinal column and pelvic girdle caused by inflexible and weak muscles.

Prevention and treatment require similar action and may involve changing the way you stand, bend, lift objects, sit, rest, sleep, and exercise. Figure 7.2 summarizes the key factors for taking care of your back and for recovering from low back pain. Study this figure carefully and complete the recommended lower-back exercises at least once a day.

Fitness Heroes

Maria Serrao was in a car accident when she was five years old and was told that she would remain in a wheelchair for the rest of her life. Many people thought that a wheelchair would limit her ability to live a healthy, normal life. Maria proved them wrong—and, while her life is far from normal, she is extremely healthy!

As a young adult, Maria began to gain weight and lose her strength. She joined a health club and started working out every day. Her stamina encouraged other gym members to work harder, and she was a role model for anyone who met her. Her fitness trainer helped her regain her strength and lose excess weight, but the trainer thought it would be impossible for Maria to participate in aerobics.

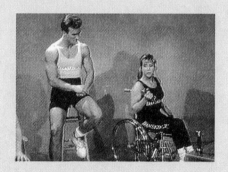

Maria disagreed. Not only did she participate fully in aerobics classes at the gym, but she created her own public access cable television show titled "Everyone Can Exercise." Her next goal is to gain national cable television access—so watch for this fitness hero on your screen! ✦

For most victims of lower-back pain, treatment involves one to three days of bedrest on a firm mattress supported by plywood, moderate application of heat and cold, and gentle massage until muscle spasms are eliminated or significantly reduced. Once this occurs, use a series of daily exercises, such as those shown in Figure 7.2 that are designed to strengthen the four key muscle groups that support your back and important abdominal muscles. Three other components are needed to complete your rehabilitation and prevention program: exercising more, decreasing your stomach fat by reducing your caloric intake, and continuing to do lower-back exercises daily in addition to 30 minutes of aerobic activity three to four days a week after recovery. Only rarely is surgery needed to correct lower-back problems.

Aid the Cooldown Phase

As we discussed in chapter 4, the final three to eight minutes of a workout should be a period of slowly diminishing intensity through the use of a slow jog or walk followed by a brief stretching period. By stretching at the end of your workout as the final phase of the cooldown, you are helping fatigued muscles return to their normal resting length and to a more relaxed state.

THE ASSESSMENT OF FLEXIBILITY

Since range of motion is joint-specific, no one test provides an accurate assessment of overall flexibility.

Figure 7.1 ✦ The Vertebral Column and Muscle Support

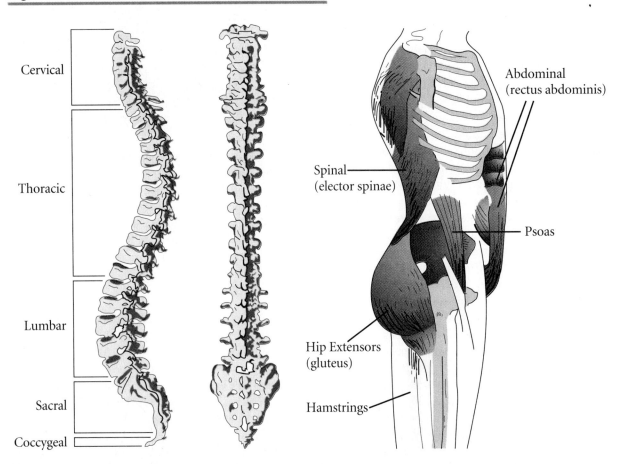

The vertebrae that make up the spinal column are designed for support, strength, and flexibility.

Adequate strength and flexibility in the muscle groups of both the back and abdomen are essential for supporting the back and maintaining posture.

Figure 7.2 ✦ Your Back and How to Care For It

Whatever the cause of low back pain, part of its treatment is the correction of faulty posture. But good posture is not simply a matter of "standing tall." It refers to correct use of the body at all times. In fact, for the body to function in the best of health it must be so used that no strain is put upon muscles, joints, bones, and ligaments. To prevent low back pain, avoiding strain must become a way of life, practiced while lying, sitting, standing, walking, working, and exercising. When body position is correct, internal organs have enough room to function normally and blood circulates more freely.

With the help of this guide, you can begin to correct the positions and movements which bring on or aggravate backache. Particular attention should be paid to the positions recommended for resting, since it is possible to strain the muscles of the back and neck even while lying in bed. By learning to live with good posture, under all circumstances, you will gradually develop the proper carriage and stronger muscles needed to protect and support your hard-working back.

How to Stay on Your Feet without Tiring Your Back

To prevent strain and pain in everyday activities, it is restful to change from one task to another before fatigue sets in. Housewives can lie down between chores; others should check body position frequently, drawing in the abdomen, flattening the back, bending the knees slightly.

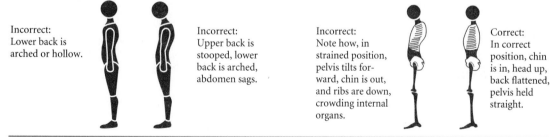

Not this way — Bend the knees and hips, not the waist.

Not this way — Use of a footrest relieves swayback.

Not this way — Hold heavy objects close to you.

Not this way — Never bend over without bending the knees.

Check Your Carriage Here

In correct, fully erect posture, a line dropped from the ear will go through the tip of the shoulder, middle of hip, back of kneecaps, and front of anklebone.

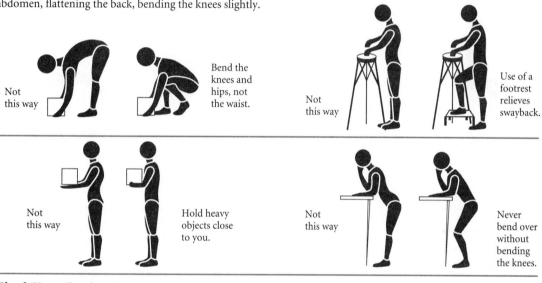

Incorrect: Lower back is arched or hollow.

Incorrect: Upper back is stooped, lower back is arched, abdomen sags.

Incorrect: Note how, in strained position, pelvis tilts forward, chin is out, and ribs are down, crowding internal organs.

Correct: In correct position, chin is in, head up, back flattened, pelvis held straight.

To Find the Correct Standing Position

Stand one foot away from wall. Now sit against wall, bending knees slightly. Tighten abdominal and buttock muscles. This will tilt the pelvis back and flatten the lower spine. Holding this position, inch up the wall to standing position, by straightening the legs. Now walk around the room, maintaining the same posture. Place back against wall again to see if you have held it.

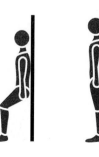

Figure 7.2 ✦ Your Back and How to Care For It *(continued)*

How to Sit Correctly

A back's best friend is a straight, hard chair. If you can't get the chair you prefer, learn to sit properly on whatever chair you get. *To correct sitting position from forward slump:* Throw head well back, then bend it forward to pull in the chin. This will straighten the back. Now tighten abdominal muscles to raise the chest. Check position frequently.

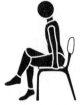 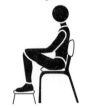 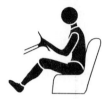 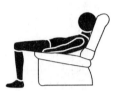

Relieve strain by sitting well forward, flatten back by tightening abdominal muscles, and cross knees.

Use of footrest relieves swayback. Aim is to have knees higher than hips.

Correct way to sit while driving, close to pedals. Use seat belt or hard backrest, available commercially.

TV slump leads to "dowager's hump," strains neck and shoulders.

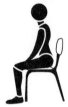 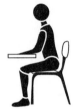 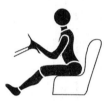 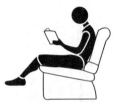

If chair is too high, swayback is increased.

Keep neck and back in as straight a line as possible with the spine. Bend forward from the hips.

Driver's seat too far from pedals emphasizes curve in lower back.

Strained reading position. Forward thrusting strains muscles of neck and head.

How to Put Your Back to Bed

For proper bed posture, a firm mattress is essential. Bedboards, sold commercially, or devised at home, may be used with soft mattresses. Bedboards, preferably, should be made of $3/4$-inch plywood. Faulty sleeping positions intensify swayback and result not only in backache but in numbness, tingling, and pain in arms and legs.

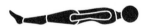 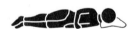 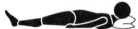 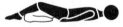

Incorrect:
Lying flat on back makes swayback worse.

Correct:
Lying on side with knees bent effectively flattens the back. Flat pillow may be used to support neck, especially when shoulders are broad.

Incorrect:
Use of high pillow strains neck, arms, shoulders.

Correct:
Sleeping on back is restful and correct when knees are properly supported.

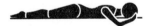  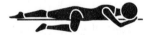

Incorrect:
Sleeping face down exaggerates swayback, strains neck and shoulders.

Correct:
Raise the foot of the mattress eight inches to discourage sleeping on the abdomen.

Incorrect:
Bending one hip and knee does not relieve swayback.

Proper arrangement of pillows for resting or reading in bed.

When Doing Nothing, Do It Right

Rest is the first rule for the tired, painful back. The following positions relieve pain by taking all pressure and weight off the back and legs. Note pillows under knees to relieve strain on spine.

For complete relief and relaxing effect, these positions should be maintained from 5 to 25 minutes.

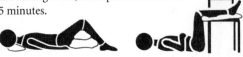 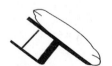

A straight-back chair used behind a pillow makes a serviceable backrest.

Figure 7.2 ✦ Your Back and How to Care For It *(continued)*

Exercise — without Getting Out of Bed

Exercises to be performed while lying in bed are aimed not so much at strengthening muscles as at teaching correct positioning. But muscles used correctly become stronger and in time are able to support the body with the least amount of effort.

Do all exercises in this position. Legs should not be straightened.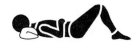

Bring knee to chest. Lower slowly but do not straighten leg. Relax.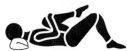

Exercise — without Attracting Attention

Use these inconspicuous exercises whenever you have a spare moment during the day, both to relax tension and improve the tone of important muscle groups.

1. Rotate shoulders forward and backward.
2. Turn head slowly side to side.
3. Watch an imaginary plane take off, just below the right shoulder. Stretch neck, follow it slowly as it moves up, around and down, disappearing below the other shoulder. Repeat, starting on left side.
4. Slowly, slowly, touch left ear to right shoulder. Raise both shoulders to touch ears, drop them as far as possible.
5. At any pause in the day—waiting for an elevator to arrive, for a specific traffic light to change—pull in abdominal muscles, tighten, hold for the count of eight without breathing. Relax slowly. Increase the count gradually after the first week. Practice breathing normally with abdomen flat and contracted. Do this sitting, standing, and walking.

Bring both knees slowly up to chest. Tighten muscles of abdomen, press back flat against the floor. Hold knees to chest 20 seconds. Then lower slowly. Relax. Repeat 5 times. This exercise gently stretches the shortened muscles of the lower back, while strengthening abdominal muscles. Clasp knees, bring them up to chest at the same time coming to a sitting position. Rock back and forth.

Rules to Live By — From Now On

1. Never bend from the waist only; bend the hips and knees.
2. Never lift a heavy object higher than your waist.
3. Always turn and face the object you wish to lift.
4. Avoid carrying unbalanced loads; hold heavy objects close to your body.
5. Never carry anything heavier than you can manage with ease.
6. Never lift or move heavy furniture. Wait for someone to do it who knows the principles of leverage.
7. Avoid sudden movements, sudden "overloading" of muscles. Learn to move deliberately, swinging the legs from the hips.
8. Learn to keep the head in line with the spine when standing, sitting, lying in bed.
9. Put soft chairs and deep couches on your "don't sit" list. During prolonged sitting, cross your legs to rest your back.
10. Your doctor is the only one who can determine when low back pain is due to faulty posture. He is the best judge of when you may do general exercises for physical fitness. When you do, omit any exercise which arches or overstrains the lower back: backward or forward bends,touching the toes with the knees straight.
11. Wear shoes with moderate heels, all about the same height. Avoid changing from high to low heels.
12. Put a footrail under the desk and a footrest under the crib.
13. Diaper a baby sitting next to him or her on the bed.
14. Don't stoop and stretch to hang the wash; raise the clothesbasket and lower the washline.
15. Beg or buy a rocking chair. Rocking rests the back by changing the muscle groups used.
16. Train yourself vigorously to use your abdominal muscles to flatten your lower abdomen. In time, this muscle contraction will become habitual, making you the envied possessor of a youthful body profile!
17. Don't strain to open windows or doors.
18. For good posture, concentrate on strengthening "nature's corset"– the abdominal and buttock muscles. The pelvic roll exercise is especially recommended to correct the postural relation between the pelvis and the spine.

Myth and Fact Sheet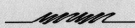

Myth	Fact
1. Stretching exercises are an excellent warmup activity.	1. Stretching exercises are only one part of a sound routine to warm up the body. To prevent injury and muscle soreness, avoid stretching cold muscles. Begin with a general warmup routine that involves large muscle groups, routines such as walking or jogging, for at least 5 minutes or until sweating is evident; then follow with 5 to 10 minutes of stretching to complete the warmup phase of your workout.
2. Stretching is only needed before vigorous activity.	2. It is important to stretch before any workout. Stretching is also an excellent cooldown activity at the end of a workout, particularly after strength training.
3. Using the body's weight to bounce into the stretch helps increase flexibility.	3. Ballistic stretching (bouncing) actually causes the muscle to shorten by stimulating a muscle spindle. The technique is unsound and may result in joint injury.
4. It is important to become as flexible as possible.	4. Joint laxity (looseness around a joint) and too much flexibility may decrease joint stability. Yoga-type exercises are often unsound and may lead to injuries associated with overstretching.
5. Strength training decreases flexibility.	5. Acquiring muscle mass does not automatically decrease joint movement. When weight-training exercises are performed correctly through the full range of motion, flexibility is improved.
6. Lost flexibility is an inevitable part of aging.	6. Inactivity causes much more loss than aging does. Now that more of the graying population remains active, some previous findings are being reconsidered.

Instead, each joint must be evaluated. This explains why so few physical-fitness batteries employ a flexibility test. Only recently have test developers begun to include flexibility as part of health-related, physical-fitness test batteries. Unfortunately, modern tests generally include only the **sit-and-reach test** that measures only lower-back and hamstring (the large muscle group located on the back of the upper leg) flexibility. Although this test is quite valuable and accurate, primarily because it involves some of the muscle groups associated with lower-back pain, a more thorough test is also needed. Take a moment to complete Lab Activity 7.1: Measuring Lower-Back and Hamstring Flexibility at the end of the chapter. Evaluate your performance using the sit-and-reach standards identified in the lab activity, and determine your flexibility rating. Repeat this test after six to eight weeks of stretching to determine the effectiveness of your flexibility-training program.

A quick evaluation of your overall flexibility level, using a less objective approach, may be even more valuable in determining your needs and the effectiveness of your stretching program. You can do this by completing the seven subjective tests described in Lab Activity 7.2: Determining Your Total Body Flexibility at the end of the chapter. If you check "yes" in any test, your flexibility is considered *good* in that joint. Strive to improve your flexibility in the areas where you checked "no." Repeat this series of tests after you have followed a stretching routine for six to eight weeks. You will discover how easy it is to increase your range of motion substantially.

Sit-and-reach test A test designed to measure the flexibility of the lower-back and hamstring muscles.

FLEXIBILITY-TRAINING PRINCIPLES

Who Should Stretch

Some individuals need to stretch more than others. Lean body types with a high range of motion may need very little stretching whereas stocky, more powerfully built athletes with limited motion need 5 to 10 minutes of flexibility exercise before making any radical moves such as bending over to touch the toes or explosive jumping or sprinting. Almost every healthy individual of any age or level of fitness can benefit from a regular stretching routine. Routines can be gentle, easy, relaxing, and safe or extremely vigorous. Daily stretching will help maintain flexibility throughout life and help prevent joint stiffness.

When to Stretch

Stretching exercises are used as part of a warmup routine to prepare the body for vigorous activity, during the cooldown phase of a workout to help muscles return to a normal relaxed state, merely to improve range of motion in key joints, and to aid in rehabilitation after injury.

Warmup and Cooldown Flexibility (stretching) exercises are often too closely associated with warm-up. Consequently, most individuals make the mistake of stretching cold muscles before beginning a workout rather than first warming the body up with some large-muscle activity such as walking or jogging for five to eight minutes or until perspiration is evident. At this point, body temperature has been elevated two to four degrees, and muscles can be safely stretched. Keep in mind that you warm up to stretch, you do not stretch to warm up. Table 7.1 provides a suggested order for stretching for those who engage in jogging, walking, cycling, swimming, racket and team sports, and strength training. Most organized aerobics classes follow a similar routine that involves a slow, gentle warmup to cause sweating, followed by careful stretching, vigorous aerobics, and a cooldown period. Joggers and runners may choose to cover the first half mile or so at a very slow pace, then do stretching exercises before completing the run, as opposed to the more common routine of stretching cold muscles prior to the jog or run. Ideally, the majority of a stretching routine should follow the jog, run, cycle, swim, strength-training, or aerobics session and take place at the end of a workout during the cooldown phase. Stretching at the end of your workout when muscle-tissue temperature is high may effectively improve range of motion and reduce the incidence of muscle soreness the following day.

Stretching to Improve Range of Motion If your main purpose is to improve body flexibility, you can safely stretch any time you desire—early in the morning, at work, after sitting or standing for long periods of time, when you feel stiff, after an exercise session, or while you are engaged in passive activities such as watching television or listening to music. Remember, you must first elevate body temperature and produce some sweating by engaging in large-muscle group activity before you stretch.

Rehabilitation from Injury When you are recovering from soft-tissue injuries, focus attention on the reduction of pain and swelling, a return to normal strength, and achieving a full, unrestricted range of motion. Unless regular stretching begins as soon as pain and swelling have been eliminated, some loss of flexibility in the injured joint is almost certain.

What Stretching Technique to Use

You can choose one of several different techniques that have been shown to increase joint flexibility effectively (see Figure 7.3 on page 136). Each method has advantages and disadvantages.

Ballistic Stretching This technique employs bouncing or bobbing at the extreme range of motion or point of discomfort. When they stretch the hamstring muscle group, for example, individuals bounce vigorously three or four times as they reach for their toes in an attempt to aid the stretch forcefully. This method has several disadvantages. A muscle that is stretched too far and too fast in this manner may actually contract and create an opposing force, causing soft-tissue injury. An injury may also occur if the force generated by the jerking motions becomes greater than the extensibility of the tissues. **Ballistic stretching** is also likely to result in muscle soreness the following day.

Static Stretching After moving slowly into the stretch, steady pressure is applied at the point of discomfort in a particular joint for 10 to 30 seconds without bouncing or jerking. Each exercise can be performed two or three times. **Static stretching** is superior to ballistic stretching since it is safe and injury-free, is not likely to result in muscle soreness, and is as effective as the other techniques.

Table 7.1 ✦ Suggested Order for a Typical Exercise Session

PROGRAM	WORKOUT ORDER	EXPLANATION
3-Mile Jog (or Run, Cycle, or Swim)		
Slow jog (1/2 mile)	1	This will elevate body temperature, produce some sweating, and warm the muscles around the joints for stretching.
Stretch (5 min)	2	Muscles can now be safely stretched.
Fast jog (2 miles)	3	The pace can now be increased to elevate the heart rate above the target level for the aerobic portion of the workout.
Cooldown jog (slow 1/2 mile)	4	This final portion of the run can be used to help the body slowly return to the preexercise state.
Cooldown stretch (6 to 10 min)	5	This concentrated, slow, stretching session will help prevent muscle soreness and improve range of motion.
Racket Sports (or Team Sports or Strength Training)		
Slow, deliberate strokes movement	1	Movements specific to the sport are used to elevate body temperature and produce sweating.
Stretch (5 min)	2	Muscles can now be safely stretched using sport-specific flexibility exercises.
Actual play or workout	3	Muscles are now prepared for vigorous, explosive movement.
Cooldown (5 min)	4	The final portion of the workout should involve a return to slow, deliberate stroking or movements of the sport.
Cooldown stretch (6 to 10 min)	5	Concentrated, slow, stretching session.

Proprioceptive Neuromuscular Facilitation (PNF).
PNF stretching is a popular two-person technique based on a contract-and-relax principle. PNF stretching requires a partner to apply steady pressure to a body area at the extreme range of motion until slight discomfort is felt. When stretching the hamstring muscle group, lie on your back with one leg raised to 90 degrees or to a comfortable stretch. Have your partner apply steady pressure in an attempt to raise your leg overhead further (see Figure 7.3 on page 137). As pressure is applied, begin to push against your partner's resistance by contracting the muscle being stretched. This isometric hamstring contraction produces no leg movement since your partner will resist whatever force you apply during the push phase. After a 10-second push, relax your hamstring muscles while your partner again applies pressure for 5 seconds to increase the stretch even further. Repeat this two or three times. The PNF method, then, involves four phases: (1) an initial, easy stretch of the muscle, (2) an isometric contraction with resistance provided by a partner, (3) relaxation for 5 seconds, and (4) a final passive stretch for 5 seconds. For variety, your partner may allow your leg to move slightly downward during the push phase. PNF stretching relaxes the muscle group being stretched, which produces greater muscle

Ballistic stretching Flexibility exercises employing bouncing and jerking movements at the extreme range of motion or point of discomfort.

Static stretching Flexibility exercises in which a position is held steady for a designated period of time at the extreme range of motion.

Proprioceptive neuromuscular facilitation (PNF) stretching A two-person stretching technique involving the application of steady pressure by a partner at the extreme range of motion for a particular exercise and steady resistance to the pressure.

length and improves flexibility. Obvious disadvantages include some discomfort, a longer workout time, and the inability to stretch without a partner.

How Much Intensity to Use

Proper stretching should take the form of slow, relaxed, controlled, and relatively pain-free movement. It is important to disregard the *no pain, no gain* mentality when you stretch since improvement occurs without undue pain. Joint pressure should produce only mild discomfort. Too much pain and discomfort is a sign you are overloading soft tissue and are at risk of injury. After experiencing mild discomfort with each stretch, relax the muscles being stretched before the next repetition. You will learn to judge each exercise by the *stretch and feel method,* easing off the push if pain becomes intense or increases as the phase progresses.

How Long to Stretch

Depending on the stretching technique you choose, the length of your workout will be determined by the number of repetitions (ballistic stretching) and/or the length of time each repetition is held in the stretched position (static and PNF stretching). The amount of time the position is held should progress from 10 seconds at first to 30 seconds after two to three months of regular stretching. A 30- to 60-second stretch appears to only slightly increase the benefits and may be impractical.

If your main purpose for stretching is to prepare your body for vigorous exercise and to maintain the existing range of motion in the major joints, 6 to 9 minutes is sufficient time. For athletes and other individuals striving to increase their range of motion, 10 to 30 minutes of careful stretching may be necessary. Several different stretching exercises may be performed for each joint.

How Flexible to Become

Just how much flexibility a person needs depends on the person. The gymnast, ballet dancer, and hurdler must be more flexible than those who merely want to maintain a high enough level to reap the health benefits, perform daily activities, and engage in regular exercise.

According to the Virginia Commonwealth University Sportsmedicine Center, orthopedic surgeons

Figure 7.3 ✦ A Comparison of Three Stretching Techniques

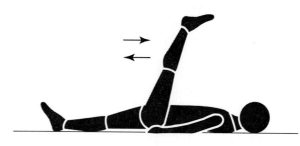

Ballistic Stretching

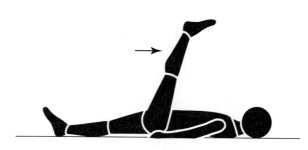

Static Stretching

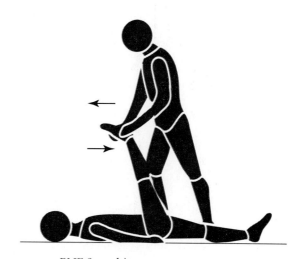

PNF Stretching

are treating more injury cases associated with excessive stretching and attempts to acquire high levels of flexibility than injuries associated with failure to stretch. This may be partially due to a renewed interest in stretching and the popularity of various forms of yoga and aerobics that tend to overemphasize flexibility or use questionable stretching exercises.

Behavioral Change and Motivational Strategies

A number of things may interfere with your flexibility-training progress. Listed below are some of these barriers (roadblocks) and strategies for overcoming them to keep you moving toward your training goals.

Roadblock	Behavioral Change Strategy
You are aware of your need to engage in flexibility training but just can't seem to stay interested long enough to avoid skipping workouts.	The first month of any exercise program is the most difficult. If you are beginning a new exercise program, it is normal to feel overloaded and anxious to complete the workout. At this point, you feel that five to ten minutes of stretching takes valuable time and you are unable to see its benefits. Try some of the following techniques to get past this critical period: 1. Arrive at the exercise site early with plenty of time to enjoy your workout. 2. After you walk or jog a few minutes, take five to ten minutes to relax, wind down, and enjoy stretching the major joints. 3. Make a mental note of how far beyond your toes you can reach, how difficult it is to reach behind your back and touch both hands, or how far forward you are able to move when stretching your calf muscle. Having these mental notes will help make you aware of improvement in future workouts. 4. Force yourself to stretch carefully prior to every workout until it becomes habit and you discover the benefits of stretching.
At the end of a workout your calves feel tight and are sometimes sore.	A feeling of tightness or even some mild soreness should only occur after your first three or four workouts. If it continues, examine every phase of your program. Are you properly warmed up prior to beginning your stretching session? Are you using static or PNF stretching exercises rather than ballistic movements? Are you stretching for three to five minutes at the end of your workout? Are you performing the correct exercises? Are you stretching both the calf muscle and the heel cord? You should find the answer to the problem in one or more of these questions.
List other roadblocks you are experiencing that seem to be limiting the effectiveness of your flexibility-training program. 1. _____ 2. _____ 3. _____	Now list the behavior change strategies that can help you overcome these roadblocks. If you need to, refer back to chapter 3 for behavior change and motivational strategies. 1. _____ 2. _____ 3. _____

How Often to Stretch

Those who are just beginning a flexibility-training program should do their routine three to four times a week. After several months, two or three workouts a week will maintain the flexibility you have acquired. As we pointed out previously, stretching should also be a part of the regular warmup routine prior to participation in aerobics, sports, or other forms of exercise.

FLEXIBILITY EXERCISES

It is important to choose at least one stretching exercise for each of the major muscle groups and to apply exercises equally to both sides of the body. Although there are hundreds of different stretches in use, many are unsafe and should be avoided. This section identifies some of the more commonly used exercises that have been shown to be potentially harmful.

What Exercises to Use

It is important to focus on a stretching routine that will increase the range of motion in particular joints of your choice. Stretching routines are also available that are designed for a specific sport or activity. After you warm up properly and are perspiring, complete each exercise gradually and slowly, beginning with a 10-second hold and adding 2 to 3 seconds to your hold time each workout until you can comfortably maintain the position at your extreme range of motion for 30 seconds. You can begin with the neck and progress downward to the shoulders and chest, trunk and lower back, groin and hips, abdomen, and upper and lower legs.

What Exercises to Avoid

As we pointed out previously, stretching can be harmful when the routine is too vigorous or too long or when bouncing at the extreme range of motion is used. The wrong choice of exercises also imposes serious risk of injury to joints. In fact, many popular stretching exercises used in the past are considered potentially harmful. Unfortunately, most people acquire their stretching knowledge by watching others. This informal, copycat approach has created a series of popular but dangerous exercises capable of damaging the knee, neck, spinal column, ankle, and lower back. Figure 7.4 on page 140 identifies 9 of the most popular "Hit List" of stretching exercises that should be avoided and offers a safe substitute that will effectively stretch the same muscle group.

Diversity Issues

Flexibility: Improving the Lives of People of All Ages

An infant or a young child has an amazing degree of flexibility. The child may place its foot behind its head or nibble on its toe—acts most adults can only admire, for, as we age, our degree of flexibility diminishes until even toe-touching becomes difficult.

Like most components of fitness, loss of flexibility occurs more rapidly and to a much higher degree among the sedentary population. Individuals of all ages, but especially the elderly, who engage in regular stretching routines can maintain a fairly high level of joint flexibility throughout life. In fact, flexibility is one of the easiest fitness components to improve. Even sedentary, inflexible individuals can greatly improve joint movement after only a few weeks of regular stretching.

Common ailments among the elderly, such as joint stiffness, pain, and inflexibility can be improved through regular exercise and stretching. In fact, stretching can improve mobility, make daily chores easier, and increase self-efficiency. Flexibility begins to decrease dramatically in sedentary college-aged men and women. Even minor injuries to the joints produce scar tissue and begin to reduce flexibility. As midlife approaches, joint stiffness becomes common, often to the point of limiting recreational pursuits and daily chores. This dramatic loss of flexibility in the aging process is primarily due to inactivity and failure to maintain an active program of stretching.

One dramatic example of the importance of maintaining adequate flexibility throughout life is low-back pain—one of the most prevalent health complaints in the United States. By middle age, approximately one in two individuals suffers from this ailment and experiences pain, discomfort, and decreased work and recreational efficiency. In most cases, low-back pain is caused by poor lower-back flexibility and inadequate abdominal muscle tone. Simply engaging in a 5- to 10-minute stretching routine three times weekly in young adulthood can maintain or improve flexibility levels and help prevent lower-back and other joint-related health problems in later years. ✦

Figure 7.4 ✦ Dangerous Popular Stretching Exercises and Suggested Replacements

OLD METHOD	NEW METHOD

Neck roll (circling)

Danger: Drawing the head backward could damage the disks in the neck area, and may even precipitate arthritis.

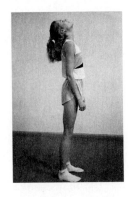

Forward neck roll

Description: Bend forward at the waist with the hands on the knees. Gently roll the head.

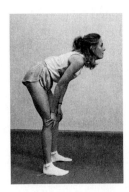

Quadricep stretch

Danger: If the ankle is pulled too hard, muscle, ligament, and cartilage damage may occur.

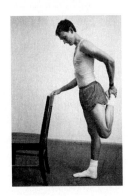

Opposite leg pull

Description: Grasp one ankle with your opposite hand. Instead of pulling, attempt to straighten the right leg.

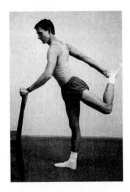

Hurdler's stretch

Danger: Hip, knee, and ankle are subjected to abnormal stress.

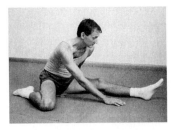

Everted hurdler's stretch

Description: Bend the right leg at the knee and slide the left foot underneath. Pull yourself forward slowly by using a towel, or by grasping the toe.

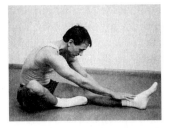

Deep knee bend (or any exercise that bends the knee beyond a right angle)

Danger: Excessive stress is placed on ligament, tendon, and cartilage tissue.

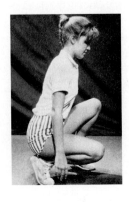

Single knee lunge

Description: Place one leg in front of your body and extend the other behind. Bend forward at the trunk as you bend the lead leg to right angles.

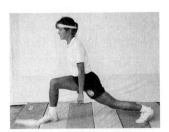

Figure 7.4 ✦ Dangerous Popular Stretching Exercises and Suggested Replacements *(continued)*

OLD METHOD	NEW METHOD

Yoga plow

Danger: This exercise could overstretch muscles and ligaments, injure spinal disks, or cause fainting.

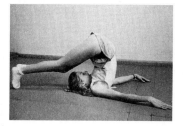

Extended one-leg stretch

Description: Lead leg extended and slightly bent at the knee. With your foot on the floor, draw the knee of the other leg toward your chest. Bend forward at the trunk as far as possible.

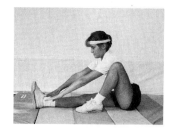

Straight-leg sit up

Danger: Produces back strain and sciatic nerve elongation. It also moves the hip flexor muscles and does not flatten the abdomen.

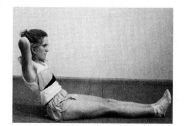

Bent-knee sit up

Description: Cross both hands on your chest, with the knees slightly bent. Raise the upper body slightly to about 25° on each repetition.

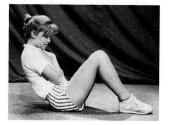

Double leg raise

Danger: Stretches the sciatic nerve beyond its normal limits, and places too much stress on ligaments, muscles, and disks.

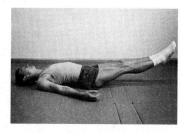

Knee-to-chest stretch

Description: Clasp both hands behind the neck. Draw the knee toward the chest, and hold that position of maximum stretch for 15–30 seconds.

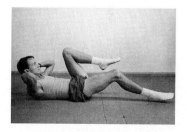

Prone arch

Danger: Hyperextension of the lower back places extreme pressure on spinal disks.

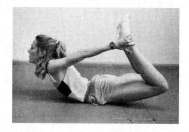

Stomach push up

Description: Lie flat on your stomach, rest on your elbows. Push slowly to raise the upper body as the lower torso remains pressured against the surface.

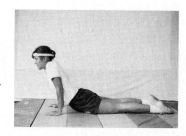

Figure 7.4 ✦ Dangerous Popular Stretching Exercises and Suggested Replacements *(continued)*

OLD METHOD	NEW METHOD

Back bends

Danger: Spinal disks can easily be damaged.

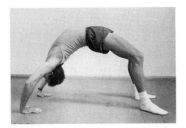

No alternate exercise has been approved.

ℐUMMARY

Factors Affecting Flexibility

A number of factors combine to place some limitation on the degree of flexibility you attain. After age, gender, heredity, and injury, your choice of lifestyle has the greatest influence on the range of motion in your joints. By engaging in a regular aerobic exercise program, stretching before and after your workout, and maintaining normal body weight and fat, you can remain relatively flexible throughout your life.

The Importance of Flexibility

Regular involvement in stretching exercises two to three times a week will increase joint flexibility, help improve performance in sports, aid in the prevention of soft-tissue injuries, help you prevent and recover from lower-back problems, and assist your muscles in returning to a relaxed status following a workout. Stretching can provide some benefit to almost everyone and make daily chores at home and at work easier and safer.

The Assessment of Flexibility

To properly evaluate your body's flexibility, one test should be used for each of the major joints. Although the sit-and-reach test is one of the most common and accurate, it only measures hamstring and lower-back flexibility. Tests are also needed to measure the range of motion in the neck, elbow, wrist, groin, trunk, hip, and shoulder.

Flexibility-Training Principles

Two to three sessions a week in addition to the stretching routine you normally perform before an aerobic workout will improve your flexibility. About 5 minutes of stretching should take place before every workout but only after body temperature has been elevated, as indicated by the presence of perspiration following some large-muscle activity such as jogging. It is important to avoid stretching cold muscles. A more concentrated 10-minute session should be used during the cooldown phase of a workout.

All three of the most common methods of stretching (ballistic, static, and PNF) have been shown to be equally effective in improving joint range of motion. Ballistic and PNF methods are more likely to result in injury and muscle soreness than static stretching is.

Stretching should produce only mild discomfort. Pain is an indication of risk of injury from overextending soft tissue. Stretching for too long a period of time in an attempt to obtain an extremely high degree of flexibility may also result in injury. Extreme flexibility is unimportant for most individuals and yoga-style contortions should be avoided.

Effective stretching involves a warmup period, stretching before and after exercise, stretching slowly and gently, holding the stretch for 10 to 30 seconds, and relaxing the body parts other than the muscle group you are stretching.

Flexibility Exercises

A sound program requires at least one exercise for each major joint and emphasis on both sides of the body. Exercises can be chosen that focus on the particular joints you identify as inflexible or important to your personal life, job, sport, or activity. Although not everyone who uses so-called banned stretching exercises will suffer an injury, it is wise to avoid those known to have the potential to damage a joint.

Lab Activity 7.1

Measuring Lower-Back and Hamstring Flexibility

INSTRUCTIONS: *The sit-and-reach test is used to determine the flexibility of your back and hamstring muscles. If a sit-and-reach box is not available, you can build one by placing a yardstick on top of a 12-inch-high box. To complete the test, follow these steps carefully:*

1. Warm up properly before the first trial by walking or jogging for one-quarter to one-half mile or until you are perspiring. Now complete your warmup by twice performing the hamstring and quadriceps exercises shown in Figure 7.4 and the lower back exercises shown in Figure 7.2. Maintain the hold position for 30 seconds.

2. Remove your shoes, sit on the floor with your hips, back, and head against a wall and both legs fully extended, feet contacting the sit-and-reach box.

3. Place one hand on top of the other so the middle fingers are together.

4. Lean forward slowly as far as possible, without bouncing, sliding your hands along the measuring scale on top of the box. Repeat this movement three times, stretching forward as far as possible a third time and hold this position for two seconds.

5. Complete two trials and record the average as your final score.

6. Determine your hamstring- and back-flexibility rating from the chart below.

PERFORMANCE STANDARDS	COLLEGE FEMALES (INCHES)	COLLEGE MALES (INCHES)
Excellent	8 or above	7 or above
Good	5 to 7	4 to 6
Average	1 to 4	1 to 3
Poor	0 or negative	0 or negative

Lab Activity 7.2

Determining Your Total Body Flexibility

INSTRUCTIONS: *You can test aspects of your flexibility subjectively alone or with a partner. The only equipment needed is a straight-backed chair and a ruler. Score each test by checking "Yes" or "No," depending on whether you can meet the standard sited.*

		Yes	No
1. **Neck** Normal neck flexibility will allow you to use your chin to sandwich your flattened hand against your chest.		____	____
2. **Elbow and Wrist** You should be able to hold your arms out straight with palms up and little fingers higher than your thumbs.	Right arm/wrist	____	____
	Left arm/wrist	____	____
3. **Groin** While standing on one leg, raise the other leg to the side as high as possible. You should be able to achieve a 90-degree angle between the two legs.	Right leg	____	____
	Left leg	____	____
While you are sitting on the floor, put the soles of your feet together and draw your heels as close to your body as possible. Try to touch your knees to the floor or to press your upright fists to the floor using your knees.		____	____
4. **Trunk** While sitting in a straight chair with your feet wrapped around the front legs, twist your body 90 degrees without allowing your hips to move.	Right twist	____	____
	Left twist	____	____
5. **Hip** While standing, hold a yardstick or broom handle with your hands shoulder-width apart. Without losing your grasp, bend down and step over the stick (with both feet, one at a time) and then back again.		____	____
6. **Shoulder** In a standing position, attempt to clasp your hands behind your back by reaching over the shoulder with one arm and upward from behind with the other. Repeat, reversing the arm positions.	Right arm top	____	____
	Left arm top	____	____

8 chapter

Nutrition

Chapter Objectives

By the end of this chapter, you should be able to:

1. Discuss the functions of the six categories of nutrients in the diet.

2. Compare carbohydrates, fats, and proteins in terms of how each provides energy to the body.

3. Describe a sound nutritional plan based on the RDA, *Dietary Guidelines for Americans,* and the nutrition pyramid.

4. Demonstrate the ability to read a food label.

5. Discuss the role of nutrition in the prevention of disease.

6. Describe the special nutritional needs of the active individual.

7. Dispel common nutritional myths.

DURING RITA'S FRESHMAN year, cafeteria food became unappealing. She had gained 9 pounds, had low energy, and was aware she was eating too much fat. She also was sick a number of times and wondered whether any of these illnesses were related to her poor eating habits. To be honest, Rita had to admit, she just didn't know enough about proper nutrition. Even if she discontinued the university meal plan, she would not know what to do.

This chapter focuses on Rita's concerns and presents an overview of sound nutrition to help her (and others like her) make appropriate choices in the cafeteria or prepare her own nutritional program. Discussion is provided on the basic food components, the energy nutrients (carbohydrates, fats, and proteins), the nonenergy nutrients (vitamins, minerals, and water), food density, dietary guidelines for good health and high energy, food labeling, nutrition-disease relationships, and special needs of the active person.

BASIC FOOD COMPONENTS

Kinds of Nutrients

Six categories of nutrients—carbohydrates, fats, and proteins (the energy nutrients), and vitamins, minerals, and water (the nonenergy nutrients)—satisfy the basic body needs:

- Energy for muscle contraction
- Conduction of nerve impulses
- Growth
- Formation of new tissue and tissue repair
- Chemical regulation of metabolic functions
- Reproduction

The body's use of these nutrients for conversion into tissue, production of energy for muscle contraction, and maintenance of chemical machinery is called **metabolism**.

THE ENERGY NUTRIENTS

Carbohydrates and fat provide the body with its two main sources of energy. All food has energy potential, measured in calories. Since one calorie is too small a unit to be convenient, nutritionists use a large, or **kilocalorie** (kcal), as a measure. One kilocalorie is equal to 1000 small calories. One kilocalorie is the amount of heat required to raise the temperature of one kilogram (about one quart) of water one degree Celsius. The energy in one peanut, for example, can add one degree of heat to two gallons of water. Only carbohydrates, fats, and protein contain calories; vitamins, minerals, and water do not.

Just how much energy do these nutrients provide? Carbohydrates and protein contain four cal per gram (g), fat contains nine cal per g, and alcohol contains seven cal per g (1 g equals one-fifth of a level teaspoon, 100 g equal one-half cup, 1 milligram [mg] equals .001 g).

Basal metabolism, or **metabolic rate**, is the number of calories expended by a resting person over a 24-hour period. Basal metabolism depends on age, gender, height, weight, and activity patterns (work and play).

Carbohydrates

Carbohydrates are organic components of various elements that provide a continuous supply of energy in the form of glucose (sugar) to trillions of body cells. **Simple carbohydrates (monosaccharides and disaccharides)** come concentrated, such as refined sugar, which is made from cane or beet sugar, molasses, and honey, and natural, such as the sugars in some fruits, vegetables, and grains. **Complex carbohydrates (polysaccharides)** are chains of sugar molecules found in fruits, vegetables, and grains. Carbohydrates are broken down into six simple carbon-sugar molecules to permit absorption into the bloodstream. After food is eaten, the blood-sugar level is elevated, and there is an increase in the amount of glucose transported to the cells. Excess sugar is converted to glycogen and stored for future use in the liver and muscles. Once maximum storage capacity is reached, excess sugars are converted to body fat and stored in **adipose** (fat) cells.

Simple carbohydrates (sugars) are consumed in four forms: sucrose, glucose, fructose, and lactose. Annual cane and beet sugar intake in the United States exceeds 100 lb per person: 20 to 25 lb of syrups (glucose and fructose) are also consumed, bringing the total to over 125 lb of sugar intake per person per year. Consumed in these large quantities, sugar contributes to dental cavities, excessive weight, and body

---

Metabolism The sum of energy expended in carrying on the normal body processes: converting nutrients into tissue, muscle contraction, and maintenance of the body's chemical machinery.

Kilocalorie A large calorie, equal to one thousand small calories; one kilocalorie is the amount of heat required to raise the temperature of one kilogram (about one quart) of water one degree Celsius.

Metabolic rate Amount of calories burned at rest.

Simple carbohydrates (monosaccharides and disaccharides) Sugars; chains of sugar molecules (one or two) found in concentrated sugar and the sugar that occurs naturally in food.

Complex carbohydrates (polysaccharides) Starch and fiber; chains of sugar molecules (three or more) found in fruits, vegetables, and grains.

Adipose tissue Fatty tissue.

Nutrition density Foods that are high in nutrients and low in calories.

Dietary fiber The undigestible portion of food after it is exposed to the body's enzymes.

Table 8.1 ◆ Sugar Content of Common Food and Drinks

Food	Size	Approximate Content in Teaspoons
Beverages	12 oz	
Sodas		5–9
Sweet cider		4¼
Jams and jellies, candies	1 tbsp	4–6
Milk chocolate	1½ oz	2½
Fudge	1 oz	4½
Hard candy	4 oz	20
Marshmallow	1	1½
Fruits and canned juices		
Dried raisins, prunes, apricot, dates	3–5	4
Fruit juice	8 oz	2½–3½
Breads		
White	1 slice	¼
Hamburger/hot dog bun	1	3
Dairy products		
Ice cream cone	Single dip	3
Sherbet	One scoop	9
Desserts		
Pie (fruit, custard cream)	1 slice	4–13
Pudding	½ cup	3–5

fat and indirectly to such degenerative diseases as diabetes and heart disease. As you can see from Table 8.1, it is not unusual for a person to consume the equivalent of 50 teaspoons of sugar per day. Sugar intake should be managed from infancy. Infants seem to be born with a preference for sweet foods, and it is not until early adulthood that the desire for sugar slowly decreases. You can reduce your own sugar intake by reading the labels for sweeteners and sugars in products you are considering (the terms *sucrose, glucose, dextrose, fructose, corn syrup, corn sweetener, natural sweetener,* and *invert sugar* all mean that the product contains sugar), substituting water and unsweetened fruit juices for sodas and punches, buying fruit canned in its own unsweetened juice, cutting back on desserts, purchasing cereals low in sugar, reducing the amount of sugar called for in recipes, and avoiding sweet snacks. If you never again consumed concentrated sugars, it would have absolutely no effect on sound nutrition.

Complex carbohydrates are your major source of vitamins (except vitamin B_{12}) and minerals, an important long-term energy source, and the only source of fiber. Complex carbohydrates burn efficiently, leave no toxic waste in the body, and do not tax the liver or raise blood-fat levels. Fruits, vegetables, and grains also have high **nutrition density**, providing a high percentage of our needed daily nutrients in a low number of calories. In the past 75 years, our intake of complex carbohydrates has declined by about 30 percent as sugar intake increased by a similar amount. Unlike sugars, complex carbohydrates are the body's chief source of fuel. Sugar, on the other hand, provides empty calories and very little long-term energy.

Complex carbohydrates should make up at least 48 percent of your total daily calories. Simple carbohydrates should be reduced from 24 percent to 10 percent of total calories.

Dietary Fiber The indigestible portion of complex carbohydrates is a nonnutritive substance that cannot be broken down by the enzymes in the human body. Six of the seven types of fiber are carbohydrate. Only lignin, found in fruit and vegetable skins and the woody portions of plants, is a noncarbohydrate.

Table 8.2 on page 150 provides an overview of key information on fiber, including water-soluble and -insoluble varieties, recommended daily intake, nutritional advantages of adequate amounts, dangers of excess intake, and the food sources for both types. Complete Lab Activity 8.1: Estimating Your Daily Fiber Intake at the end of the chapter to discover whether your diet contains enough fiber.

Blood-Glucose Control Blood-glucose levels are carefully regulated by the pancreas. When blood-sugar levels are too high, the pancreas releases a hor-

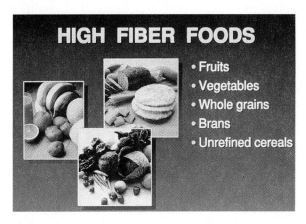

(Photo Courtesy of the American Heart Association.)

Table 8.2 ✦ All About Fiber

Water-Insoluble	Cellulose, forming the cell walls of many plants, is the most abundant insoluble fiber. Cellulose and lignin (from the woody portion of plants, parts of fruit and vegetable skins, and whole grains) cannot be broken down, digested, or made to provide calories for the body.
Water-Soluble	The fiber in food that can be broken down and digested to provide calories for the body is referred to as water-soluble. Dried beans and peas (8 grams per ½ cup), oat bran, and the flesh of fruits and vegetables are excellent sources of water-soluble fiber.
Dietary fiber	Undigested residue after the action of the body's enzymes; much more concentrated than crude fiber. (1 gram of crude fiber = 2–3 grams of dietary fiber.) Dietary fiber (water insoluble) is reported on most labels that list fiber content.
Crude fiber	Remaining portion of food that cannot be dissolved or broken down into a liquid when exposed to acids and alkalis in the laboratory. This fiber, consisting of cellulose and lignin, was reported on product labels and tables for many years. Due to inaccurate measurement, the crude fiber was reported at levels two to three times lower than dietary fiber.
Daily Needs	25–35 grams. It is important to increase your daily intake slowly if you are unaccustomed to adequate fiber to avoid frequent bowel movements and diarrhea. Add several grams daily over a period of a few weeks to give your system a chance to adjust.
Nutritional Advantages of Consuming Adequate Fiber	*Insoluble* fiber increases transit time (digestion and elimination of food) and decreases the amount of time the bacteria in the food has to act on intestinal walls. It helps prevent colon and rectal cancer and *diverticulosis* (outpouchings in the wall of the large intestine), provides bulk to the stools, helps eliminate constipation, helps maintain normal bowel movement, and helps to control and maintain normal body weight and fat. *Water-soluble* fiber is associated with lower cardiovascular disease, lower blood cholesterol, and lower blood pressure.
Dangers of Excess Fiber	Excess fiber binds to some trace minerals and causes excretion prior to the absorption of these minerals. Excessive fiber intake causes poor absorption of nutrients, interferes with the absorption of some drugs, reduces the ability to digest and absorb food by speeding up digestive time, and causes irritation of the intestinal wall. The high phosphorus content of high-fiber foods may create special problems for some individuals, such as those with kidney problems.
Food Sources	Complex carbohydrates (fruits, vegetables, and grains) are the sole source of fiber. Both water-insoluble and water-soluble fiber are contained in some food sources, such as in the skin of fruits and vegetables (insoluble) and in the flesh of fruits and vegetables (soluble). Raw fruits and vegetables are a major source of insoluble fiber such as in dried beans and peas (8 grams per ½ cup). Oat bran and grains are a major source of soluble fiber.
	Many hot and cold cereals (unprocessed bran, 100 percent bran, shredded wheat, oatmeal) contain 2–5 grams of fiber per serving. Legumes provide about 8 grams per portion (½ cup of garbanzo beans, kidney beans, or baked beans). Fruits provide about 2 grams per serving (one small apple, banana, orange; two small plums, a medium peach, ½ cup strawberries, ten large cherries). Vegetables also provide about 2 grams per serving (broccoli, brussels sprouts, two stalks of celery, small corn cob, lettuce, green beans, small potato, tomato), and 1 gram of fiber is provided by ten peanuts, ¼ cup walnuts, 2½ teaspoons of peanut butter, and a pickle. Additional foods with fiber are breads (whole wheat, whole grain), crackers, and flours (wheat germ, wild rice, cornmeal, buckwheat, millet, rice, raisin, and popcorn). Cooking does not significantly reduce the fiber content of foods.

Source: Greenberg, Jerry, and Dintiman, George B. *Exploring Health: Expanding the Boundaries of Wellness.* Englewood Cliffs, NJ: Prentice-Hall, 1992.

Figure 8.1 ✦ Controlling Blood Glucose Levels

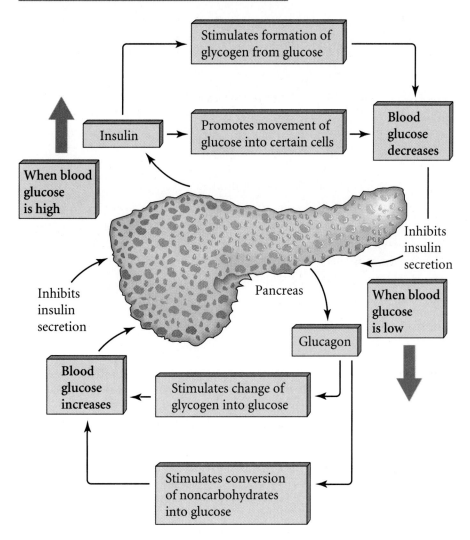

Source: From David C. Nieman, et al., *Nutrition,* Revised First Edition, Copyright © 1992 Wm. C. Brown Communications, Inc., Dubuque, IA. All rights reserved. Reprinted by permission.

mone called **insulin**, which promotes the movement of glucose into certain cells, dropping blood-sugar levels. When levels are too low, the pancreas secretes a hormone called **glucagon**, which stimulates the changing of stored glycogen into glucose and the conversion of noncarbohydrates into glucose to raise the blood-sugar level (see Figure 8.1). The pancreas of individuals suffering from **Type I** (insulin-dependent) **diabetes mellitus** fails to produce insulin so it must be injected to control blood-glucose levels. The pancreas of most individuals suffering from adult-onset, **Type II** (noninsulin-dependent) **diabetes mellitus** produces insulin; glucose uptake at the cellular level, however, does not occur normally and blood-sugar levels remain high. For most individuals, the

Insulin A natural hormone produced in the pancreas gland that aids in the digestion of sugars and other carbohydrates; it is secreted when blood sugar is too high.

Glucagon A natural hormone secreted by the pancreas that stimulates the metabolism of sugar; it is secreted when blood sugar is too low, a condition that causes the release of liver glycogen and its transformation into glucose.

Diabetes mellitus A disease caused by insufficient production of insulin by the endocrine portion of the pancreas; **Type I** (insulin dependent) or **Type II** (noninsulin dependent).

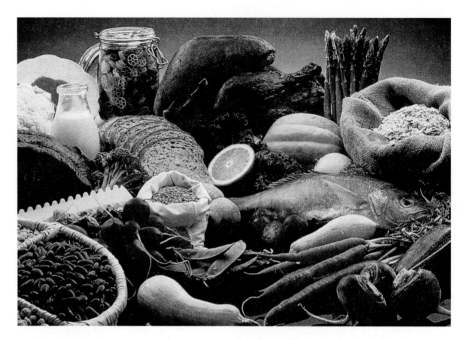

To maintain sound nutrition, choose lower fat foods whenever possible. (Photo Courtesy of the American Heart Association.)

pancreas does its job and, in conjunction with proper diet, maintains blood glucose at normal levels regardless of what we eat and how much we exercise.

Fats

Fat is a critical nutrient that provides a tremendous source of energy to the human body. Fat also stores and transports vitamins A, D, E, and K; carries linoleic acid (an essential fatty acid); increases the flavor and palatability of foods; provides sustained relief from hunger; and helps to keep protein from being used as energy. The fatty tissue in our bodies supports organs, cushions them from injury, and aids in the prevention of heat loss. Fat is in most body tissue, with bone marrow containing 96 percent, liver 2.5 percent, and blood 0.5 percent. Unfortunately, too much body fat and high blood-fat levels can shorten life and increase vulnerability to numerous chronic and degenerative diseases, such as cardiorespiratory disease and cancer.

The fat in food is classified as **saturated, polyunsaturated**, and **monounsaturated. Cholesterol** is used in the synthesis of sex hormones, vitamin D, and bile salts. It is also associated with artery clogging and heart disease (see chapter 5). Cholesterol is a **nonessential nutrient**. Blood levels depend on the cholesterol consumed in your diet and that produced by the liver (see Table 8.3). The intake of saturated fat stimulates the liver to produce more cholesterol.

The average person in the United States consumes over 55 lb of **visible fat** and over 130 lb of **invisible fat** each year. Dietary fat contributes approximately 42 percent of the total calories although the recent favorable pattern of fat intake shows that more

Saturated fat Fat that contains glycerol and saturated fatty acids, found in high quantities in animal products (such as meat, milk, butter, and cheese) and in low quantities in vegetable products; high intake is associated with elevated blood cholesterol levels.

Polyunsaturated fat Fat containing two or more double bonds between carbons; found heavily in vegetable oils, nuts (such as almonds, pecans, walnuts, and filberts), fish, and margarines.

Monounsaturated fat Fat containing one double bond between carbons, found in foods such as avocados, cashews, and peanut and olive oils.

Cholesterol One of the sterols, or fat-like chemical substances, manufactured in the body and consumed from foods of animal origins only; high intake is associated with elevated blood cholesterol levels and heart disease.

Nonessential nutrient Nutrients the body can manufacture in sufficient quantities without there being any of that substance in your diet.

Table 8.3 ✦ Cholesterol Content of Selected Foods

Food	Serving Size	Cholesterol (mg)
Milk		
Skim milk	1 C	7
Whole milk	1 C	25
Ice cream	¼ C	50
Meat		
Beef, lean, cooked	3 oz	110
Chicken, flesh only, cooked	3 oz	90
Egg, whole (50 g)	1	255
Egg white (33 g)	1	0
Egg yolk (17 g)	1	255
Fish fillet, cooked	3 oz	60
Heart, cooked	3 oz	130
Kidney, cooked	3 oz	320
Lamb, lean, cooked	3 oz	110
Liver, cooked	3 oz	260
Lobster, cooked	3 oz	170
Mutton, lean, cooked	3 oz	130
Oysters, raw	3 oz (15)	165
Pork, lean, cooked	3 oz	140
Shrimp, flesh only, cooked	3 oz	105
Veal, lean, cooked	3 oz	180
Caviar	1 oz	85
Cheddar cheese	1 oz	30
Creamed cottage cheese	¼ C	9
Cream cheese	1 oz	35
Fat		
Butter	1 tsp	12
Margarine, all vegetable	1 tsp	0
Margarine, ⅔ animal fat, ⅓ vegetable fat	1 tsp	3
Lard or other animal fat	1 tsp	5

Source: Hamilton, Eva May, and Whitney, Eleanor. *Nutrition Concepts and Controversies.*
St. Paul, MN: West, 1979. Used by permission.

fat is being consumed from plants and less from animal sources. Since saturated fat intake stimulates the production of cholesterol, it is important to reduce cholesterol intake to less than 300 milligrams daily and total saturated fat to less than 10 percent of daily calories. Both dietary saturated fat and cholesterol contribute to elevated blood-cholesterol levels.

The five kinds of foods containing the highest percentage of fat are hamburgers and meatloaf (63 percent); hot dogs, ham, and luncheon meats (58 percent); whole milk (54 percent); doughnuts, cakes, and cookies (54 percent); and beefsteak and roasts (50 percent). Another major source of saturated fat in our diet is the food eaten in fast-food restaurants. Most hamburgers, hot dogs, and chicken and fish sandwiches served by major fast-food chains contain more than 50 percent fat and are very high in calories.

Visible fat Fat content of food that can be seen, such as the fat in butter and oils.

Invisible fat Hidden fat in food that cannot be seen such as the fat in dairy products, egg yolks, and meat.

Even McDonald's McLean Deluxe Sandwich contains 320 calories and 10 g of fat (90 cal) for a total of 28 percent fat. Other popular sandwiches and their percent of calories from fat include: McDonald's Filet-O-Fish (440 calories, 53 percent fat), Burger King's Broiler Chicken Sandwich (379 calories, 42 percent fat), Burger King's Double Whopper with Cheese (935 calories, 59 percent fat), Wendy's Grilled Chicken Sandwich (340 calories, 34 percent fat), Wendy's Big Classic (570 calories, 52 percent fat), Kentucky Fried Chicken's Lite 'n Crispy Drumsticks (242 calories, 52 percent fat), and Kentucky Fried Chicken's Chicken Sandwich (482 calories, 50 percent fat).

Protein

Protein, from the Greek word *proteios*, or *primary*, is critical to all living things. In the human body, it is used to repair, rebuild, and replace cells; aid in growth; balance fluid, salt, and acid-base; and provide needed energy when carbohydrates and fats are insufficient or unavailable. Protein is produced in the body through building blocks called **amino acids.** Some of these amino acids are produced in the body; others are derived only from food sources. **Nonessential amino acids** can be manufactured by the body if not obtained from the diet. **Essential amino acids**, 8 to 10 of which must be present in the body in the proper amount and proportion to the nonessential acids for normal protein metabolism to proceed, cannot be manufactured by the body and must be acquired through diet. All 22 amino acids must be present simultaneously (within several hours) in order for the body to synthesize them into proteins that will be used for optimal maintenance of body growth and function.

Humans obtain protein from both animal and plant foods. In general, animal protein is superior to plant protein because it contains all the essential amino acids in the proper proportions. If one essential amino acid is missing or present in the incorrect proportion, protein construction may be blocked.

Eggs are the complete protein by which all other protein is judged. Milk, cheese, other dairy products, meat, fish, and poultry compare favorably with eggs as excellent sources of protein. Although eggs contain about 213 milligrams (mg) of cholesterol and 5 g of fat (60 percent), they are a low-calorie (75-cal) source of protein, vitamin A, riboflavin, vitamin B_{12}, iron, zinc, phosphorus, calcium, potassium, and other nutrients. It is still advisable to consume no more than two to three eggs per week, never more than one per

day, to eliminate or substitute other food products in recipes calling for eggs as an ingredient, and to purchase small eggs rather than medium, large, or extra large. The American Heart Association guideline of no more than 300 mg of cholesterol per day is difficult to follow if you start the day with an egg rather than with cold or hot cereal.

Protein containing all essential amino acids is termed a **complete**, or a high-quality, **protein**; protein from most vegetable sources are low in some amino acids and will not support growth and development when used as the only source of protein. This sort of protein is called **incomplete**, or low-quality, **protein**. Terms such as **low** and **high biological value** are also used to describe the quality of protein.

Approximately 54 g of protein are recommended daily for college-aged males and 46 to 48 g for females. To determine your specific protein needs multiply your body weight in kilograms (kg) by .8 g. A 132-lb woman, for example, weighs 60 kg (132 divided by 2.2) and needs 48 g (60 × .8 = 48) of protein daily. Larger individuals, pregnant and lactating women, adolescents, and those who are ill may need slightly more protein. Physically active individuals generally do not require additional protein unless the weather is hot and profuse sweating that produces additional nitrogen loss occurs. Those living in extremely hot climates may also need slightly more protein. Approximately 12 to 15 percent of the total daily calories in the U.S. diet should come from protein.

It is not difficult for most people to obtain their recommended daily intakes (RDIs) of protein. Meat contains about seven grams per ounce; milk has eight grams per glass; and protein is plentiful in eggs and dairy products and present in small quantities in vegetables and grains. Two glasses of milk; one ounce of cheese; and three ounces of beef, chicken, or fish provide all the protein the average person needs in one day.

Vegetarian Diets Believing that vegetables are healthier than meats, that it is morally wrong to consume meat, or that meat is contaminated with growth-enhancing drugs, more and more people in the United States are resorting to some form of vegetarianism.

There are three basic kinds of vegetarians: the **vegan**, the **lactovegetarian**, and the **ovolactovegetarian**. All vegetarians must plan their diets carefully since it is more difficult for them to consume adequate protein, iron, and vitamin B_{12} intake than it is for people who are not vegetarians. Since dairy products and eggs are excellent protein sources, lacto- and ovolactovegetarians have much less difficulty than strict vegans do. Vegans must use complementary protein combinations of vegetables and grains to include proper amounts of protein in their diets. Traditional complementary protein diets include combinations of soy beans or tofu with rice (China and Indochina); peas with wheat (the Middle East); beans with corn (Central and South America); and rice with beans, black-eyed peas, or tofu (United States and the Caribbean). Other protein combinations readily available to U.S. vegans include peanut butter and whole-grain bread, whole-wheat bread, black beans, and black bean and rice soup. These combinations of complete proteins are excellent substitutes for meat, egg, and dairy proteins.

Because fruits, vegetables, and grains contain no cholesterol, little saturated fat, and high fiber, vegans tend to escape heart disease for ten years longer than meat eaters do. Vegetarians may also be able to avoid certain kinds of digestive system cancers; however, vegans are especially prone to dangerous deficiencies in iron, calcium, and vitamin B_{12} (available only in animal products). In order to combat serious nutrient shortages, vegans should follow certain daily dietary recommendations and include in their diets:

- Two cups of legumes daily for proper levels of calcium and iron.

- One cup of dark greens daily to meet iron requirements (for women).

- At least one gram of fat daily for proper absorption of vitamins.

- A supplement of fortified plant foods (like soy or nut milks or a multiple vitamin and mineral) to obtain vitamin B_{12}.

The Energy Systems Practically all energy your muscles use is formed by the chemical reactions of two unique pathways of energy formation: the **glycolysis** and the **citric acid cycle.**

The majority of energy formed by glycolysis is derived from glucose, and since it is anaerobic, it can be produced quickly. The glucose used to fuel glycolysis comes from blood glucose, glycogen (stored form of glucose), glycerol (small fraction of stored fat molecules), and several amino acids. Most college-aged people have approximately 1000 cal of stored glycogen in the muscles and 300 stored in the liver (liver glycogen can be used to supply glucose to muscles). Short, intense anaerobic exercises such as sprinting, weight training, pull ups, diving, and push ups, are fueled by the glycolysis energy cycle.

The citric acid cycle uses three different types of fuel: glucose fragments produced by glycolysis, fatty acids, and certain amino acids. Fatty acids drawn from the body's fat stores are by far the largest supplier of energy in this aerobic cycle. Only in the aerobic cycle where oxygen is present can fat be burned as fuel. Activities such as walking, jogging, running, lap swimming, aerobic dance, cycling, basketball, and soccer are fueled by fat in the citric acid cycle. These aerobic activities are ideal for weight and fat loss. Fat cannot be burned in the anaerobic cycle since oxygen is not present.

Amino acids The basic component of most proteins.

Nonessential amino acids Amino acids that can be manufactured by the body if they cannot be acquired from food sources.

Essential amino acids Amino acids that cannot be manufactured by the body and therefore must be acquired from food sources.

Complete protein Food source containing all essential amino acids in the correct proportions.

Incomplete protein Food source that does not contain all essential amino acids or contains several in incorrect proportions.

Low biological value A protein source such as corn and wheat that does not contain all eight essential amino acids or contains some in low proportions.

High biological value A protein source such as meat that contains all eight essential amino acids in the correct proportions.

Vegan A strict vegetarian who consumes only fruits, vegetables, and grains.

Lactovegetarian An individual who eats fruits, vegetables, grains, and dairy products and avoids meat products.

Ovolactovegetarian An individual who eats fruits, vegetables, grains, dairy products, and eggs but avoids meat products.

Glycolysis energy cycle The anaerobic energy pathway fueled primarily by glucose.

Citric acid energy cycle The aerobic energy pathway fueled primarily by fat, small quantities of glucose fragments, and certain amino acids.

Nonenergy Nutrients: Vitamins, Minerals, and Water

Vitamins

Vitamins are essential in helping chemical reactions take place in the body and are required in very small amounts. Water-soluble vitamins (vitamin C and the B-complex vitamins) need to be consumed in the proper amounts over a five- to eight-day period since they are easily dissolved in water, not stored for long periods of time, and eliminated in the urine (see Table 8.4 on page 157 and 8.5 on page 158). Fat-soluble vitamins (vitamins A, D, E, and K) are stored in large amounts in fatty tissues and the liver and are absorbed through the intestinal track as needed.

Regardless of the claims, vitamin C does not cure or prevent the common cold. Large supplements of other vitamins and minerals are being examined for their disease-fighting potential and their ability to assist in medical treatment. It is important to realize three important things about taking supplements: (1) The best way to obtain adequate vitamins and minerals is from food, not from supplements. Food has the added benefit of containing fiber and water. (2) The vast majority of people in the United States get all the vitamins and minerals they need from their diets and do not need supplements. (3) Vitamin and mineral toxicity problems are found predominantly in those who take supplements.

Minerals

Minerals are present in all living cells. They serve as key components of various hormones, enzymes, and other substances that aid in regulating chemical reactions within cells. Mineral elements play a part in the body's metabolic processes, and deficiencies can result in serious disorders. *Macrominerals,* such as sodium, potassium, calcium, phosphorus, magnesium, sulfur, and chlorides, are needed by the body in large amounts. *Trace minerals* are needed in small amounts. A minimum of 14 trace minerals must be ingested for optimum health. Iron, iodine, copper, fluoride, and zinc are the ones most important for body function. The body is composed of about 31 minerals, 24 of

Megavitamin intake Consuming 10 to 100 times the RDA for a particular vitamin.

which are considered essential for sustaining life (see Table 8.6 on page 159 and Table 8.7 on page 160).

Iron is one of the body's most essential minerals. Approximately 85 percent of our daily iron intake is used to produce new hemoglobin (the pigment of the red blood cells that transports oxygen); the remaining 15 percent is used for the production of new tissue or held in storage. Iron needs also vary according to age and gender. Table 8.8 on page 161 summarizes these variables. Iron deficiency results in loss of strength and endurance, rapid fatigue during exercise, shortening of the attention span, loss of visual perception, impaired learning, and numerous other physical disorders. Although the importance of sufficient dietary iron is common knowledge, many women may not get enough iron in their diet. In the United States, iron intake has been reduced by the removal of iron-containing soils from the food supply and the diminished use of iron cooking utensils. Whereas animals can ingest iron from muddy water and soil, humans must rely solely on food.

Iron deficiency anemia, a major health problem in the United States, is common in older infants, children, women of childbearing age, pregnant women, and low-income people. People must also be aware, however, that too much iron can be dangerous. Iron toxicity is rare, but a condition called *iron overload* occurs when the body is overwhelmed with too much iron given by vein (by blood transfusion) or when too much iron is absorbed because of hereditary defects, heavy supplementation, and alcohol abuse (which increases absorption). Iron overload can cause tissue and liver damage. Rapid ingestion of large amounts of iron can also cause sudden death. Iron overdose is the second most common cause of accidental poisoning in small children. High blood-iron levels may also be related to heart disease in men.

Iron is more easily absorbed from meat, fish, and poultry (heme iron) than it is from vegetables (non-heme iron). Twice the volume of vegetable iron is absorbed when vegetables and meats are consumed during the same meal.

Supplementation Some people take large doses of vitamins and minerals in the belief that these are neessary to correct dietary deficiencies or to prevent or cure a variety of ills. More commonly, the multiple vitamin/mineral pill is taken as an *insurance policy* against improper nutrition. Unfortunately, consuming too many vitamins and minerals, especially fat-soluble vitamins, which the body stores for long periods of time, can be toxic. The **megavitamin** approach

text continues on page 161

Table 8.4 ✦ Summary of Information on Fat-Soluble Vitamins

Name	RDA for adults*	Sources	Stability	Comments
Vitamin A (retinol; α-, β-, γ-carotene)	M: 1000 RE F: 800 RE	Liver, kidney, milk fat, fortified margarine, egg yolk, yellow and dark green leafy vegetables, apricots, cantaloupe, peaches.	Stable to light, heat, and usual cooking methods. Destroyed by oxidation, drying, very high temperature, ultraviolet light.	Essential for normal growth, development, and maintenance of epithelial tissue. Essential to the integrity of night vision. Helps provide for normal bone development and influences normal tooth formation. Toxic in large quantities.
Vitamin D (calciferol)	M: 5 μg F: 5 μg	Vitamin D milk, irradiated foods, some in milk fat, liver, egg yolk, salmon, tuna fish, sardines. Sunlight converts 7-dehydrocholesterol to cholecalciferol.	Stable to heat and oxidation.	Really a prohormone. Essential for normal growth and development; important for formation of normal bones and teeth. Influences absorption and metabolism of phosphorus and calcium. Toxic in large quantities.
Vitamin E (tocopherols and tocotrienols)	M: 10 α-TE F: 8 α-TE	Wheat germ, vegetable oils, green leafy vegetables, milk fat, egg yolk, nuts.	Stable to heat and acids. Destroyed by rancid fats, alkali, oxygen, lead, iron salts, and ultraviolet irradiation.	Is a strong antioxidant. May help prevent oxidation of unsaturated fatty acids and vitamin A in intestinal tract and body tissues. Protects red blood cells from hemolysis. Role in reproduction (in animals). Role in epithelial tissue maintenance and prostaglandin synthesis.
Vitamin K (phylloquinone and menaquinone)	M: 80 μg F: 65 μg	Liver, soybean oil, other vegetable oils, green leafy vegetables, wheat bran. Synthesized in intestinal tract.	Resistant to heat, oxygen, and moisture. Destroyed by alkali and ultraviolet light.	Aids in production of prothrombin, a compound required for normal clotting of blood. Toxic in large amounts.

*M = male; F = female; RE = retinol equivalents; α-TE = alphatocopherol equivalents.

Source: Mahan, Kathleen L., and Arlin, Marian. *Food Nutrition and Diet Therapy.* Philadelphia: W. B. Saunders, Company, 1992, p. 105. Used by permission.

Table 8.5 ✦ Summary of Information on Water-Soluble Vitamins

NAME	RDA FOR ADULTS*	SOURCES	STABILITY	COMMENTS
Thiamin	M: 1.5 mg F: 1.1 mg	Pork, liver, organ meats, legumes, whole-grain and enriched cereals and breads, wheat germ, potatoes. Synthesized in intestinal tract.	Unstable in presence of heat, alkali, or oxygen. Heat stable in acid solution.	As part of cocarboxylase, aids in removal of CO_2 from alpha-keto acids during oxidation of carbohydrates. Essential for growth, normal appetite, digestion, and healthy nerves.
Riboflavin	M: 1.7 mg F: 1.3 mg	Milk and dairy foods, organ meats, green leafy vegetables, enriched cereals and breads, eggs.	Stable to heat, oxygen, and acid. Unstable to light (especially ultraviolet) or alkali.	Essential for growth. Plays enzymatic role in tissue respiration and acts as a transporter of hydrogen ions. Coenzyme forms FMN and FAD.
Niacin (nicotinic acid and nicotinamide)	M: 19 mg NE F: 15 mg NE	Fish, liver, meat, poultry, many grains, eggs, peanuts, milk, legumes, enriched grains. Synthesized by intestinal bacteria.	Stable to heat, light oxidation, acid, and alkali.	As part of enzyme system, aids in transfer of hydrogen and acts in metabolism of carbohydrates and amino acids. Involved in glycolysis, fat synthesis, and tissue respiration.
Vitamin B_6 (pyridoxine, pyridoxal, and pyridoxamine)	M: 2.0 mg F: 1.6 mg	Pork, glandular meats, cereal bran and germ, milk, egg yolk, oatmeal, and legumes. Synthesized by intestinal bacteria.	Stable to heat, light, and oxidation.	As a coenzyme, aids in the synthesis and breakdown of amino acids and in the synthesis of unsaturated fatty acids from essential fatty acids. Essential for conversion of tryptophan to niacin. Essential for normal growth.
Folate	M: 200 μg F: 180 μg	Green leafy vegetables, organ meats (liver), lean beef, wheat, eggs, fish, dry beans, lentils, cowpeas, asparagus, broccoli, collards, yeast. Synthesized in intestinal tract.	Stable to sunlight when in solution; unstable to heat in acid media.	Appears essential for biosynthesis of nucleic acids. Essential for normal maturation of red blood cells. Functions as a coenzyme: tetrahydrofolic acid.
Vitamin B_{12}	2 μg	Liver, kidney, milk and dairy foods, meat, eggs. Vegans require supplement.	Slowly destroyed by acid, alkali, light, and oxidation.	Involved in the metabolism of single-carbon fragments. Essential for biosynthesis of nucleic acids and nucleoproteins. Role in metabolism of nervous tissue. Involved with folate metabolism. Related to growth.
Pantothenic acid	Level not yet determined but 4–7 mg believed safe and adequate.	Present in all plant and animal foods. Eggs, kidney, liver, salmon, and yeast are best sources. Possibly synthesized by intestinal bacteria.	Unstable to acid, alkali, heat, and certain salts.	As part of coenzyme A, functions in the synthesis and breakdown of many vital body compounds. Essential in the intermediary metabolism of carbohydrate, fat, and protein.
Biotin	Not known but 30–100 μg believed safe and adequate.	Liver, mushrooms, peanuts, yeast, milk, meat, egg yolk, most vegetables, banana, grapefruit, tomato, watermelon, and strawberries. Synthesized in intestinal tract.	Stable.	Essential component of enzymes. Involved in synthesis and breakdown of fatty acids and amino acids through aiding the addition and removal of CO_2 to or from active compounds, and the removal of NH_2 from amino acids.
Vitamin C (ascorbic acid)	60 mg	Acerola (West Indian cherry-like fruit), citrus fruit, tomato, melon, peppers, greens, raw cabbage, guava, strawberries, pineapple, potato.	Unstable to heat, alkali, and oxidation, except in acids. Destroyed by storage.	Maintains intracellular cement substance with preservation of capillary integrity. Cosubstrate in hydroxylations requiring molecular oxygen. Important in immune responses, wound healing, and allergic reactions. Increases absorption of nonheme iron.

*M = male; F = female; NE = niacin equivalents

Source: Mahan, Kathleen L. , and Arlin, Marian, *Food Nutrition and Diet Therapy.* Philadelphia: W.B. Saunders, Company, 1992, pp. 105–106. Used by permission.

Table 8.6 ✦ Macronutrients Essential at Levels of 100 mg/day or More

MINERAL	LOCATION IN BODY AND SOME BIOLOGIC FUNCTIONS	RDA* OR ESADDI† FOR ADULTS	FOOD SOURCES	COMMENTS ON LIKELIHOOD OF A DEFICIENCY
Calcium	99% in bones and teeth. Ionic calcium in body fluids essential for ion transport across cell membranes. Calcium is also bound to protein, citrate, or inorganic acids.	800 mg 1200 mg for women 19–24 yr	Milk and milk products, sardines, clams, oysters, kale, turnip greens, mustard greens, tofu.	Dietary surveys indicate that many diets do not meet recommended dietary allowances for calcium. Since bone serves as a homeostatic mechanism to maintain calcium level in blood, many essential functions are maintained, regardless of diet. Long-term dietary deficiency is probably one of the factors responsible for development of osteoporosis in later life.
Phosphorus	About 80% in inorganic portion of bones and teeth. Phosphorus is a component of every cell and of highly important metabolites, including DNA, RNA, ATP (high energy compound), and phospholipids. Important to pH regulation.	800 mg 1200 mg for women 19–24 yr	Cheese, egg yolk, milk, meat, fish, poultry, whole-grain cereals, legumes, nuts.	Dietary inadequacy not likely to occur if protein and calcium intake are adequate.
Magnesium	About 50% in bone. Remaining 50% is almost entirely inside body cells with only about 1% in extracellular fluid. Ionic Mg functions as an activator of many enzymes and thus influences almost all processes.	350 mg for male, 280 mg for female	Whole-grain cereals, tofu, nuts, meat, milk, green vegetables, legumes, chocolate.	Dietary inadequacy considered unlikely, but conditioned deficiency is often seen in clinical medicine, associated with surgery, alcoholism, malabsorption, loss of body fluids, certain hormonal and renal diseases.
Sodium	30 to 45% in bone. Major cation of extracellular fluid and only a small amount is inside cell. Regulates body fluid osmolarity, pH, and body fluid volume.	500–3000 mg	Common table salt, seafoods, animal foods, milk, eggs. Abundant in most foods except fruit.	Dietary inadequacy probably never occurs, although low blood sodium requires treatment in certain clinical disorders. Sodium restriction necessary practice in certain cardiovascular disorders.
Chloride	Major anion of extracellular fluid, functioning in combination with sodium. Serves as a buffer, enzyme activator; component of gastric hydrochloric acid. Mostly present in extracellular fluid; less than 15% inside cells.	750–3000 mg	Common table salt, seafoods, milk, meat, eggs.	In most cases dietary intake has little significance except in the presence of vomiting, diarrhea, or profuse sweating, when a deficiency may develop.
Potassium	Major cation of intracellular fluid, with only small amounts in extracellular fluid. Functions in regulating pH and osmolarity, and cell membrane transfer. Ion is necessary for carbohydrate and protein metabolism.	2000 mg	Fruits, milk, meat, cereals, vegetables, legumes.	Dietary inadequacy unlikely, but conditioned deficiency may be found in kidney disease, diabetic acidosis, excessive vomiting, diarrhea, or sweating. Potassium excess may be a problem in renal failure and severe acidosis.
Sulfur	Most dietary sulfur is present in sulfur-containing amino acids needed for synthesis of essential metabolites. Functions in oxidation-reduction reactions. Also functions in thiamin and biotin, and as inorganic sulfur.	Need for sulfur is satisfied by essential sulfur-containing amino acids.	Protein foods such as meat, fish, poultry, eggs, milk, cheese, legumes, nuts.	Dietary intake is chiefly from sulfur-containing amino acids and adequacy is related to protein intake.

*RDA = recommended dietary allowance.   †ESADDI = estimated safe and adequate daily dietary intake.

Source: Mahan, Kathleen L., and Arlin, Marian. *Food Nutrition and Diet Therapy.* Philadelphia: W.B. Saunders Company, 1992, p. 137. Used by permission.

Table 8.7 ✦ Micronutrients Essential at Levels of a Few mg/day

MINERAL	LOCATION IN BODY AND SOME BIOLOGIC FUNCTIONS	RDA* OR ESADDI† FOR ADULTS	FOOD SOURCES	COMMENTS ON LIKELIHOOD OF A DEFICIENCY
Iron	About 70% is in hemoglobin; about 26% stored in liver, spleen and bone. Iron is a component of hemoglobin and myoglobin, important in oxygen transfer; also present in serum transferrin and certain enzymes. Almost none in ionic form.	10 mg for male, 15 mg for female	Liver, meat, egg yolk, legumes, whole or enriched grains, dark green vegetables, dark molasses, shrimp, oysters.	Iron-deficiency anemia occurs in women in reproductive years and in infants and preschool children. May be associated in some cases with unusual blood loss, parasites, and malabsorption. Anemia is last effect of deficient state.
Zinc	Present in most tissues, with higher amounts in liver, voluntary muscle, and bone. Constituent of many enzymes and insulin; of importance in nucleic acid metabolism.	15 mg for male, 12 mg for female	Oysters, shellfish, herring, liver, legumes, milk, wheat bran.	Extent of dietary inadequacy in this country not known. Conditioned deficiency may be seen in systemic childhood illnesses and in patients who are nutritionally depleted or have been subjected to severe stress, such as surgery.
Copper	Found in all body tissues; larger amounts in liver, brain, heart, and kidney. Constituent of enzymes and of ceruloplasmin and erythrocuprein in blood. May be integral part of DNA or RNA molecule.	1.5–3 mg	Liver, shellfish, whole grains, cherries, legumes, kidney, poultry, oysters, chocolate, nuts.	No evidence that specific deficiencies of copper occur in the human. Menkes' disease is genetic disorder resulting in copper deficiency.
Iodine	Constituent of thyroxine and related compounds synthesized by thyroid gland. Thyroxine functions in control of reactions involving cellular energy.	150 μg	Iodized table salt, seafoods, water and vegetables in nongoitrous regions.	Iodization of table salt is recommended especially in areas where food is low in iodine.
Manganese	Highest concentration is in bone; also relatively high concentrations in pituitary, liver, pancreas, and gastrointestinal tissue. Constituent of essential enzyme systems; rich in mitochondria of liver cells.	2.5–5.0 mg	Beet greens, blueberries, whole grains, nuts, legumes, fruit, tea.	Unlikely that deficiency occurs in humans.
Fluoride	Present in bone and teeth. In optimal amounts in water and diet, reduces dental caries and may minimize bone loss.	1.5–4.0 mg	Drinking water (1 ppm), tea, coffee, rice, soybeans, spinach, gelatin, onions, lettuce.	In areas where fluoride content of water is low, fluoridation of water (1 ppm) has been found beneficial in reducing incidence of dental caries.
Molybdenum	Constituent of an essential enzyme xanthine oxidase and of flavoproteins.	75–250 μg	Legumes, cereal grains, dark green leafy vegetables, organs.	No information.
Cobalt	Constituent of cyanocobalamin (vitamin B_{12}), occurring bound to protein in foods of animal origin. Essential to normal function of all cells, particularly cells of bone marrow, nervous system, and gastrointestinal system.	2.0 μg of vitamin B_{12}	Liver, kidney, oysters, clams, poultry, milk.	Primary dietary inadequacy is rare except when no animal products are consumed. Deficiency may be found in such conditions as lack of gastric intrinsic factor, gastrectomy, and malabsorption syndromes.
Selenium	Associated with fat metabolism, vitamin E, and antioxidant functions.	70 μg— male 55 μg— female	Grains, onions, meats, milk, vegetables variable—depends on selenium content of soil.	Keshan disease is a selenium-deficient state. Deficiency has occurred in patients receiving long-term TPN without selenium.
Chromium	Associated with glucose metabolism.	0.05–0.2 mg	Corn oil, clams, whole-grain cereals, meats, drinking water variable.	Deficiency found in severe malnutrition, may be factor in diabetes in the elderly and cardiovascular disease.
Tin Nickel Vanadium Silicon	Now known to be essential but no RDA or ESADDI established.			

*RDA = recommended dietary allowance. †ESADDI = estimated safe and adequate daily dietary intake.
Source: Mahan, Kathleen L., and Arlin, Marian. *Food Nutrition and Diet Therapy.* Philadelphia: W.B. Saunders Company, 1992, pp. 137–138. Used by permission.

Table 8.8 ✦ Recommended Dietary Allowances for Iron

	AGE (YEARS)	RDA (MG)
Infants	0.0–0.5	6
	0.5–1.0	10
Children	1–3	10
	4–6	10
	7–10	10
Males	11–14	12
	15–18	12
	19–24	10
	25–50	10
	51+	10
Females	11–14	15
	15–18	15
	19–24	15
	25–50	15
	51+	10
	Pregnant	30
	Lactating	
	1st 6 mo	15
	2nd 6 mo	15

Source: Reprinted with permission from *Recommended Dietary Allowances,* 10th ed. Copyright © 1989 by the National Academy of Sciences. Courtesy of the National Academy Press, Washington, DC.

may result in **hypervitaminosis**. The body also has an adequate reserve storage system for key vitamins and minerals (see Table 8.9 on page 162) to prevent health problems. This reserve capacity helps prevent deficiencies when you fail to eat right for a few days or weeks, but it should not be relied on for long periods of time.

With very few exceptions, individuals who experience toxicity problems from overdose of a specific vitamin or mineral are involved in heavy supplementation. It is extremely difficult to produce toxic reactions from food intake alone. See Table 8.10 on page 162 to help decide whether you should consider use of supplementation.

Water

The most critical food component is water. Though it has no nutritional value, water is necessary for energy production, temperature control, and elimination. Although water is present in all foods, experts recommend a minimum of 6 to 8 glasses of it daily, exclusive of other fluids, and 12 to 15 glasses when you are trying to lose weight. For a more detailed discussion of daily water needs, see the section entitled "Special Needs of the Active Individual" later in this chapter.

FOOD DENSITY

You can easily determine whether a food item or meal is nutritionally dense by examining the calorie and nutrient content. A high-density food or meal is one that provides more nutrients than calories or in other words is low in calories and high in the percentage of key vitamins and minerals you need daily. A good cold cereal with skim milk, for example, provides about 190 calories and 20 to 30 percent of practically all vitamins, minerals, carbohydrates, and protein for the day. Since the cold-cereal breakfast contains only 190 calories and about 8 percent of a 120-lb woman's daily energy needs, the meal is said to be nutritionally dense. Fruits, vegetables, and grains are examples of foods that are dense for a given nutrient or group of nutrients. Potato or corn chips and cake are examples of low-density foods that supply a high percentage of your daily calories and a low percentage of key nutrients.

Cold or hot cereal is an excellent way to start the day. Read the labels and choose cereals that contain no sugar, fat, or sodium and at least two grams of protein and three grams of fiber.

DIETARY GUIDELINES FOR GOOD HEALTH

Describing a practical plan for healthy eating is not as easy as it may sound. Complicated tables and elaborate analysis are impractical for most people. Although some recordkeeping is needed, a good system should allow some quick, daily spot checking without time-consuming analysis. A basic understanding of RDAs, the nutrition pyramid, and the dietary recommendations for people in the United States provides such a method.

Recommended Dietary Allowances (RDAs)

Every five years, the Food and Nutritional Board of the National Academy of Sciences' National Research

Hypervitaminosis The toxic side effects that result from the consumption of excess vitamins.

Table 8.9 ✦ Extent of Body Reserves of Nutrients and Nutrient/Health Consequences of Depletion

Nutrient	Approx. time to deplete	Potential Health Implications
Amino acids	3–4 hours	Although you awake each morning with your amino acids depleted, no health consequences occur.
Calcium	2500 days	The majority of the body's calcium storage is in the skeletal system; drawing on this storage supply for long periods of time will adversely affect the bones.
Carbo-hydrates	12–15 hours	Short term depletion causes no problems since the body can switch to protein and fat for energy. Long-term use of protein for energy can cause serious health problems.
Fat	25–50 days	Adipose tissue provides approximately 100,000–150,000 kcal of energy and is the body's greatest reserve source of fuel.
Iron	125 days (women) 750 days (men)	Women possess a smaller reserve capacity due to monthly loss of iron in blood during menstruation.
Sodium	2–3 days	After prolonged sweating without food intake, muscle cramps, heat exhaustion and heat stroke may occur.
Vitamin C	60–120 days	Most excess intake of this water-soluble vitamin is excreted in urine.
Vitamin A	90–360 days	Excess intake of this fat-soluble vitamin is stored in the fat cells.
Water	4–5 days	Death.

Council reviews the recommended dietary allowances (RDAs) of certain essential nutrients that supply the body with the known nutritional needs for maintaining health in people in the United States. The margin of safety is substantial, and it is estimated that two-thirds of the recommended amounts is adequate for most healthy people. Failing to meet the allowances for one day does not mean you have a deficient diet; the RDAs, however, should average out over a five- to eight-day period. Separate RDAs are

Table 8.10 ✦ Situations in Which Vitamin and Mineral Supplements May Be Beneficial

Situation	Supplement type
Oral contraceptive use	Folic acid, vitamin B_6
Pregnancy	Iron, folic acid
Diagnosed deficiency disease (for example, anemias)	As indicated
Vegan diets	B_{12}, vitamin D, zinc, iron
Osteoporosis	Calcium, vitamin D, fluoride
Chronic dieting	Multivitamin and mineral
Use of drugs that interfere with the micronutrients (for example, antihypertensives and antibiotics)	As indicated by type of drug
Diseases that produce malabsorption (for example, cystic fibrosis, celiac disease)	Multivitamin and mineral or as indicated
Inadequate diets due to food allergies, alcoholism, or a narrow selection of food types	Multivitamin and mineral or as indicated by type of deficiency signs

Source: From *The Science of Human Nutrition* by Judith Brown. Copyright © 1990 by Harcourt Brace & Company, reproduced by permission of the publisher.

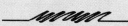

Myth and Fact Sheet

Myth	Fact
1. A candy bar or cola before exercise gives you extra energy.	1. If you eat large amounts of sugar at one time, such as an entire candy bar, the blood releases too much insulin, starting a series of complex chemical reactions. As a result, too much glucose is removed from the blood and stored in the fat cells and liver. This process can leave you with less energy than you would have had without eating the candy bar or drinking an entire can of cola. Sugar also draws fluid from other body parts into the gastrointestinal tract and may contribute to dehydration, distention of the stomach, cramps, nausea, and diarrhea. To avoid these problems, dilute concentrated fruit juices with twice the recommended water, add an equal volume of water to commercial drinks, and eat only small quantities of sugar. Sugar is absorbed faster than the muscles can use it, thus, frequent small amounts are preferable to single doses. Your blood-glucose level will reach a peak about half an hour after consumption, and then rapidly decline. Eating large quantities of sugar causes more rapid decline and greater shortage of glucose for energy.
2. Honey provides quick energy for exercise.	2. For years, honey has been used before, during, and after exercise for quick energy and rapid recovery. Since 40 percent of the sugar in honey is fructose, which is rapidly converted to glycogen, it has been stated that honey will quickly restore glycogen reserves. Unfortunately, there is no evidence to support this theory. There are no quick-energy foods, and honey has the same limitations and advantages of any sugar.
3. Starchy foods are fattening and should be avoided.	3. Starch is the main energy source of complex carbohydrates. Their reputation as fattening is due to the fact that they are normally eaten with fat, such as butter on bread and sour cream on potatoes.
4. Gelatin improves physical fitness.	4. Plain, dry gelatin added to water is almost pure protein. The dessert-type gelatin contains about 4 g of protein and 34 g of carbohydrate. Athletes consider gelatin a good source of protein and a precursor for the formation of phosphocreatine, which helps provide anaerobic energy. The theory advanced is that gelatin may help form phosphocreatine in the muscle. Findings of recent researchers indicate no beneficial effect on performance or on fitness.
5. Wheat germ oil (vitamin E) improves fitness.	5. Recent research suggests that vitamin E may help prevent early heart disease. There is no evidence to support any claims for improved fitness levels.
6. Alcohol keeps you warm and improves performance.	6. The initial increase in warmth comes from dilation of blood vessels near the skin. Actually, after you consume alcoholic drinks, heat loss increases, and you are more susceptible to chilling.
7. Milk cuts your wind and brings on early fatigue.	7. Drinking milk or putting it on cereal does not result in early fatigue or loss of fitness. Skim milk with no fat is still a sound, high-density, nutritional choice.
8. Exercise, particularly swimming, should be avoided following a meal.	8. People have avoided exercise after eating for years, believing that it hindered digestion, brought on stomach cramps, and contributed to drowning. Exercise does slow acid secretion and the movement of food from the stomach during activity and for about an hour later. After this time, there is actually increased digestive action. In the final analysis, over a 12- to 18-hour period, exercise has little effect on the speed of digestion. Performance could be hindered, although that is unlikely, because of the discomfort of overeating or a feeling of lethargy. Stomach cramps while you are swimming are highly unlikely, even if you swim immediately after eating. It may be wise to wait about 45 minutes if you are a beginning swimmer and are tense about the water.

Figure 8.2 ✦ USDA's Food Guide Pyramid. A guide to daily food choices, food groups, and number of servings to consume of each.

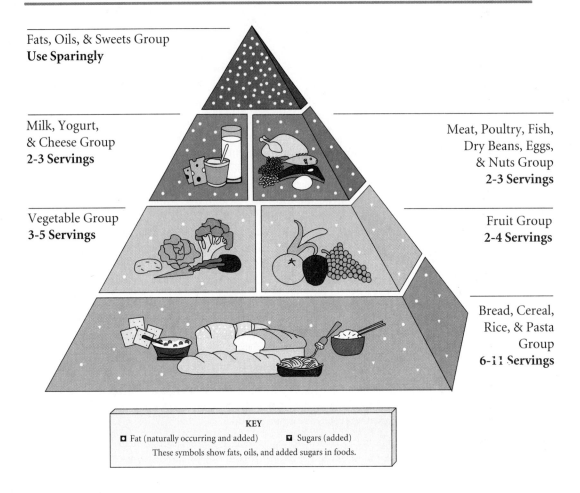

Fats, Oils, & Sweets Group
Use Sparingly

Milk, Yogurt,
& Cheese Group
2-3 Servings

Meat, Poultry, Fish,
Dry Beans, Eggs,
& Nuts Group
2-3 Servings

Vegetable Group
3-5 Servings

Fruit Group
2-4 Servings

Bread, Cereal,
Rice, & Pasta
Group
6-11 Servings

KEY
▫ Fat (naturally occurring and added)   ◼ Sugars (added)
These symbols show fats, oils, and added sugars in foods.

provided for infants, children, males, females, and pregnant and lactating women.

The most recent RDAs are shown in Table 8.11. Unless computer software and/or elaborate record-keeping is used, the RDA does not provide a practical means of evaluating your daily nutrition. A much easier approach involves the use of the nutrition pyramid and general dietary recommendations.

The Nutrition Pyramid

After decades of use, the basic four food group plan was recently discarded in favor of the **nutrition pyra-**

Nutrition pyramid New dietary guidelines emphasizing fruits, vegetables, and grains and deemphasizing meats, dairy products, sweets, fats, and oils.

mid shown in Figure 8.2. The pyramid contains five food groups and emphasizes complex carbohydrates (fruits, vegetables, and grains). The small space at the top of the pyramid, not a sixth food group, singles out fats, oils, and sweets as items that should be used sparingly or not at all. Neither the meat nor the dairy industry are happy with their tiny spaces on the pyramid although the number of servings represent the daily needs of most people in the United States. Variety, moderation, and balance, the three key elements of sound nutrition, are met by consuming the recommended number of servings from the five food groups over a five- to seven-day period. Recommended serving sizes are relatively small. A sandwich with two pieces of bread, for example, provides two servings of grains; one egg, two to three ounces of meat, or a small piece of fresh fruit is one serving. Those who follow the nutritional pyramid will consume less total fat, saturated fat, cholesterol, sugar, salt, and calories and more fruits, vegetables, grains, and dietary fiber.

Table 8.11 ✦ Recommended Dietary Allowances [a]

Category	Age (years) or Condition	Weight[b] (kg)	Weight[b] (lb)	Height[b] (cm)	Height[b] (in)	Protein (g)	A (μg RE)[c]	D (μg)[d]	E (mg α-TE)[e]	K (μg)	C (mg)	Thiamin (mg)	Riboflavin (mg)	Niacin (mg NE)[f]	B6 (mg)	Folate (μg)	B12 (μg)	Calcium (mg)	Phosphorus (mg)	Magnesium (mg)	Iron (mg)	Zinc (mg)	Iodine (μg)	Selenium (μg)
Infants	0.0–0.5	6	13	60	24	13	375	7.5	3	5	30	0.3	0.4	5	0.3	25	0.3	400	300	40	6	5	40	10
	0.5–1.0	9	20	71	28	14	375	10	4	10	35	0.4	0.5	6	0.6	35	0.5	600	500	60	10	5	50	15
Children	1–3	13	29	90	35	16	400	10	6	15	40	0.7	0.8	9	1.0	50	0.7	800	800	80	10	10	70	20
	4–6	20	44	112	44	24	500	10	7	20	45	0.9	1.1	12	1.1	75	1.0	800	800	120	10	10	90	20
	7–10	28	62	132	52	28	700	10	7	30	45	1.0	1.2	13	1.4	100	1.4	800	800	170	10	10	120	30
Males	11–14	45	99	157	62	45	1000	10	10	45	50	1.3	1.5	17	1.7	150	2.0	1200	1200	270	12	15	150	40
	15–18	66	145	176	69	59	1000	10	10	65	60	1.5	1.8	20	2.0	200	2.0	1200	1200	400	12	15	150	50
	19–24	72	160	177	70	58	1000	10	10	70	60	1.5	1.7	19	2.0	200	2.0	1200	1200	350	10	15	150	70
	25–50	79	174	176	70	63	1000	5	10	80	60	1.5	1.7	19	2.0	200	2.0	800	800	350	10	15	150	70
	51+	77	170	173	68	63	1000	5	10	80	60	1.2	1.4	15	2.0	200	2.0	800	800	350	10	15	150	70
Females	11–14	46	101	157	62	46	800	10	8	45	50	1.1	1.3	15	1.4	150	2.0	1200	1200	280	15	12	150	45
	15–18	55	120	163	64	44	800	10	8	55	60	1.1	1.3	15	1.5	180	2.0	1200	1200	300	15	12	150	50
	19–24	58	128	164	65	46	800	10	8	60	60	1.1	1.3	15	1.6	180	2.0	1200	1200	280	15	12	150	55
	25–50	63	138	163	64	50	800	5	8	65	60	1.1	1.3	15	1.6	180	2.0	800	800	280	15	12	150	55
	51+	65	143	160	63	50	800	5	8	65	60	1.0	1.2	13	1.6	180	2.0	800	800	280	10	12	150	55
Pregnant						60	800	10	10	65	70	1.5	1.6	17	2.2	400	2.2	1200	1200	320	30	15	175	65
Lactating	1st 6 Months					65	1300	10	12	65	95	1.6	1.8	20	2.1	280	2.6	1200	1200	355	15	19	200	75
	2nd 6 Months					62	1200	10	11	65	90	1.6	1.7	20	2.1	260	2.6	1200	1200	340	15	16	200	75

[a]The allowances, expressed as average daily intakes over time, are intended to provide for individual variations among most normal persons as they live in the United States under usual environmental stresses. Diets should be based on a variety of common foods in order to provide other nutrients for which human requirements have been less well defined. See the RDA publication for detailed discussion of allowances and of nutrients not tabulated.

[b]Weights and heights of Reference Adults are actual medians for the U.S. population of the designated age, as reported by NHANES II. The use of these figures does not imply that the height-to-weight ratios are ideal.

[c]Retinol equivalents. 1 retinol equivalent = 1 μg retinol or 6 μg β-carotene.

[d]As cholecalciferol, 10 μg cholecalciferol = 400 IU of vitamin D.

[e]α-Tocopherol equivalents. 1 mg d-α tocopherol = 1 α-TE.

[f]1 NE (niacin equivalent) is equal to 1 mg of niacin or 60 mg of dietary tryptophan.

Source: Food and Nutrition Board, National Research Council Recommended Dietary Allowances, Revised 1989, 10th Edition. Washington, DC: National Academy of Sciences.

Fitness Heroes 〰〰〰

Bob Gold is a nationally renowned health educator who should have known better. In spite of the research he conducted, the books he wrote, and the courses he taught, Bob ignored his own advice. He spent approximately 35 years being extremely overweight, inactive, and a workaholic. When he was younger, he even smoked cigarettes. Bob also had a family history of heart disease. When Bob experienced chest pains at age 35, no one was surprised. The diagnosis was three clogged coronary arteries, and the treatment soon began.

Over several years, Bob ingested nitroglycerine tablets to dilate his arteries, underwent angioplasty, and had open-heart surgery. His excessive weight also caused his congenitally deformed hip to need replacement.

Finally, Bob decided that he wanted to see his children grow up. He needed to completely change his lifestyle. He sought referral to diet and exercise programs and began exercising at least four days a week. While he still works long hours, he takes breaks for exercise and socializing. He is now down to his recommended weight, his body fat was recently measured at 8 percent, and he is leading a healthy life. Bob is a true fitness hero, demonstrating that fitness is within everyone's grasp. ✦

Dietary Guidelines

The U.S. Department of Agriculture and the U.S. Department of Health and Human Services have listed seven dietary guidelines that have implications for good health:

1. Eat a variety of foods.
2. Maintain ideal weight.
3. Avoid too much fat, especially saturated fat, and cholesterol.
4. Eat foods with adequate starch and fiber.
5. Avoid too much sugar.
6. Avoid too much sodium.
7. If you drink alcohol, do so in moderation.

An awareness of these guidelines is also helpful for daily nutritious eating.

Table 8.12 compares the current U.S. dietary intake of food and drink with the proposed dietary goals or recommendations. In most areas, our current dietary intake in percent of daily calories fails to meet the proposed goals. There is too much total fat in our total daily calories (42 percent instead of 30 percent), saturated fat (16 percent instead of 10 percent), and concentrated sugar (25 percent instead of 10 percent) and too little total carbohydrates (46 percent instead of 58 percent) and complex carbohydrates (22 percent instead of 48 percent). In addition, we consume too much cholesterol (500 to 1000 mg instead of less than 300 mg), salt (6 to 19 g instead of 4 g), and alcohol; too many carbonated drinks; too much coffee and tea; too many total calories; and not enough water. It is obvious that our eating habits are much more influenced by taste than they are by concern for our own health. To compare your nutritional practices to the standards in Table 8.12 complete Lab Activity 8.2: Do You Meet the U.S. Government Dietary Recommendations? at the end of the chapter.

Food Labeling

The Food and Drug Administration (FDA) is responsible for food labeling, excluding meat, poultry, and alcoholic beverages, in the United States, while the Federal Trade Commission (FTC) regulates the advertising of food products and takes action, through the FDA, against unsubstantiated food claims. Although fresh fruits, vegetables, and meats were not subject to labeling requirements in the past, most of them now contain labels. Foods with a *standard of identity,* those that filed a specific recipe with the FDA, were also once exempt from listing ingredients unless special items, such as extra spices and flavors, were added. Catsup, ice cream, mustard, and mayonnaise all fell into this category. Before 1994, over 60 percent of all food and beverages sold in the United States contained a nutrition label; about one-half of these were voluntarily provided by manufacturers.

The new law that went into effect in May, 1994 requires the large majority of food products to be labeled and to follow strict guidelines (see Figure 8.3 on page 168). New food labels, previously called the U.S. RDAs, are now called **recommended daily intakes (RDIs)**. With the new labels, the daily recommended values (DRVs) have been determined by the FDA for parts of the diet not covered by the 1989 RDA labels, such as carbohydrates, fats, and dietary fiber.

Table 8.12 ✦ Summary of Dietary Recommendations to the American Public

	CURRENT DIETARY INTAKE	PROPOSED DIETARY GOALS
Calories	Excess calories are consumed by the average person	Per lb. weight: Active: 17; moderately active: 12–13; sedentary: 10–11
Carbohydrate	46% of daily calories	58% of daily calories
Simple	24%	10%
Concentrated sugar, sugar in fruits, vegetables, and grains		5% 5%
Complex fruits, vegetables, and grains	22%	48%
Protein	12% of daily calories	12%
Total Fat	42%	30%
Saturated	16%	10%
Monounsaturated	13%	10%
Polyunsaturated	13%	10%
Cholesterol	500–1000 milligrams	less than 300 mg
Salt*	6–18 grams	less than 4 grams (1100–3300 mg)
Dietary Fiber	11 grams	25–35 g
Fluid		
Water	2–3 glasses†	6–8 glasses, 10–12 if on any type of diet
Alcohol	—	Less than 10% of daily calories, 1–2 drinks
Carbonated Drinks	—	No more than 1–2 daily
Coffee or Tea	—	No more than 1–2 daily

*Salt substitutes that contain potassium chloride may not be wise choices. Some evidence indicates that it is the chloride in salt (sodium chloride), not the sodium, that is associated with high blood pressure in some individuals. Salt substitutes containing potassium also contain chloride.

†Results of four-year survey of students at Virginia Commonwealth University, 1986–1990.

Source: Greenberg, Jerry, and Dintiman, George B. *Exploring Health: Expanding the Boundaries of Wellness.* Englewood Cliffs, NJ: Prentice-Hall, 1992, p. 176.

The major general and specific changes are:

General

- Practically all products must contain a label.

- Specific listings on the label concerning health claims must be accurate and must keep pace with changing health concerns in the United States.

- Names of nutrient allowances have been changed to percent of *daily value* (DV). RDIs and DRVs are used as reference values to show how the nutrients contribute toward a sound diet.

> **Recommended daily intakes (RDIs)** The levels of intake of essential nutrients considered adequate to meet the known nutritional needs of healthy persons in the United States.

Figure 8.3 ✦ The Nutrition Label

Serving Size

Is your serving the same size as the one on the label? If you eat double the serving size listed, you need to double the nutrient and calorie values. If you eat one-half the serving size shown here, cut the nutrient and calorie values in half.

Calories

Are you overweight? Cut back a little on calories! Look here to see how a serving of the food adds to your daily total. A 5'4", 138-lb. active woman needs about 2,200 calories each day. A 5'10", 174-lb. active man needs about 2,900. How about you?

Total Carbohydrate

When you cut down on fat, you can eat more carbohydrates. Carbohydrates are in foods like bread, potatoes, fruits and vegetables. Choose these often! They give you more nutrients than **sugars** like soda pop and candy.

Dietary Fiber

Grandmother called it "roughage," but her advice to eat more is still up-to-date! That goes for both soluble and insoluble kinds of dietary fiber. Fruits, vegetables, whole-grain foods, beans and peas are all good sources and can help reduce the risk of heart disease and cancer.

Protein

Most Americans get more protein than they need. Where there is animal protein, there is also fat and cholesterol. Eat small servings of lean meat, fish and poultry. Use skim or low-fat milk, yogurt, and cheese. Try vegetable proteins like beans, grains and cereals.

Vitamins & Minerals

Your goal here is 100% of each for the day. Don't count on one food to do it all. Let a combination of foods add up to a winning score.

Nutrition Facts

Serving Size 1/2 cup (114g)
Servings Per Container 4

Amount Per Serving

Calories 90   Calories from Fat 30

	% Daily value*
Total Fat 3g	**5%**
Saturated Fat 0g	**0%**
Cholesterol 0mg	**0%**
Sodium 300mg	**13%**
Total Carbohydrate 13g	**4%**
Dietary Fiber 3g	**12%**
Sugars 3g	
Protein 3g	

Vitamin A 80%	•	Vitamin C 60%
Calcium 4%	•	Iron 4%

* Percent Daily Values are based on a 2,000 calorie diet. Your daily values may be higher or lower depending on your calorie needs:

		Calories	2,000	2,500
Total Fat	Less than		65g	80g
Sat Fat	Less than		20g	25g
Cholesterol	Less than		300mg	300mg
Sodium	Less than		2,400mg	2,400mg
Total Carbohydrate			300g	375g
Fiber			25g	30g

Calories per gram:
Fat 9 • Carbohydrate 4 • Protein 4

More nutrients may be listed on some labels.

Total Fat

Aim low: Most people need to cut back on fat! Too much fat may contribute to heart disease and cancer. Try to limit your **calories from fat.** For a healthy heart, choose foods with a big difference between the total number of calories and the number of calories from fat.

Saturated Fat

A new kind of fat? No – saturated fat is part of the total fat in food. It is listed separately because it's the key player in raising blood cholesterol and your risk of heart disease. Eat less!

Cholesterol

Too much cholesterol – a second cousin to fat – can lead to heart disease. Challenge yourself to eat less than 300 mg each day.

Sodium

You call it "salt," the label calls it "sodium." Either way, it may add up to high blood pressure in some people. So, keep your sodium intake low – 2,400 to 3,000 mg or less each day.*

*The AHA recommends no more than 3,000 mg sodium per day for healthy adults

Daily Value

Feel like you're drowning in numbers ? Let the Daily Value be your guide. Daily Values are listed for people who eat 2,000 or 2,500 calories each day. If you eat more, your personal daily value may be higher than what's listed on the label. If you eat less, your personal daily value may be lower.

For fat, saturated fat, cholesterol and sodium choose foods with a low % **Daily Value**. For total carbohydrate, dietary fiber, vitamins and minerals, your daily value goal is to reach 100% of each.

g = grams (About 28 g = 1 ounce)
mg = milligrams (1,000 mg = 1 g)

Key Words: *Fat Free:* Less than 0.6 g of fat per serving; *Low Fat:* 3g of fat or less per serving; *Lean:* Less than 10 g of fat, 4 g of saturated fat and 96 mg. of cholesterol per serving; *Light (Lite):* 1/2 less calories or no more than 1/2 the fat of the higher-calorie, higher-fat version; or no more than 1/2 the sodium of the higher-sodium version; *Cholesterol Free:* Less than 2 mg. of cholesterol and 2g or less of saturated fat per serving. **To Make Health Claims About...The Food Must be...**Heart Disease and Fats: Low in fat, saturated fat and cholesterol; Blood Pressure and Sodium: Low in sodium; Heart Disease and Fruits, Vegetables, and Grain Products: A fruit, vegetable, or grain product low in fat, saturated fat and cholesterol, that contains at least 0.6 g soluble fiber, without fortification, per serving.

Source: Food and Drug Administration, American Heart Association, 1993.

- A *dictionary of terms* with consistent and uniform definitions has been developed for terms such as *free, low, high, source of, light, reduced, less, more, fat free, low fat, no cholesterol,* and *high fiber.*

- Definitions must be specific for fatty acid and cholesterol content.

Specific

- Cholesterol content

- Saturated fat content

- Total dietary fiber

- Total calories from fat, saturated fat, complex carbohydrates, and sugars

- Polyunsaturated and monounsaturated fats and water-soluble and -insoluble fibers are required if a health claim is made for the product.

- Thiamin, niacin, riboflavin, and other nutrients are optional in listings since the concern about deficiencies is no longer valid.

Nutrition labeling reform was long overdue to eliminate misleading and false advertising by manufacturers who seemed to change their lines only when the majority of people in the United States became aware of a specific nutritional practice. Public knowledge of the hazards of dietary cholesterol and sodium prompted such changes. Unfortunately, manufacturers produce and advertise as low-cholesterol products, foods that actually contain saturated fat, which is known to elevate blood cholesterol levels. That practice and numerous other attempts at deception that have been used should be eliminated by the new labeling regulations. False claims, such as "95 percent fat-free" and "2 percent fat," which referred to the weight of the fat content and not the percent of total calories from fat, will also be eliminated.

Table 8.13 ✦ Nutrition Risk Factors Associated with the Development of Diseases and Disorders

DISEASE OR DISORDER	NUTRITION RISK FACTORS
Heart disease and atherosclerosis ("hardening of the arteries")	Diets high in animal fat and cholesterol; obesity
Cancer*	Diets high in fat and low in vitamin A, beta-carotene, dietary fiber, and certain types of vegetables
Diabetes (in adults)	Obesity
Cirrhosis of the liver	Excessive alcohol consumption, malnutrition
Infertility	Underweight, obesity, zinc deficiency (in men)
Health problems of pregnant women and newborns	Maternal underweight, obesity, malnutrition, and excessive use of vitamin and mineral supplements or alcohol
Growth retardation in children	Diets low in calories, protein, iron, zinc
Tooth decay	Frequent consumption of sweets, diets low in fluoride
Iron-deficiency anemia	Diets low in iron
Constipation	Diets low in fiber and fluids
Obesity	Excessive calorie intake
Underweight	Deficient calorie intake
Hypertension	Diets high in sodium, excessive alcohol consumption, obesity
Osteoporosis	Diets low in calcium and vitamin D

*The development of most types of cancer, notably excluding leukemia, have been associated with nutrition risk factors.

Source: From *The Science of Human Nutrition* by Judith E. Brown, copyright © 1990 by Harcourt Brace & Company, reproduced by permission of the publisher.

Reform is of little value, however, unless people develop the habit of reading food labels before making selections. The dietary guidelines discussed in the previous section will help focus on the key aspects for making quick decisions about products. For many products, it is only necessary to look for a reasonable portion size; the number of calories; and zero grams of fat, cholesterol, salt, sodium, and sugar. Since it is difficult to avoid these health-related ingredients, which also occur naturally in some food, it is wise to purchase processed foods (any food item that is packaged) with these ingredients absent or in very low quantity.

NUTRITION-DISEASE RELATIONSHIPS

Scientific evidence associating diet with numerous diseases has increased in the past decade. Although cause-and-effect relationships are still rather uncommon, dietary risk factors have been identified for a number of diseases and disorders (see Table 8.13), and the consumption of various nutrients has been associated with the prevention of some diseases.

High-fat diets have been linked to cardiorespiratory disease and cancer; high sodium and alcohol intake to a small percentage of the hypertense population; and high-calorie intake and obesity to high blood pressure, diabetes, cardiorespiratory disease, and cancer. On the other hand, diets high in complex carbohydrates (fruits, vegetables, and grains) that contain vitamin A, beta-carotene, dietary fiber, and cruciferous vegetables have been tied to the prevention of cancer (colon, stomach, and so forth), diverticulitis, and constipation; and low-fat diets with the prevention of cardiorespiratory disease and certain types of cancer. The prevention of osteoporosis is associated with adequate intake of calcium, vitamin D, and fluoride; weight-bearing exercise; and hormone therapy (see chapter 14). There have been numerous other dietary connections made with disease prevention.

Consumers must resist the temptation, however, to consume very large amounts of a nutrient identified as having the potential for disease prevention until supportive evidence is found.

SPECIAL NEEDS OF THE ACTIVE INDIVIDUAL

Active individuals who follow the nutritional plan already presented in this chapter have a few special nutritional needs. There are only four other areas of concern for those who exercise three to seven times weekly:

1. Eating enough calories for energy and body repair in order to benefit fully from the conditioning program.

2. Eating a sufficient amount of carbohydrates and fats to spare the body from burning protein.

3. Drinking sufficient fluid to prevent dehydration, heat-related illness, and early fatigue.

4. Replacing electrolytes (potassium, sodium, and chloride) lost in perspiration.

5. Considering the use of iron supplements (for women).

Eating Enough Calories

If you are neither losing nor gaining weight, you are taking in the correct number of calories daily to maintain your present weight and fat level. Weigh yourself at exactly the same time of day and under the same conditions, preferably in the morning on rising. If no weight gain or loss is occurring, there is no real need for complicated recordkeeping of caloric intake and expenditure, unless you wish to lose or gain weight.

You can estimate the number of calories you need from Table 8.14. Multiply your body weight times the calories recommended per pound for your activity level. This is only an estimate of your needs. Your body has an infallible computer that accurately registers your caloric intake daily; the output is body-weight changes.

Your source of calories is also an important factor in providing sufficient energy for exercise. The percent of calories from carbohydrates, fats, and protein, shown in Table 8.12 is sufficient for most exercising individuals. Increasing your complex carbohydrate (fruits, vegetables, and grains) intake from 48

Table 8.14 ✦ Approximate Number of Calories Needed Daily Per Pound of Body Weight

AGE RANGES	7–10	11–14	15–22	23–35	36–50	51–75
Males						
Very Active	21–22	23–24	25–27	23–24	21–22	19–20
Moderately Active	16–17	18–19	20–23	18–29	16–17	11–15
Sedentary	11–12	13–14	15–18	13–14	11–12	10–11
Females						
Very Active	21–22	22–23	20–21	20–21	18–19	17–18
Moderately Active	16–17	18–19	16–18	16–17	14–15	12–13
Sedentary	11–12	13–14	11–12	11–12	9–10	8–9

Sedentary—No physical activity beyond attending classes and desk work.

Moderately Active—Involved in a regular exercise program at least three times weekly.

Very Active—Involved in a regular aerobic exercise program 4–6 times weekly, expending more than 2,500 calories per week during physical activity.

percent to 60 percent of total calories will increase your energy level. Total fat intake should be decreased by 10 to 12 percent.

Protein Sparing

Eating sufficient fruits, vegetables, and grains is extremely critical for the exercising individual. When the body does not have adequate carbohydrate available for energy, it will convert dietary protein and lean protein mass (muscle) to glucose to supply the nervous system. When this occurs, loss of lean muscle tissue takes place throughout the body, including major organs such as the heart. Failing to spare protein for long periods of time can seriously jeopardize health and is suspected of having caused death from heart-rhythm disturbances in some dieters. A high percentage of complex carbohydrates in your diet will spare protein, provide a high level of energy, and protect your health.

Carbohydrate Loading or Supercompensation

The body has an adequate supply of energy available in the form of glucose and glycogen for performing regular exercise or competing in a sport. Glucose (sugar in the blood available for energy) and glycogen (the chief storage form of carbohydrate) are available in the blood, muscles, and liver and provide sufficient energy for most anaerobic workouts.

Individuals who compete in marathons, triathlons, and other endurance contests lasting several hours need additional energy and can benefit from a technique called **carbohydrate loading**, or **supercompensation**. New evidence indicates that the depletion stage may be unnecessary. By merely increasing carbohydrate intake three to four days before an important exercise activity or competition, liver and muscle glycogen stores will more than double. Such an increase provides approximately 3060 calories of energy—enough for practically any endurance event. Two large, high-carbohydrate meals (300 g, 1200 cal-

Carbohydrate loading (supercompensation) An attempt to reduce carbohydrate intake to near zero for two to three days (depletion stage) before resorting to a high-carbohydrate diet for three to four days (loading phase) to raise glycogen stores in skeletal muscle and the liver to increase energy levels on the day of competition.

Diversity Issues

Dietary Patterns

Dietary patterns vary considerably from one country to another and among various ethnic and religious groups in the United States. In some countries, low protein intake and malnutrition result in numerous diseases and restricted growth and development. In other countries, the high intake of fruits, vegetables, and grains coupled with a low meat, dairy, and egg consumption provides a healthy advantage to residents.

Unfortunately, individuals who immigrate to the United States sometimes have difficulty finding their native foods and continuing their native customs and they eventually get caught up in the typical U.S. diet: high-fat, high-sugar, and high-calorie. Vegetarian immigrants from India, for example, may have trouble finding foods in U.S. supermarkets that meet their dietary needs for protein, because many of the grains, rice, and beans they are used to eating can be difficult to find here. Asian immigrants, too, might find it difficult to adjust if they do not live close to a specialty Asian market. While native foods can be difficult to find, they can also be expensive.

There is a need in many communities to assist foreign services to provide education and guidance in this critical area of nutrition. Those who are interested might contact some of the community agencies or churches that assist with resettlement of immigrants to the United States. These agencies are interested in expertise in other languages and knowledge of nutrition in order to provide key information to immigrants. By learning where to purchase some of their native foods and how to substitute domestic items to ensure sound nutrition, immigrants could improve their general health and incorporate their cultural customs into their new American way of life. ◆

ories per meal) are recommended daily for three or four days.

Replacing Fluids (Water)

Water needs depend on the individual and on factors such as body weight, activity patterns, sweat loss,

Behavioral Change and Motivational Strategies

People in the 1990s are more educated about nutrition than previous generations have been. Unfortunately, knowledge about proper nutrition does not readily translate into sound eating behavior. Busy schedules, lack of money, fad diet and nutrition information, easy access to fast-food restaurants, youthful feelings of indestructibility, culture and religion, and many other factors help explain why, in spite of this knowledge, the typical diet of people in the United States is too high in saturated fat, cholesterol, total fat, calories, sodium, and sugar and too low in complex carbohydrates (fruits, vegetables, and grains) and water. These problems are very much related to present and future health, behavior, mood, and energy level. With only minimum effort, some of these problems can be corrected.

Roadblock	Behavioral Change Strategy
Some people just do not seem to like water and therefore consume less than three of the recommended six to eight glasses daily. Most liquid consumed is coffee, tea, or high-calorie (150 cal per 12-oz serving) soft drinks, juices, milk, beer, and other alcoholic drinks. Avoiding water allows more room for calories and salt, sugar, and fat.	You can change your liquid consumption patterns slowly and reacquire your taste for water. For a seven-day period, try: 1. Placing your favorite glass in the bathroom and drinking one full glass of water immediately on rising in the morning and just before bedtime. You are now already drinking more water than most people do. 2. Not passing a water fountain, even if you are not thirsty. Take at least five swallows (about three oz). 3. Placing a cold pitcher of water in the front of your refrigerator so it is the first thing you see. 4. Drinking at least one glass of water with each meal.
So much of what we eat is processed food, which is typically high in sodium. There seems to be no way of avoiding the problem.	Although high sodium intake may not be as much of a health hazard as originally suspected, it is a good idea to cut back. About one-third of the salt you consume comes from processed food, one-third from table salt, and the rest occurs naturally in food. There are a number of things you can do: 1. Restrict your visit to fast-food restaurants to no more than once a month. 2. Avoid or use very little table salt, substituting herbs and spices such as lemon and orange. Use a salt substitute that does not contain sodium potassium. Plan on three or four weeks to become adjusted to not adding table salt to your food. 3. Read food labels and purchase products with no or low salt. 4. Avoid luncheon meats, smoked meats, hot dogs, sausage, and high-salt cheeses.
Although you are aware of the association between high total fat, high saturated fat, high-cholesterol diets, and heart disease, it is just too difficult to avoid high fat in the diet.	It does seem that way, particularly if you eat on the run and do not have time to plan meals. There are some specific things you can do that are certain to reduce the percent of calories you consume from fat daily: 1. Take the time to glance at the label of every product you purchase. If it does not say it has zero grams of fat, do not buy it. 2. If you eat ice cream, purchase one of the brands that use artificial fat; the taste is excellent and the product is nearly fat- and cholesterol-free. 3. Pack a lunch every day consisting of fruit, vegetables, and a low-calorie sandwich. This will keep you from skipping a meal or running to a fast-food restaurant during the day.

Roadblock	Behavioral Change Strategy
	4. Reduce your intake of invisible fat by reducing your consumption of chocolate, eggs, red meat, poultry skin, and dairy products.
	5. Cut the skin off the raw poultry before cooking, avoid frying, and choose cooking methods that do not require the use of oils.
	6. Use paper towels to soak up the fat when you cook hamburger and other meats.
List some roadblocks that interfere with your following sound nutritional practices.	Now, cite behavior-change strategies that can help you overcome the roadblocks you just listed. If you need to, refer back to chapter 3 for behavior change and motivational strategies.
1. _____	1. _____
2. _____	2. _____
3. _____	3. _____

loss through expired air and urine, and the amount of liquid consumed through other foods and drinks (see Figure 8.4 on page 174).

The active individual needs a minimum of six to eight glasses (1.5 to 2 quarts) of water daily—much more in hot, humid weather. It is not unusual to lose one to two liters of water per hour when exercising in extremely hot, humid weather. Drinking too much water generally poses no problem; water is rarely toxic, and the kidneys merely excrete it efficiently. The kidneys are also capable of conserving water when the body is deprived by excreting more highly concentrated urine. If the color of your urine is darker than a manila folder, you need to consume additional water (not fluid from other drinks). Surveys by the authors of Virginia Commonwealth University undergraduate students suggest that the college-aged generation is becoming a waterless society as soft drinks, coffee, tea, cocoa, beer, wine coolers, and juices dominate palates. The average daily intake of water, as shown in a June 1990 survey by the authors, was slightly less than two glasses. These findings were almost identical to the results of a similar survey conducted by the authors in 1980. More soda, coffee, tea, and beer were consumed than water. It bears stating again that the body needs plain water for heat regulation and proper functioning of systems.

If you exercise in hot, humid weather, thirst sensations will underestimate your needs. By the time you are thirsty, a water deficit has been created that cannot be undone for several hours. Forced drinking (hydrating), even when no thirst sensation exists, will minimize water deficit, keep body temperature one or two degrees lower in hot weather, result in more efficient performance, and delay fatigue. The most beneficial approach is to force down an extra 16 to 32 ounces of water less than 15 minutes before you begin to exercise. Earlier consumption may fill the bladder and make you uncomfortable during the activity.

Water will not interfere with your performance; drink it freely before, during, and after your workout. It is the single most important substance in preventing heat-related illnesses and in restoring the body to normal following exercise in hot, humid weather. For the quickest absorption of fluid, drink plain water chilled to about 40 degrees Fahrenheit. (For additional discussion on water and its role in preventing heat exhaustion, muscle cramps, and heat stroke, see chapter 12.)

Maintaining Electrolyte Balance

Electrolytes lost through sweat and water vapor from the lungs must be replaced. It is the proper balance of each electrolyte that prevents dehydration, cramping, heat exhaustion, and heat stroke. Too much salt without adequate water, for example, actu-

Electrolytes Chemical compounds (water, sodium, potassium, and chloride) in solution in the human body capable of producing electric current; important in the prevention of cramps, heat exhaustion, and heat stroke.

Figure 8.4 ✦ Water Intake and Loss

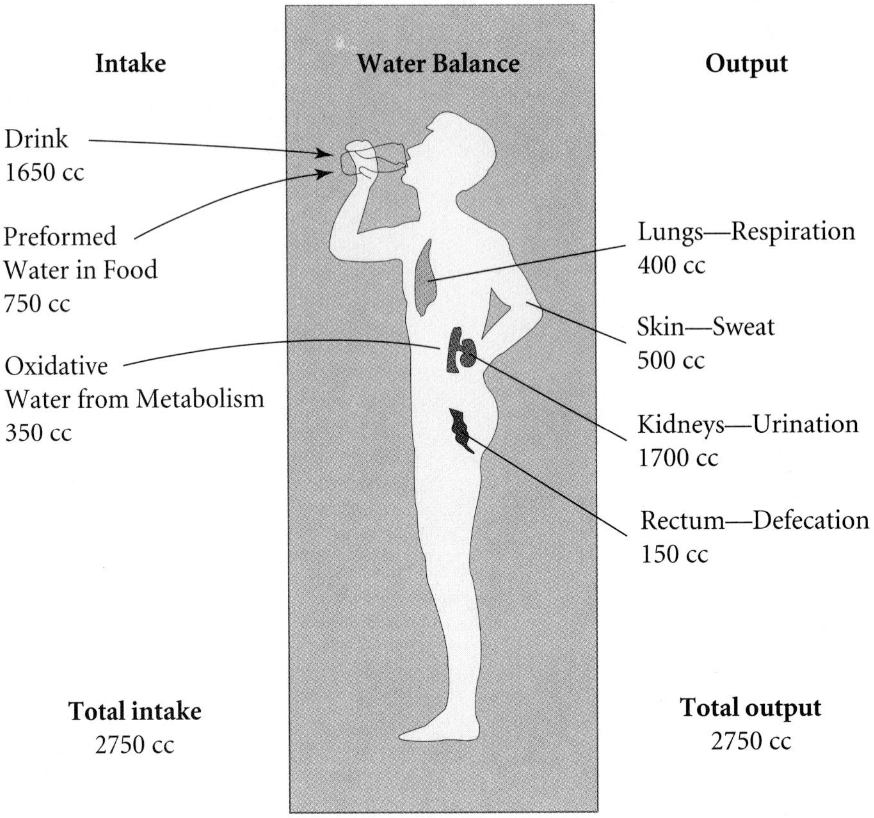

Source: David C. Nieman et al., *Nutrition,* Revised First Edition, Copyright © 1992 Wm. C. Brown Communications, Inc. All rights reserved. Reprinted by permission.

ally draws fluid from the cells, precipitates nausea, and increases urination and potassium loss. A salt supplement is therefore rarely needed in spite of the weather or intensity and duration of exercise. The salt that occurs naturally in food, salt in processed food, and that used from the salt shaker will provide sufficient sodium even for active individuals.

Potassium is critical to maintaining regular heartbeat, and it also plays a role in carbohydrate and protein metabolism. Profuse sweating over several days can deplete potassium stores by as much as 3 mg per day. The average diet provides only 1.5 to 2.5 mg daily. If you sweat profusely and exercise almost daily, you may need five to eight servings of potassium-rich foods each day. Excellent sources of potassium include orange juice, skim milk, bananas, dried fruits, and potatoes. A potassium supplement is not recommended since too much potassium is just as dangerous as too little.

Ionic chloride is part of hydrochloric acid and serves to maintain the strong acidity of the stomach. Loss of too much chloride upsets the acid-base balance of the body. Adding chlorine to public water provides this valuable element and makes water safe for human consumption.

Water alone will not restore electrolyte balance. One alternative is to use commercially prepared, concentrated electrolyte drinks, providing you alter their contents. Some of these drinks contain too much sugar and should be diluted with twice the normal amount of water to increase absorption time and prevent a rapid drop in blood-glucose level shortly after consumption.

While it is useful before and after exercise, the addition of electrolytes to water is of minimal value during a workout. Research suggests that electrolyte replacement is also secondary in importance to water replacement during rehydration after exercise. Fruit juices have the same pitfalls as commercial electrolyte drinks, and the concentrated varieties should be diluted with at least twice the amount of water suggested on the container.

Replacing Iron

Iron deficiency can lead to loss of strength and endurance, early fatigue during exercise, shortening of attention span, loss of visual perception, and impaired learning. Check the results of Lab Activity 8.2: Do You Meet the U.S. Government Dietary Recommendations? to see if you are consuming enough iron. Adolescent girls are more apt to be iron-deficient than women are at any other age. Consequently, food intake may be restricted and this will lead to iron deficiency. During menstruation, female athletes of all ages should discuss the need for an iron supplement with their physician.

SUMMARY

Basic Food Components

Six categories of nutrients satisfy the basic body needs: the energy nutrients (carbohydrates, fats, and proteins) and the nonenergy nutrients (vitamins, minerals, and water).

Carbohydrates and fats provide the main sources of energy (kcal) to perform work. Simple carbohydrates found in concentrated sugar provide empty calories to the diet and very little nutrition in terms of key vitamins and minerals. Complex carbohydrates (fruits, vegetables, and grains) are our only source of fiber and a major supplier of long-term energy. Complex carbohydrates are nutritionally dense foods, providing low calories and a high percentage of our daily needs in vitamins and minerals. Both water-insoluble (dietary) and water-soluble fibers provide important health benefits.

Dietary fat is a critical nutrient and a source of high energy for the human body. Fat is classified as saturated, polyunsaturated, or monounsaturated. Cholesterol, a type of fat, is found in animal sources and also manufactured by the human liver.

Protein can be obtained from both animal and plant foods. In the human body, protein is used for the repair, rebuilding, and replacement of cells; growth; fluid, salt, acid-base balance; and energy in the absence of sufficient dietary carbohydrate and fat. Protein from meat, eggs, and dairy products is termed *complete* since it contains all the essential amino acids in the correct proportion. The correct combinations of various vegetables and grains also make up complete protein sources. With proper planning, vegetarians can easily obtain sufficient protein in their diet without consuming meat, eggs, or dairy products.

Vitamins help chemical reactions take place in the body and are needed in only small amounts. A balanced diet provides the necessary vitamins and minerals needed daily for most people.

Minerals are present in all living cells and serve as components of hormones, enzymes, and other substances aiding chemical reactions in cells. Macro-minerals are needed in large amounts whereas 14 trace minerals are required in small quantities for optimum health. Your daily mineral needs can also be obtained through a balanced diet.

Although it has no nutritional value, water is necessary for all energy production, temperature control, and elimination. A minimum of six to eight glasses of water should be consumed daily, exclusive of all other beverages.

Food Density

A food is said to be nutritionally dense if it contains a low percentage of the daily caloric needs and a high percentage of key nutrients such as protein, vitamins, and minerals. Complex carbohydrates are the most nutritionally dense foods; foods high in fat are the least dense.

Dietary Guidelines for Good Health

You can be assured of sound nutrition by planning your diet around the nutrition pyramid. The recommended servings from each of five key food groups and the limited use of the sixth group (fats, oils, and sweets) will provide you with excellent nutrition. The pyramid offers a less complicated approach to sound nutrition for the lay person than RDA tables and complicated calculations do.

Dietary recommendations have also been made in terms of percent of total calories to guide your intake of carbohydrates, protein, fat, and alcohol. Specific guidelines in grams or milligrams are also available for fiber, salt, and cholesterol.

Nutrition and Disease

The evidence associating nutritional practices with various diseases and disorders and linking sound nutrition to the prevention of some of these diseases continues to mount. Diets that are high in complex carbohydrates and low in fat, cholesterol, sodium, and calories offer the greatest advantage.

Special Needs of the Active Individual

Physically active individuals who follow the nutritional guidelines presented in this chapter have only a few special needs. Sufficient calories must be consumed to support activity levels and to prevent weight and muscle loss; adequate carbohydrates and fat must be consumed to prevent the loss of lean muscle mass; water intake should increase dramatically; electrolyte balance must be maintained; and care must be take to obtain sufficient dietary iron.

Lab Activity 8.1

Estimating Your Daily Fiber Intake

INSTRUCTIONS: *Record all the fiber-containing foods you eat for a period of three days in Column 1. Remember that you must only keep records of the amount and portion size of all fruits, vegetables, and grains eaten.*

To help you estimate the grams of fiber in each food item consumed, turn to Table 8.2. Now record the number of grams of dietary fiber you consume in each food daily in the last column. Divide the total grams by three to determine your average daily intake.

✦ **Record of Daily Fiber Intake**

DAY	FOOD ITEM	SIZE OR AMOUNT	GRAMS OF FIBER
1	Fruits:		
	Vegetables:		
	Grains:		
2	Fruits:		
	Vegetables:		
	Grains:		
3	Fruits:		
	Vegetables:		
	Grains:		

Total grams of dietary fiber in three days _____

Average grams per day _____

Recommended daily intake = 35g

Additional daily fiber needed _____

- Are you consuming at least 35 g of dietary fiber daily? _____ Yes _____ No

- If you responded "no," on the reverse side of this sheet list three or four ways you can alter your meal and snacking to increase fiber intake.

Lab Activity 8.2

Do You Meet the U.S. Government Dietary Recommendations?

INSTRUCTIONS: *The first step toward developing healthy eating habits is to identify your current behavior. This requires careful recording of everything you eat and drink for a three- to four-day period. Estimate the portion size and secure the calories, fiber, salt, cholesterol, and fat content from the tables in this chapter and in Appendix B. Reproduce copies to complete your three- to four-day log.*

✦ **Food and Drink Diary of** _____ **Date** _____

TIME	FOOD/DRINK QUANTITY	ESTIMATED				
		CALORIES	FIBER	SALT	CHOL.	FAT
Breakfast						
Between meal						
Lunch						
Between meal						
Dinner						
Evening						

1. Record the percentage of your daily calories that come from the following:

   Simple carbohydrates _____

   Complex carbohydrates _____

   Protein _____

   Saturated fat _____

   Polyunsaturated fat _____

   Monounsaturated fat _____

2. Are you consuming too much salt? Cholesterol?

3. Are you consuming enough water?

4. Summarize the strengths and weaknesses of your diet in terms of food and fluid intake. What steps can you take toward a healthier diet?

9

Exploring Weight Control

Chapter Objectives

By the end of this chapter, you should be able to:

1. Identify the major causes of obesity and overfatness in the United States.

2. Evaluate and determine your ideal weight and percent of body fat.

3. Define overweight, overfat, and obesity.

4. Describe a sound, long-term weight-loss program.

5. Discuss the role of exercise in weight and fat management.

6. Differentiate between anorexia nervosa and bulimia.

7. Identify the key behaviors linked to weight and fat loss, and describe how to use several behavior-modification techniques to achieve your desired weight.

SUSAN HAS ALWAYS been preoccupied with her weight. As far back as she can remember, she was too fat. For years she considered it purely a genetic problem. After all, her father is obese and her mother is stocky. She thinks perhaps the cards are stacked against her. As an adult, she has tried every diet described in *Good Housekeeping, Redbook,* or that appeared on the bestseller list. Perhaps there is nothing she can do about it. According to the literature, diets don't work and she hates to exercise. Why diet for a lifetime when you need to lose only eight to ten pounds?

Is there any hope for women and men like Susan? This chapter provides the answers to these and other questions about weight control.

During the late nineteenth century in the United States, human muscle power provided 33 percent of the energy needed to run the farms, homes, and factories. Today, muscular effort contributes only 0.05 percent of the energy. Most people in the United States work in office-bound, service-oriented jobs and use business machines, pens, and pencils to accomplish their tasks. The jobs we do and the types of energy needed for those jobs have changed over the past 100 years. The human body has remained the same, however, as we became victims of a technology-oriented lifestyle. As a result, approximately 50 million men and 60 million women between the ages of 18 and 79 and 10 to 20 percent of the school-aged population are overweight and overfat. The incidence of overfatness and obesity among the U.S.'s elementary-school children has increased by 50 percent over the past 15 years. This alarming trend will result in a significant increase in the number of obese adults in the future. With each passing decade, the typical U.S. adult accumulates additional pounds of excess fat and loses some lean muscle tissue until, by middle age, over 50 percent of adult men and women in the United States are overfat or obese.

In the past 15 years, the average weight of U.S. adults has increased 7 to 10 pounds. At all ages we are growing several pounds heavier each decade. Although our average height is also increasing, the majority of this weight gain is fat, not muscle. This trend must be brought under control since obesity is associated with a number of disorders including atherosclerosis, hypertension, diabetes, heart/lung difficulties, early heart attack, and numerous other chronic and degenerative diseases and disorders. The death rate for obese men between the ages of 15 and 69 is 50 percent higher than that of normal-weight persons and 30 percent higher than those classified as merely overweight. For every 10 percent a person is above normal weight, it is estimated that life span is decreased by one year. Unfortunately, the quality of life also declines dramatically in obese individuals.

This chapter examines the critical aspects of weight control: causes of obesity, assessment, safe weight-loss methods, the role of exercise in weight and fat management, underweight and eating disorders, and the role of behavioral modification techniques in helping young people to manage body weight and fat during late teenage and early adulthood.

CAUSES OF OBESITY

Inactivity and overeating are the two most common causes of obesity and overfatness. Physical activity can do much to offset weight gain and regulate the tendency to put on unwanted pounds. Weight gain of genetically obese mice, for example, is drastically reduced by treadmill exercise. In humans, extremely high caloric intake can also be offset by a vigorous exercise program and result in little or no weight gain.

Social, genetic, and psychological factors may also result in overeating and obesity. It has been found that in only a small percentage of cases are glandular or other physiological disorders related to weight problems although many obese people blame these factors. Sedentary living and excessive eating are the two greatest perpetuators of obesity; both can be controlled.

Set Point Theory

The human body regulates its own functions with tremendous precision. Body weight is one of these functions. Each individual appears to have an ideal biological weight (the **set point**) and will defend it against pressure to change. Those who do succeed in losing or gaining weight generally return to their set point weight in a few months or years. Within 24

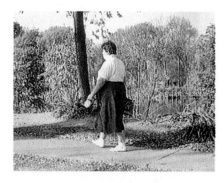

A regular exercise program, such as walking, can be a person's greatest defense against weight gain. (Photo Courtesy of Cable News Network.)

Set point A theory postulating that each individual has an ideal weight (the set point) and that the body will attempt to maintain this weight against pressure to change it.

hours of beginning a very low-calorie diet, for example, metabolic rate (amount of calories burned at rest) slows by 5 to 20 percent as a means of conserving energy, making it more difficult to lose weight. The body is convinced it is starving, and the calorie conservation is a way of hanging on to the energy for a longer period of time. In addition, once excess fat cells become depleted, they signal the central nervous system to alter feeding behavior by increasing caloric intake so that the set point can be maintained. In other words, some experts feel that an internal thermostat regulates body fat and weight and triggers an increase in food intake when fat and weight are lowered too much. Overcoming the set point is difficult. Willpower and other factors that aid in tolerating the discomfort of hunger are poor matches for a computer-like system that never quits.

Research suggests that one of the ways to take it off and keep it off may be to lower the thermostat. *Yo-yo* dieting (the cycle of losing and regaining weight and fat) may have the opposite effect and actually result in a higher setting on the thermostat with the body then defending an even higher weight. This may explain why people who complete several cycles of losing and regaining ten pounds find it nearly twice as hard to lose weight and twice as easy to gain weight on their next attempt. With each yo-yo cycle, the individual also acquires extra body fat and loses some muscle mass. Regular, aerobic exercise 4 to 5 times weekly combined with a sound nutritional plan appears to lower the thermostat over time and allows loss of weight and maintenance of that lower weight.

Early Eating Patterns

Most experts agree that the eating habits formed in infancy and childhood carry over into the adult years. Rats who are exposed to unlimited milk, for example, continue to eat much more and exercise less after they are weaned than rats who receive only limited milk. In other words, rats who are overfed prior to weaning become sedentary adult rats who overeat, become fat, and suffer from early cardiorespiratory disease. By contrast, rats who eat less prior to weaning, continue to eat less, exercise more, live longer, and experience less cardiorespiratory disease. The response in humans is similar. Children who are inactive and overeat are also more likely to continue these behaviors later in life and become overfat adults.

Environmental forces appear to influence eating patterns more than physiological forces such as hunger. Negative eating behavior may begin in infancy. Some experts feel that bottle feeding, for example, may predispose infants to obesity. Approximately three times more bottle-fed than breast-fed babies are *overfat*. Bottle feeding fails to provide the solace of breast feeding and tends to produce anxiety, which may provoke overeating. Breast-fed babies also learn to stop feeding when the richest portion of the milk gives way to more watery milk. The bottle does not provide such a natural mechanism so bottle-fed babies require more calories to satisfy their hunger.

Perhaps a more important problem is feeding babies solid foods too early, which may contribute to the production of excess fat cells. Experts recommend that parents start feeding their infants solid foods at the age of five months rather than earlier, except for cases of very large or fast-developing babies. This is no easy task for sleep-deprived mothers who long for the day the baby sleeps through the night without waking for a feeding.

There is little danger that a growing child will be obese if the child itself decides when to stop eating at a meal. Forcing children to clean the plate is a mistake and is the same as forcing a child to overeat. Making sweets plentiful, using them as rewards, and placing emphasis on the fat baby also compounds the problem, shortens life span, encourages premature heart disease, forms undesirable eating habits that will be continued throughout life, and destines the child to a life of restricted eating because of having a high number of fat cells formed in early life. A lean child with a great deal of energy and vitality is healthier and more likely to be healthy later in life.

There is no stage in life when excess fat is desirable; however, the earlier in life a child is obese, the

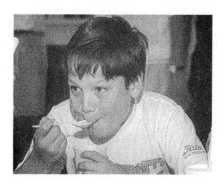

Overweight children are likely to grow into overweight adults. (Photo Courtesy of Cable News Network.)

greater the chance is that the child will eventually be of normal weight. The later in life a child is obese, the less likely it is that he or she will ever return to normal weight. It is estimated that an obese adolescent, for example, has approximately a 1 in 16 chance of returning to normal weight as an adult. The fatter you are at any age, the less likely you will ever return to normal weight. It is therefore advisable to start children off right and avoid overstuffing. If their mechanism for pushing up from the table when they are full is destroyed, they are certain to need plenty of real push ups in the adult years to control weight.

Fat Cells

Our fat cells are formed early in life and increase in both size and number until the end of adolescence. Calorie restriction will decrease only the size of fat cells, not the number. With a large number of fat cells formed, a return to an overfat condition is quite easy. This partially explains why adults who were fat babies often have difficulty keeping their weight down. These extra adipose cells also affect metabolism and result in the need for fewer calories to maintain normal weight than are needed by someone who generally remains at normal weight. Unlike muscle, fat requires little energy to maintain and additional fat weight will not increase metabolic rate.

The number of fat cells in the human body grows rapidly during three stages of development: (1) the last trimester of pregnancy (in the unborn child), (2) the first year of life, and (3) the adolescent growth spurt. Fat is acquired by increasing the size of existing adipose cells (**hypertrophy**) and by new fat-cell formation prior to adulthood (**hyperplasia**). It is doubtful that new fat cells are formed after age 21 (approximately) unless someone becomes extremely obese.

There is a wide variation in the number of fat cells in different people. A nonobese person has approximately 25 to 30 billion fat cells while an extremely obese person may have as many as 260 billion. A formerly obese adult may never be cured because weight loss does not reduce the number of existing cells, it only reduces their size.

Hypertrophy The enlargement of existing fat cells.

Hyperplasia New fat-cell formation.

Genetics

It is now clear that the genes we inherit influence our weight. Children of overfat or obese parents, particularly the biological mother, are much more likely to be overfat or obese. It is important to keep in mind, however, that environment is still critical. Genetics may merely predispose you or provide you with the tendency to become fat—a problem that regular exercise and proper nutrition can overcome.

Environmental Factors

Although heredity plays an important role, environment is also critical. Sound exercise and eating and drinking habits can overcome the genetic tendency to be either thin or fat.

One of the clearer causes of obesity and overfatness in children is watching television. People on television programs eat about eight times per hour and commercials generally advertise high-calorie, high-fat foods. Television watchers pick up on these cues and tend to eat more often and more high-fat, high-calorie foods. In addition, television is a passive activity. Almost any activity will burn more calories. While it is a good idea to restrict the number of television-watching hours for all children and teenagers, it is absolutely necessary to do so for the overfat child.

Other environmental influences, such as eating and exercise habits of parents, food availability, and nutritional knowledge, may not be as important as was once believed. Experts feel that genetic influences account for about 70 percent of the differences in body-mass index (BMI) that are found later in life and that childhood environment has less influence than was once thought. This does not mean that environment has no influence on obesity. Nongenetic factors are important determinants of body fat. These factors are reversible and capable of overcoming some of the genetic factors that make us fat.

Metabolic Factors

Even small changes in metabolic rate translate into large increases in body fat and weight. A 10 percent decline in metabolism, for example, could result in an annual weight gain of about 15 lb for the average individual. Aerobic exercise increases metabolic rate both during and after the exercise session. The afterburn continues for from 20 minutes to several hours, depending on the duration and intensity of the workout. Coffee, tea, cocoa, colas, other caffeine-contain-

Diversity Issues

Fat Control

Fat is the primary energy reserve of the body. The natural distribution and amount of fat varies considerably between men and women. Some experts identify the appropriate body fatness in women as 20 to 27 percent compared to 12 to 15 percent in men. Achieving a body fat below the level of essential fat represents no health advantage for either sex and may actually be detrimental to health.

Weight and fat management is a much more difficult task for women than for men because about 12 percent of fat in women is essential fat (as opposed to 4 to 7 percent in men), which includes an extra 5 to 9 percent of sex-specific fat in the breasts, pelvic region, and thighs. The childbearing role and the fact that women generally possess smaller bodies requiring fewer calories also makes it much more difficult for a woman to lose fat and weight as rapidly than for a man.

Fat accumulates in different sites on men and women. In general, men tend to possess fat receptors in the abdominal area and fat inhibitors in the buttocks, hips, and upper legs. This partially explains why most men develop the beer belly and rarely accumulate fat in other areas. Women tend to possess fat receptors in the hips, buttocks, and thighs, and often have fat inhibitors in the abdomen. Various patterns of obesity exist in both sexes with most obese individuals distributing fat throughout the body. Android

(excessive fat in the lower body) and gynoid (excessive fat in the abdomen) obesity may result in both men and women. The so-called pear (fat accumulation in the hips and lower body common in women) and apple (fat accumulation in the abdominal area common in men) shapes have also been examined by researchers. Apple shapes with large fat accumulation around the midsection and chest may impose a greater risk for heart disease than does the pear shape.

Because most women need significantly fewer calories to maintain their lower body weight, it is more difficult to enter into a large negative calorie balance daily and lose weight rapidly. A 120-lb woman may need only 1800 calories daily, for example. A 1000-calorie deduction leaves only 800 calories to obtain adequate nourishment and energy—a nearly impossible task. A 200-lb man, however, may require as much as 3000 calories daily to maintain weight. A 1000-calorie deficit daily still leaves a total of 2000 calories—enough for sufficient nourishment and energy.

We all must become more tolerant of our bodies and accept the fact that our percent of body fat will increase slightly with age and that aging will alter the shape and appearance of our bodies regardless of our best exercise and eating efforts. Overemphasis on thinness and a youthful body is dangerous for both sexes and often leads to self-concept problems and serious eating disorders. ✦

ing food and drink, and amphetamines and other drugs increase metabolic rate. In midafternoon, metabolism tends to slow, making this an excellent time for aerobic exercise to boost metabolic rate. As one ages, metabolism also slows until at age 50 metabolic rate may have decreased by as much as 15 to 25 percent in a sedentary individual. In those who have remained active through a combination of aerobic exercise and strength training, metabolic rate slows only slightly. Loss of muscle mass is one of the leading causes of reduced metabolic rate with aging.

BODY COMPOSITION

Many people have an ideal image of their bodies that they would someday like to achieve. For some, such an image may be unrealistic. Regardless of your motivation to change, there are several methods derived from research or actuarial tables that may help you set realistic goals for a better-looking body.

A simple method of estimating proper body weight is to use the Metropolitan Life Insurance

Table 9.1 ✦ Metropolitan Life Insurance Height-Weight Table

| MEN | | | | | | WOMEN | | | | |
| HEIGHT | | FRAME | | | HEIGHT | | FRAME | | | |
Feet	Inches	Small	Medium	Large	Feet	Inches	Small	Medium	Large
5	2	128–134	131–141	138–150	4	10	102–111	109–121	118–131
5	3	130–136	133–143	140–153	4	11	103–113	111–123	120–134
5	4	132–138	135–145	142–156	5	0	104–115	113–126	122–137
5	5	134–140	137–148	144–160	5	1	106–118	115–129	125–140
5	6	136–142	139–151	146–164	5	2	108–121	118–132	128–143
5	7	138–145	142–154	149–168	5	3	111–124	121–135	131–147
5	8	140–148	145–157	152–172	5	4	114–127	124–138	134–151
5	9	142–151	148–160	155–176	5	5	117–130	127–141	137–155
5	10	144–154	151–163	158–180	5	6	120–133	130–144	140–159
5	11	146–157	154–166	161–184	5	7	123–136	133–147	143–163
6	0	149–160	157–170	164–188	5	8	126–139	136–150	146–167
6	1	152–164	160–174	168–192	5	9	129–142	139–153	149–170
6	2	155–168	164–178	172–197	5	10	132–145	142–156	152–173
6	3	158–172	167–182	176–202	5	11	135–148	145–159	155–176
6	4	162–176	171–187	181–207	6	0	138–151	148–162	158–179

Weights at ages 25 to 29 based on lowest mortality. Weights in pounds according to frame (in indoor clothing weighing 5 lb for men or 3 lb for women; shoes with 1-inch heels). For frame size standards, see Table 9.2.

Source: Reproduced with permission of Metropolitan Life Insurance Company. Source of basic data: Society of Actuaries and Association of Life Insurance Medical Directors of America, *1979 Build Study,* 1980. Copyright © 1983 Metropolitan Life Insurance Company. All rights reserved. Reproduced by permission.

height-weight standards shown in Table 9.1. Charts of so-called ideal weight for men and women are based on data associating average weights by height and age with long life. Prior to 1980 figures indicated that those who weighed less than their recommended weight on the charts lived up to 20 percent longer than other people. The charts, which became the national guide for determining overweight and obesity for the general public, worked on the theory that "the greater the weight, the greater the risk of death." The validity of such data is now being questioned since it is evident that less-than-average weights may involve health risks even greater than those associated with overweight and that the U.S. preoccupation with *thin* may not be much of a health advantage.

Authorities do not dispute that people who are much heavier than average (more than 20 percent above ideal weight on the charts) obtain health benefits from weight reduction. Even small amounts of weight loss, for example, may aid the diabetic patient. For those in normal health who are at average or near average weight, there may be no health benefit to losing weight. The key factor that determines what is too much or too little is body fat, not total body weight.

Determining Ideal Body Weight from Height-Weight Charts

Check your ideal weight on to Table 9.1. Frame size can be determined by wrapping your thumb and middle finger around your opposite wrist. If the thumb and finger do not meet, you have a large frame. If they just meet or barely overlap, you have a medium frame, and if they overlap, you have a small frame. For a much more accurate indicator of frame size, follow the directions in Table 9.2 to obtain the exact width of your elbow.

Since height-weight charts provide only a rough guide to the determination of ideal weight, use the lowest weight to the midpoint from Table 9.1 as the range for your desirable body weight. See how your actual weight compares. If you fall 20 percent below or above the range for your height, you are roughly classified as underweight or overweight; 30 percent above classifies you as obese. Keep in mind that this table provides only a rough guide to desirable weight and it is not uncommon for an individual to fall considerably above a weight range and still possess normal or even below-normal body fat. This is particu-

Table 9.2 ✦ Approximating Frame Size

MEN		WOMEN	
Height in 1" heels	*Elbow breadth*	*Height in 1" heels*	*Elbow breadth*
5'2"–5'3"	2½"–2⅞"	4'10"–4'11"	2¼"–2½"
5'4"–5'7"	2⅝"–2⅞"	5'0"–5'3"	2¼"–2½"
5'8"–5'11"	2¾"–3"	5'4"–5'7"	2⅜"–2⅝"
6'0"–6'3"	2¾"–3⅛"	5'8"–5'11"	2⅜"–2⅝"
6'4"	2⅞"–3¼"	6'0"	2½"–2¾"

Extend your arm and bend the forearm upward to a 90-degree angle. Keep fingers straight and turn the inside of your wrist toward your body. If you have a caliper, use it to measure the space between the two prominent bones on *either* side of your elbow. Without a caliper, place thumb and index finger of your other hand on these two bones. Measure the space between your fingers against a ruler or tape measure. Compare it with these tables that list elbow measurements for *medium-framed* men and women. Measurements lower than those listed indicate you have a small frame. Higher measurements indicate a large frame.

Source: 1979 Build Study. Society of Actuaries and Association of Life Insurance Medical Directors of America, 1980. Copyright © 1983 Metropolitan Life Insurance Company. All rights reserved. Reproduced by permission.

larly common in muscular men and women. Conversely, it is entirely possible to fall within the desired range and still possess excess body fat.

Determining Percent of Body Fat

A more important consideration in goal setting for a better-looking and healthier body involves not body weight but the amount of adipose tissue you possess. Weight control is simply another name for fat control, and measurement of body fat is essential in setting goals for your body.

The average percent of body fat is approximately 25 percent for females and 20 percent for males. Individuals are considered obese if they possess more than 30 percent (men) or 35 percent (women) body fat (see Table 9.3).

Since about half of all body fat lies just beneath the skin, it is possible to pinch certain body parts, measure the thickness of two layers of skin and the connected fat, and estimate the total percent of fat on the body.

You can measure the thickness of four skinfold sites with a caliper. Considerable practice is needed, however, before accurate measurements can be taken. Take a moment to complete Lab Activity 9.1: Determining Your Percent of Body Fat at the end of this chapter to develop your skills and determine your estimated percent of body fat.

There are other methods of estimating percent of body fat. **Electrical impedance** is a quick method. Electrodes are attached to the wrist and ankle of the reclining subject. In less than two minutes, a printout provides your percent of body fat, total amount of fat weight, ideal percent of fat, and ideal body weight. It is necessary to follow certain nutritional and exercise rules for 24 hours before the test. **Hydrostatic weighing** is probably the most accurate method of estimating body fat. In the test the subject sits on a scale in a

Table 9.3 ✦ Fatness Ratings of College-Aged Men and Women

RATING	MEN	WOMEN
Very low fat	5 to 7.9	12 to 14.9
Low fat	8 to 10.9	15 to 17.9
Ideal fat	11 to 14.9	18 to 21.9
Above ideal fat	15 to 17.9	22 to 24.9
Over fat	18 to 22.9	25 to 27.9
High fat	23+	28+

Electrical impedance A quick, accurate means of determining an individual's percent of body fat that uses electrodes attached to wrists and ankles to electronically determine the percent.

Hydrostatic weighing A method of measuring body fat by submerging an individual in water.

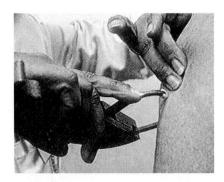

Measurement of body fat using skinfold calipers. (Photo Courtesy of Cable News Network.)

tank of water, exhales as completely as possible, and is submerged for approximately 10 seconds while weight is recorded. The proportions of lean body mass and fat mass are determined from calculations that involve weight underwater, weight out of water, and known densities of lean and fatty tissues.

SAFE WEIGHT-LOSS PROCEDURES

Hunger and Appetite

Hunger is generally considered physiological, an inborn instinct, whereas **appetite** is a psychological, or a learned, response. This helps to explain why it is so common to have an appetite and eat when you are not hungry; conversely, some very thin people or those with eating disorders may experience hunger without appetite. Hunger is an active experience, whereas appetite is passive.

The feeling of fullness or satisfaction that prompts us to stop eating is called *satiety,* one of the key regulators of eating behavior. Some experts feel that eating behavior is always in operation except when the satiety signal turns it off. Just how that happens is unknown although a number of theories have been advanced. The **glucostatic theory** of hunger regulation suggests that blood glucose levels and the exhaustion of liver glycogen may account for the starting and stopping of eating. The liver stores about 75 grams (g) of glycogen or 300-plus energy units (calories). When liver glycogen levels fall significantly, feelings of hunger may occur. The **lipostatic theory** suggests that hunger is regulated in some way by the number of fat-storing enzymes on the surfaces of fat cells. The messenger that the cells send to the brain in this theory has not been identified. The **purinegic theory** is relatively new and untested and proposes that the circulating levels of purines, mole-

cules found in DNA and RNA, govern hunger. Exactly where and how the brain receives these messages is also unknown. The **hypothalamus gland** appears to be important in regulating eating. Damage to this area can produce eating disorders and severe weight loss or gain.

Eating behavior appears to occur in response to numerous signals. The possibility also exists that an inherited, internal regulatory defect is at least partially responsible for obesity, rather than its being a purely learned behavior or genetically caused.

It is obvious that there is much to be learned about the causes of obesity. There are many other theories. A summary of research currently in progress to discover the answers to these and other questions appears in Figure 9.1. An understanding of the difference between hunger and appetite and the factors suspected of controlling food intake will help you control your body weight and fat.

Controlling Appetite From the limited information available, it is known that two basic approaches to controlling appetite are somewhat effective: (1) keeping the stomach full of low-calorie food and drink and (2) raising the body's blood-sugar level. Increasing your fluid intake (particularly your water consumption) and consuming complex carbohydrates such as raw fruits and vegetables both between meals and at mealtimes will keep the stomach relatively full. New raw grain products are also available

---

Hunger A physiological response of the body indicating a need for food involving unpleasant sensations.

Appetite The desire to eat; pleasant sensations aroused by the thoughts of the taste and enjoyment of food.

Glucostatic theory A theory about hunger regulation suggesting that blood-glucose levels determine whether one is hungry or satiated through the exhaustion of liver glycogen.

Lipostatic theory A theory about hunger control suggesting that the size of fat stores signals us to eat.

Purinegic theory A theory about hunger suggesting that the circulating levels of purines, molecules found in DNA and RNA, govern hunger.

Hypothalamus gland A portion of the brain that regulates body temperature and other functions; thought to be important in the regulation of food intake.

Figure 9.1 ✦ Hunger and Appetite: Some of the Factors Suspected of Controlling Food Intake

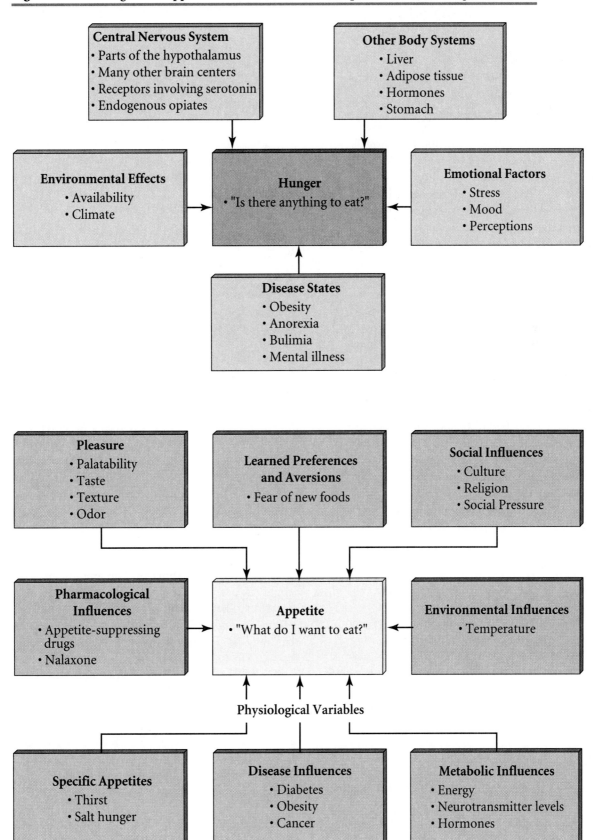

Source: Adapted from T.W. Castonguay et al., "Hunger and Appetite: Old Concepts/New Distinctions," *Nutrition Reviews* 41 (April 1983): 101–110. Copyright ILSI-Nutrition Foundation. Used with permission.

Fitness Heroes

Margie McCarthy was a dedicated student. She created demanding study schedules for herself and, with added encouragement from her family, got excellent grades in high school. In college, however, Margie's regimented lifestyle became her downfall. She awoke every morning at 6 AM and worked out, attended classes, and studied for the rest of the day. While controlling her schedule, she also started dieting. Eventually, she became obsessed with her eating habits and she developed anorexia nervosa. She felt that by controlling her weight, she could gain control over her life.

Her bout with anorexia was one of the most difficult times in Margie's life. Her weight fell to 65 pounds, her skin dried out, she became short-winded, her hair fell out, and her eyes were always dry. In addition, the stress of studying and getting through college made everything worse.

When Margie finally recognized that she had a problem, she enlisted the help of family, friends, and a psychotherapist. It took years of therapy for Margie to recover, but she is now a successful career woman planning her wedding. She focuses on exercise and nutrition to control her weight, but says that her anorexic impulses sometimes return when she feels that life is getting out of control. She combats the impulses by walking, riding an exercise bike, and eating a balanced diet, and is now leading a happy and productive life. ✦

that are equally effective. Small amounts of candy, such as one or two chocolate squares, 20 to 30 minutes before a meal, or when you have the urge to snack, is another technique you can use. Slow eaters (those taking 20 minutes or more) also experience this elevated blood-sugar level and are less likely to overeat.

Calorie Counting

If you are overfat according to the guidelines in this chapter, you may want to consider an exercise and diet regimen to lose body fat and weight. When you set goals for body-fat loss, you can expect to lose about .5 millimeters (mm) of body fat per week with an appropriate combination of diet and exercise. For

example, if you are now classified as *above average fat*, it is realistic to expect to reach the *average fat* category after a 10-week program.

As a first step in losing body fat, turn to Lab Activity 9.2: Determining Your Caloric Needs at the end of the chapter to determine how many calories you need to maintain your present weight. These figures will help you decide how much to increase your daily energy expenditure and reduce your daily caloric intake to meet your weight- and fat-loss goals. You can then reduce your caloric intake and increase your exercise expenditure to produce a slow, safe weight and fat loss.

How Exercise Helps

A pleasant occurrence often accompanying weight losses of over 5 to 10 lb is enhanced self-concept and increased energy levels. Remember that the weight you choose as a target is one that, once reached, must be maintained for the rest of your life. It is not just weight loss per se, but the acceptance of a healthy lifestyle that is most likely to keep your *thin self* going in the future. Regular vigorous exercise is an essential part of this healthy, holistic lifestyle.

If you expect to lose body fat and weight and then maintain this lower level, you need both to restrict your caloric intake and to engage in regular exercise. By remaining physically active, you will be able to consume more calories daily. The alternative is to remain mildly hungry most of your life. There are numerous other reasons why both diet and exercise should be included in a weight-loss or weight-management program.

Exercise Depresses Appetite The amount of body weight and fat lost during an exercise program is greater than what can be attributed to the number of calories expended. This suggests that exercise acts on the body to further increase energy expenditure through changes in metabolism or to decrease energy intake through changes in appetite. It is also a well-established principle that physical activity decreases appetite. Physical inactivity and high body fat and decreases in appetite and regular aerobic exercise are all strongly associated. The food intake of elementary school-aged children has also been shown to decrease by scheduling the recess period before, rather than after, lunch.

Exercise Maximizes Fat Loss and Minimizes Loss of Lean Muscle Tissue There is a difference between weight loss in terms of pounds and fat loss in terms of adipose tissue. A diet without exercise can result in about 70 to 80 percent fatty-tissue loss and 20 to 30 percent lean-muscle loss. With the combination of exercise and diet, fatty-tissue loss can be increased to 95 percent and lean-muscle loss kept to 5 percent or less of total weight loss.

Exercise Burns a High Number of Calories and Increases Metabolic Rate Exercise burns calories both during an exercise session and for 20 minutes to several hours after exercise ceases (afterburn). A three-mile run or walk will expend 250 to 300 cal depending on the individual. For the next 20 minutes (for the walker) to several hours (for the jogger or runner), an additional 25 to 40 calories per hour will be burned due to an increase in metabolic rate. The total caloric benefit of a three-mile run then may be as high as 500 calories. Four to five such workouts weekly would produce a body weight/fat loss of about three lb monthly, 36 lb per year.

Strength-training programs involving weights add muscle mass and increase metabolism permanently. Keep in mind that fat is a dormant tissue and requires very few calories to maintain. Muscle tissue, on the other hand, requires considerable calories to maintain. It is estimated that for every pound of muscle you add, metabolic rate increases 30 to 50 cal per 24-hour period. If you add five lb of muscle over a six-month period, your metabolic rate may increase as much as 200 calories daily. This translates into about 6000 cal monthly and nearly two lb of fat (3500 cal = one lb of fat). This is obviously a very significant change.

The best system of controlling body weight is changing your eating habits and beginning an exercise program you enjoy and are likely to continue throughout life. If you change your behavior in these two areas, you will go through life at your ideal body weight and fat. Body weight is carefully regulated by complex forces, but the formula for weight loss is simple. If you eat more calories than you burn through activity, a positive caloric balance exists and produces weight gain. If you burn up more calories than you eat, a negative caloric balance exists and weight and fat loss will occur.

Table 9.4 on pages 192 and 193 shows the number of calories used per hour in various activities. It does not reflect the additional effects of afterburn or the changes in metabolic rate that occur from muscle-weight gain. Walking, bicycling, swimming, dancing, jogging, and other aerobic activities are all effective means of exercise for weight loss. Some types of physical activity and sports are relaxing and enjoyable. Other activities are superior in weight loss and aerobic benefits.

When you choose a particular exercise program, consider that:

1. You are more likely to continue exercising in activities you enjoy.
2. Activities that expend a high number of calories per minute are the best ones for weight loss.
3. Lifelong physical-recreational sports that provide heart-lung benefits are superior.
4. The choice you make should allow you to start at your present fitness level and progress to higher levels later.

Exercise Brings Needed Calcium to the Bones As a result of normal aging and weight loss, bones lose calcium and other minerals and become brittle. It takes adequate calcium in your diet (see chapter 8) plus weight-bearing exercise (walking, jogging, running, aerobic dance) to increase the amount of calcium that reaches the bones and thereby helps prevent osteoporosis.

Exercise Changes the Way Your Body Handles Fats Exercise helps lower and maintain serum cholesterol and triglycerides. HDL (high-density lipoprotein, the good cholesterol) increases, and the ratio of HDL to total cholesterol improves. High HDL counts and a high ratio of HDL to total cholesterol (1:4 or higher) have been associated with a lower incidence of heart attacks.

SPECIAL DIETS

There are numerous reasons why the average diet lasts only 5 to 7 days: boredom, monotony, lack of energy, fatigue, depression, complicated meal planning and purchasing, and failure to lose weight and fat fast enough. These problems are less likely to occur for individuals on a sound diet. Unfortunately, diet choices are often restricted to magazine, book, or television publicity that promises some *secret* easy method of shedding pounds and fat. These and practically all other diets simply do not work, are potentially dangerous, and should be avoided. Safe, effective, and long-term management of body weight and fat involves a lifelong plan of proper nutrition and regular exercise. Quick weight-loss approaches provide only a temporary fix with over 90 percent of those who try any of them regaining the lost weight within 6 to 12 months. In the meantime, the body may have been exposed to extreme health hazards.

Table 9.4 ✦ Activity Rating Chart (Calories Burned per Hour)

ACTIVITY	110 LB.		120 LB.		130 LB.		140 LB.		150 LB.	
	M	F	M	F	M	F	M	F	M	F
Sleeping, reclining	–	45	–	50	–	54	–	58	68	62
Very light: sitting, standing, driving	–	65	–	72	–	77	–	83	102	88
Light: walking on level, shopping, golf, table tennis, carpentry, light housekeeping	–	130	–	143	–	153	–	166	197	177
Moderate: walking, weeding, cycling, skiing, tennis, dancing	–	205	–	226	–	242	–	262	292	279
Heavy: walking uphill, shoveling, basketball, swimming, climbing, football, jogging, running	–	400	–	440	–	472	–	512	571	544

Courtesy of Safeway, Inc. 1994.

– = Data unavailable

Snacking

Between-meal and late-evening snacking is a leading cause of overfatness. It is not uncommon to consume over 1000 calories between 8 PM and midnight; nearly one-third of a pound of fat. Yet it is unrealistic to expect people to avoid snacking altogether. In fact, planned snacking on the right foods can help you control hunger and eat less. Snacks likely to be low in calories are those that are thin and watery, such as tomato juice, crisp but not greasy (celery, carrots, radishes, cucumbers, broccoli, cauliflower, apples, berries, and other fresh fruits and vegetables and raw grains), and bulky (salad greens). Prepare a tray of these nutritious, low-calorie snacks and place it in the front of your refrigerator. Most snackers are compulsive and consume the first thing they see.

Characteristics of the Ideal Diet Plan

This ten-point plan is nothing more than sound nutrition and exercise advice, and it should be followed throughout life. Although you can always find a diet book on the bestseller list, the fact remains that most diets fail and the large majority of individuals who lose weight return to their overweight or overfat condition within a very short time. A lifetime plan for proper eating and exercise offers you the best chance for success and safety.

1. Consume a minimum of 1200 calories daily.

2. Drink a minimum of 10 glasses of water daily when you diet.

3. Eat sufficient protein daily. Consult the recommended dietary allowance (RDA) table in chapter 8 to determine your exact needs.

4. Eat at least 100 g (400 cal) of carbohydrate and 10 g of fat (90 cal) daily to spare protein. Unless your carbohydrate and fat intake are sufficient to meet your daily needs, dietary protein and lean protein mass (muscle) will be converted to glucose to nourish the nervous system. Failing to spare protein for weeks at a time can prove fatal. Fat is also very important for satiety.

5. Never skip a meal, even if you are not hungry. Choose a variety of foods from the nutrition pyramid in chapter 8.

6. Gear your program to a weight loss of between one and two pounds weekly and stay with it until you reach your goal.

7. Premeasure each food portion, keep records of your food and drink intake, identify problem areas, and take steps to change.

8. Avoid laxatives, stimulants, and diuretics, and use a multiple vitamin and mineral daily.

9. Combine dieting with exercise in an activity or aerobic program you enjoy; exercise a minimum of three times weekly, for at least 30 minutes each time.

10. Plan to stay with your new eating and exercise routine for a minimum of 12 months.

UNDERWEIGHT CONDITIONS AND EATING DISORDERS

The problems of gaining weight are just as complex as those associated with weight loss. Hunger, appetite, and satiety irregularities; psychological factors; or

| 160 LB. | | 170 LB. | | 180 LB. | | 190 LB. | | 200 LB. | | 210 LB. | | 220 LB. | | 230 LB. | |
M	F	M	F	M	F	M	F	M	F	M	F	M	F	M	F
72	66	77	70	81	75	86	78	90	83	95	–	99	–	104	–
110	95	116	100	123	107	129	112	137	118	143	–	150	–	158	–
212	190	223	200	238	213	250	224	264	237	276	–	290	–	305	–
314	300	331	316	353	336	370	353	391	373	409	–	430	–	452	–
613	584	647	616	689	656	722	688	764	728	798	–	840	–	882	–

metabolic problems can cause dangerous underweight. For some individuals who need additional weight and muscle for sports and others who merely want to be and appear stronger, gaining a pound is just as difficult as losing a pound is for others.

Gaining Weight

A drug-free muscle-weight-gain program requires considerable dedication to both diet and exercise. Sound approaches strive to add no more than a half-pound of muscle per week, two pounds per month. This is about as quick as the body can add lean muscle tissue. Faster approaches involving too many calories are almost certain to add adipose tissue.

A sound strength-training program, such as weight training, is an absolute must for muscle-weight gain (see chapter 6). It may be necessary to train for several hours six times weekly, alternating muscle groups each day.

The nutritional support for a sound weight-gain program involves an increase in food (about 400 to 500 additional calories daily) that provides high calories in as small volume as possible to keep you from getting uncomfortably full, a slight increase in total protein intake (14 to 15 percent of daily calories), and a slight reduction in total fat intake (18 to 20 percent of daily calories). Extra calories should come from complex carbohydrates (65 to 68 percent of daily calories) to provide long-term energy and for **protein sparing**. Most individuals who have difficulty gaining weight do not eat enough calories to support their vigorous workout schedule. Using protein or amino acid tablets is not a good idea as they are hazardous and a waste of money. In the majority of cases, individuals consume more protein than they need already; adding more in the form of supplements is unnecessary.

Eating Disorders

The current overemphasis on flat stomachs, lean thighs, firm buttocks, and slimness is at least partially responsible for aggravating two serious eating disorders that can lead to death: **anorexia nervosa** and **bulimia**. Both disorders are known only in developed nations and are most common in higher economic groups.

Anorexia The number of cases of anorexia nervosa is increasing and now occurs in almost 1 of every 100 women, 19 out of 20 of whom are young women. The disease is four to five times more common in identical than in fraternal twins, suggesting an inherited predisposition to the disease. Unfortunately, our culture encourages anorexia nervosa.

Protein sparing Consuming sufficient amounts of dietary carbohydrate and fat on a daily basis to prevent the conversion of dietary and lean muscle protein to glucose.

Anorexia nervosa An eating disorder that involves lack or loss of appetite to the point of self-starvation and dangerous weight loss.

Bulimia An eating disorder found most often in women involving eating binges followed by self-induced vomiting or the use of laxatives to expel the unwanted food.

Myth and Fact Sheet

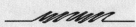

Myth	Fact
1. Overweight and obese people are always big eaters.	1. In both children and adults, studies show that the major cause of heaviness is inactivity followed by overeating. The major problem for the majority of over-fat people in the United States is inactivity. A regular exercise program is still the best health-insurance policy and the best approach to weight and fat loss.
2. The major part of excess weight and fat is water.	2. This is not true. Do not restrict your water intake in any way. Water is essential to the proper function of every body system. Fluid retention is common while dieting since water remains in the spaces freed by the disappearance of fat. This fluid generally remains for two to three weeks and often obscures actual weight loss. Drink water freely at all times, particularly when you are restricting your calories. The majority (about 80 percent) of excess weight is fat, not water.
3. Beer helps me relax and avoid food calories.	3. Alcohol in any form is high in calories (7 cal per g, 150 cal per beer, mixed drink, or four-ounce glass of wine). Since alcohol is a depressant, it encourages relaxation, and relaxation improves appetite. In addition, there is generally high-calorie snack food available when alcohol is served.
4. Candy and other sweets help me curb my appetite.	4. In very small amounts, such as one or two squares of a chocolate bar, one or two pieces of hard candy, or three or four ounces of soda, blood-sugar levels are raised and give you the impression you are not hungry. In larger amounts, however, high blood sugar levels rapidly fall, leaving you with little energy and hungry enough to eat several more high-calorie candy bars.
5. There's nothing wrong with resorting to quick weight-loss diets.	5. You should lose weight at the rate of no more than one to two pounds weekly. Very low calorie diets that produce rapid weight loss have a number of pitfalls: (1) They are dangerous and possibly life-threatening. (2) Rapid weight loss is usually followed by rapid weight gain. (3) Your percent of body fat increases each time you lose and reacquire the weight. (4) Sufficient carbohydrate is often not consumed to spare protein resulting in lean-tissue loss even from the heart muscle itself. Sufficient cardiac tissue loss to the heart might cause serious rhythm problems.
6. Cellulite can be eliminated with special foods and exercise.	6. From a medical point of view, there is no such thing as cellulite as a particular form of fat. Fat is merely fat although the size and appearance of fat cells vary in different body parts and in different people. The lumpy, dimple-like deposits called cellulite tend to be most visible in women and often appear on the thighs, back of legs, and buttocks. These deposits are merely large fat cells that show through the somewhat thinner skin of women. Thicker-skinned males tend not to develop this appearance unless they become extremely fat. Prevention is easier than treatment and focuses on proper nutrition, maintaining normal weight and fat, and avoiding rapid weight-loss attempts or yo-yo dieting.
7. It is better to remain fat than to lose weight and end up with wrinkled skin.	7. You are partially correct. It is better to stay somewhat fat rather than lose then regain body weight rapidly. If you lose weight and fat slowly through a combination of diet and exercise and lose only 10 to 15 pounds, skin wrinkling is unlikely. It is also helpful to include weight training as part of your exercise routine. As your fat cells shrink, the added muscle mass will help your skin fit you better in some areas, such as the back of the arm. If you have more than 15 pounds to lose, work with your physician on a 6- to 12-month program.

Myth	Fact
8. Sit ups will remove fat from the stomach.	8. It requires reduced calories, regular exercise, and abdominal exercises to flatten your stomach. With calorie restriction, the fat cells in the stomach will shrink, and your stomach will get smaller. Your sit-up routine (see chapter 6) will strengthen the underlying muscle tissue. Both adipose and muscle tissue need changing; you cannot convert fatty tissue to muscle tissue, nor will muscle tissue change to fat when you become sedentary.
9. Laxatives help you lose weight.	9. The use of laxatives causes gastrointestinal trouble and can result in dehydration and undernourishment. It is better to be fat than to endanger your health. It is impossible to defecate away unwanted pounds safely.
10. Weight-reducing pills are a safe approach to depressing the appetite.	10. The use of drugs and drug combinations to depress appetite is dangerous and sometimes fatal. Drug usage is an attempt to cause weight loss by increasing metabolic rate, curbing the appetite, or causing fluid loss. Amphetamines and diuretics are the two most commonly used diet pills. Amphetamines toy with the thyroid gland, cause nervousness, speed up metabolism, and require increasingly stronger dosages as tolerance develops; diuretics result in rapid fluid loss. Both are dangerous, ineffective approaches to weight loss.
11. Reducing aids such as vibrators, body wraps, rubber suits, steam baths, and massage effectively remove fat from the body.	11. Each of these popular gimmick approaches to weight loss results in little calorie burning and is totally ineffective. To lose weight and fat, you must engage in exercise that burns a high number of calories, such as aerobics. You then enter a negative calorie balance and lose weight and fat.

A typical case involves a young woman from a middle-class family who values appearance more than self-worth and self-actualization. Typically, family ties are strong and the patient is efficient, eager to please her parents, and somewhat of a perfectionist. An absentee or distant father is also common. The characteristic behavior of anorexia is obsessive and compulsive, resembling addiction. Patients may become obsessed with the idea that they are, or will become, fat. They may fear the transition from girlhood to womanhood resulting in a more curvaceous figure, and become determined to stave it off by controlling their weight. This starvation approach is then carried to the extreme of undernourishment until total adolescent adult body weight is dangerously low. Even at that extreme, patients may still feel fat and continue to starve themselves, sometimes literally to death.

Young female anorexics generally develop **amenorrhea**. Females must reacquire 17 to 22 percent body fat before the menstrual cycle resumes. Young male anorexics lose their sex drive and become impotent. Thyroid hormone secretions, adrenal secretions, growth hormones, and blood pressure-regulating hormones reach abnormal levels. The heart pumps less efficiently as cardiac muscle weakens; the chambers diminish in size, and blood pressure falls. Heart rhythm disturbances and sudden stopping of the heart may occur due to lean-tissue loss and mineral deficiencies, producing sudden death in some patients. Other health problems include anemia, gastrointestinal problems, atrophy of the digestive tract, abnormal function of the pancreas, blood lipid changes, dry skin, decreased core temperature, and disturbed sleep.

Early treatment is essential if permanent damage is to be avoided. Without treatment, about 10 percent of the patients die of starvation. Forced feeding may temporarily improve health, but the condition can

Amenorrhea Loss of at least three consecutive menstrual cycles when they are expected to occur.

Behavioral Change and Motivational Strategies

Some of the more critical eating behaviors associated with weight gain that have high potential for behavior change include: drinking high-calorie drinks instead of water, consuming too much sugar, consuming too many foods high in saturated fat, binge eating, between-meal snacking, overeating at lunch and dinner, skipping breakfast or lunch, and failing to plan snacks. Exercise behaviors rated important and having the potential to be changed include: weekend leisure inactivity, long hours spent watching television, and no regular exercise program.

It is important to remember that you are in complete control of your own eating and exercise behavior. You have the power to alter behavior that is contributing to overfatness. Here is a table that includes some of the most common behavioral principles of weight loss. It should help you prepare specific motivational strategies to eliminate roadblocks.

Behavioral Principles of Weight Loss

1. Stimulus Control
   A. Shopping
      1. Shop for food after eating
      2. Shop from a list
      3. Avoid ready-to-eat foods
      4. Don't carry more cash than needed for shopping list
   B. Plans
      1. Plan to limit food intake
      2. Substitute exercise for snacking
      3. Eat meals and snacks at scheduled times
      4. Don't accept food offered by others
   C. Activities
      1. Store food out of sight
      2. Eat all food in the same place
      3. Remove food from inappropriate storage areas
      4. Keep serving dishes off the table
      5. Use smaller dishes and utensils
      6. Avoid being the food server
      7. Leave the table immediately after eating
      8. Don't save leftovers
   D. Holidays and Parties
      1. Drink fewer alcoholic beverages
      2. Plan eating habits before parties
      3. Eat a low-calorie snack before parties
      4. Practice polite ways to decline food
      5. Don't get discouraged by an occasional setback
2. Eating Behavior
   1. Put fork down between mouthfuls
   2. Chew thoroughly before swallowing
   3. Prepare foods one portion at a time
   4. Leave some food on the plate
   5. Pause in the middle of the meal
   6. Do nothing else while eating (read, watch television)

3. Reward
   1. Solicit help from family and friends
   2. Help family and friends provide this help in the form of praise and material rewards
   3. Utilize self-monitoring records as basis for rewards
   4. Plan specific rewards for specific behaviors (behavioral contracts)
4. Self-monitoring
   Keep diet diary that includes:
   1. Time and place of eating
   2. Type and amount of food
   3. Who is present/How you feel
5. Nutrition Education
   1. Use diet diary to identify problem areas
   2. Make small changes that you can continue
   3. Learn nutritional values of foods
   4. Decrease fat intake; increase complex carbohydrates
6. Physical activity
   A. Routine Activity
      1. Increase routine activity
      2. Increase use of stairs
      3. Keep a record of distance walked each day
   B. Exercise
      1. Begin a very mild exercise program
      2. Keep a record of daily exercise
      3. Increase the exercise very gradually
7. Cognitive Restructuring
   1. Avoid setting unreasonable goals
   2. Think about progress, not shortcomings
   3. Avoid imperatives like "always" and "never"
   4. Counter negative thoughts with rational restatements
   5. Set weight goals

Source: Reprinted with permission from *American Journal of Clinical Nutrition* 41 (1985): 823.
Copyright © 1985, American Society for Clinical Nutrition Inc.

Roadblock	Behavioral Change Strategy
Snacking before bedtime is a major problem. You just seem to get hungry after nine o'clock in the evening and often devour everything in sight.	You have identified one of the major eating habits contributing to weight and fat gain. To reduce the number of calories consumed between your evening meal and bedtime, try: 1. Going to bed by 10:00 PM or earlier; the longer you stay up, the more likely you are to eat and drink. 2. Preparing a tray of fruits and vegetables for snacking and placing it in the front of your refrigerator for easy access. 3. Taking a two- or three-mile walk several hours after your evening meal. 4. Drinking two or three glasses of water two hours after your evening meal.
You find that you are able to control snacking during the day but overeat at mealtime until you are stuffed and uncomfortable.	Try some of the following suggestions to reduce your intake at mealtime: 1. Eat one or two chocolate squares or drink three or four ounces of fruit juice about 30 minutes before mealtime to raise your blood-sugar level. 2. Drink two eight-oz glasses of water at mealtime before you eat anything. 3. Measure food quantities, and prepare only the amount you want to eat. 4. Eat a small amount of desert first, followed by your salad. 5. Take small portions and eat slowly, taking at least 30 minutes to complete the meal. 6. Never skip breakfast or lunch and never let yourself get too hungry; this is the main cause of overeating at the evening meal. 7. Take a walk or exercise an hour before mealtime.
You just cannot seem to find the time to exercise, and by the time the work day is over, you are too exhausted to even consider it.	Lack of time is the number one excuse of the sedentary individual. In most cases, even for extremely busy people, a 30-minute exercise session can be worked into the schedule. Evaluate each of the following to determine which suggestion may work for you: 1. Walk two or three miles each noon during your lunch break just before you eat. 2. Exercise moderately about two hours after your evening meal just prior to bedtime. 3. Consider getting up one hour earlier for a 30-minute exercise session followed by a shower. 4. Look into programs that aid muscle toning that you can perform at your desk and in your automobile.
Circle the behaviors in the table that you feel contribute to your weight problem or to a potential weight problem in the future.	Now prepare a list of some of the things you might try in order to eliminate the barriers and alter your behavior. Refer to the specific strategies discussed in this chapter, and if you need to, refer back to chapter 3 for behavioral-change and motivational strategies. 1. _____ 2. _____ 3. _____

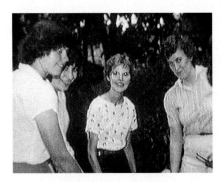

This woman developed anorexia nervosa in college because controlling her weight made her feel more in control of her life. (Photo Courtesy of Cable News Network.)

reappear unless proper psychological and medical therapy is initiated and is then successful. Treatment is directed at restoring adequate nutrition, avoiding medical complications, and altering the psychological and environmental patterns that have supported or permitted the emergence of anorexia. About 5 percent of those in treatment eventually reach 25 percent of their desired weight, and 50 to 75 percent resume normal menstrual cycles. After treatment ends, about 66 percent fail to eat normally and 7 percent die (of which 1 percent commit suicide).

Bulimia Bulimia is more common than anorexia nervosa and occurs in males as well as females. Ten to 20 percent of all college students are estimated to be bulimic. Only 5 percent of these students meet the criteria for anorexia nervosa, and less than 1 percent are actively anorexic. The typical profile of victims is similar to those suffering from anorexia nervosa, although they tend to be slightly older and healthier, malnourished but closer to normal weight. The bulimic binge is generally not a response to hunger, and the food is not consumed for nutritional value. As the binge-vomit cycle is repeated, medical problems grow. Fluid and electrolyte imbalance may lead to abnormal heart rhythm and kidney damage. Infections of the bladder and kidneys may cause kidney failure. Vomiting results in irritation and infection of the pharynx, esophagus, and salivary glands; erosion of the teeth; and dental caries. In some cases, the esophagus or the stomach may rupture.

Bulimic patients are more cooperative and somewhat easier to treat than anorexic patients since they seem to recognize that the behavior is abnormal. Most treatment programs attempt to help people gain control over their binge eating and encourage a minimum of 1500 calories daily. Lithium and other drugs have been shown to reduce the incidence of bulimic episodes by 75 to 100 percent. Most patients can also be helped by antidepressant medication.

*S*UMMARY

Causes of Obesity

Overfatness and obesity is caused by a number of factors with both genetics and environment playing key roles. Although it is a disadvantage to inherit the tendency to become fat, environment can overcome this predisposition. Inactivity and overeating are still the two major behaviors associated with weight and fat gain.

The body appears to defend its biological weight, referred to as *set point*, by resisting attempts to lose weight. Lowering the set point requires regular aerobic exercise and reduced caloric intake for 6 to 12 months or until it is evident that the body is now defending the lower weight and fat levels.

Overeating in infancy, bottle feeding instead of breast feeding, and early consumption of solid foods prior to the age of five months may contribute to the development of excess fat cells and overeating later in life.

Fat cells increase in number only until growth ceases, at which time one becomes fat only through the enlargement of existing adipose cells. Adults who become obese may develop some new fat cells.

Small changes in metabolism result in large increases or decreases in weight over a period of 6 to 12 months. Only a small percentage of individuals with weight problems suffer from an underactive thyroid gland. If this condition is suspected, it is wise to see a physician.

Body Composition

There are a number of ways to determine ideal body weight and percent of body fat. Height-weight tables should only be used as a guide to ideal weight since they provide no indication of percent of body fat, the key factor in determining health risks.

By measuring the thickness of two layers of skin and the underlying fat, you can secure an estimate of total body fat and identify ideal body weight. A number of different skinfold sites can be used. Electrical impedance and underwater weighing are more accurate techniques; however, special equipment is needed.

Safe Weight-Loss Procedures

Hunger is a physiological, inborn instinct designed to control food intake whereas appetite is a psychological, learned response. Although numerous theories have been advanced to explain how food intake is controlled, the exact signals that cue us to consume food have not been positively identified.

Calories count, and the body handles the matter with computer-like precision storing one lb of fat for every 3500 excess cal consumed.

Exercise is essential to the control of body weight and fat. Regular aerobic exercise depresses appetite, minimizes fat loss, maximizes the loss of lean-muscle tissue, burns a high number of calories, brings need- ed calcium to the bones, and changes the way the body handles dietary fat.

Special Diets

The majority of special diets fail. In many cases, this occurs within 5 to 7 days. Approximately 90 percent of those who succeed in losing weight will regain the weight within one year.

Dieting is extremely dangerous and can prove fatal if certain nutritional guidelines are not followed. The best approach is to develop sound exercise and eating habits that can be followed throughout life.

Underweight and Eating Disorders

Weight gain is just as difficult as weight loss. A complete program of muscle-weight gain requires sound nutritional support and an organized weight-training program that involves up to six, two-hour workouts weekly.

The number of cases of anorexia nervosa and bulimia continue to increase in the United States. As long as U.S. society places such high value on thinness, this trend will continue. Both disorders are extremely difficult to treat and can produce numerous health consequences and even death.

Lab Activity 9.1

Determining Your Percent of Body Fat

INSTRUCTIONS: *One way to determine your percent of body fat is to measure the thickness of four skin-folds. The procedure for measuring skinfold thickness is to grasp a fold of skin and* subcutaneous *(just under the skin) fat firmly with the thumb and forefinger, pulling it away and up from the underlying muscle tissue. Attach the jaws of the calipers one centimeter below the thumb and forefinger. All measurements should be taken on the right side of the body with the subject standing. Working with a partner, practice taking each other's measurements in the four areas described below.*

Triceps With the arm resting comfortably at the side, take a vertical fold parallel to the long axis of the arm midway between the tip of the shoulder and the tip of the elbow.

Biceps With the arm in the same position, take a vertical fold halfway between the elbow and top of the shoulder on the front of the upper arm.

Subscapula Just below the scapula (shoulder blade), take a diagonal fold across the back.

Suprailiac Just above the hip bone, take a diagonal fold following the natural line of the iliac crest.

Record the information below to complete your evaluation (for example, John is a 20-year-old who weighs 185 pounds. His four skinfold measurements were 16, 12, 42, and 15; follow his evaluation to help you understand the procedure):

1. Total of the four skinfold measures in millimeters
   (16, 12, 42, 15 = 85 millimeters)   85 mm

2. Percent of body fat based on this total from the table on page 202.
   Moving down in the first vertical column to 80 and over to the 17
   to 29 age group for males in column two, we find that John has
   about 24.8% fat.   24.8%

3. According to the percent of body fat from Table 9.3 on page 187,
   John's ideal fat percentage is 14.9% or less.   14.9%

4. Percent of fat to lose to reach the ideal percent from Table 9.3. John
   possesses about 10% too much fat (24.8 – 14.9 = 10) and therefore
   needs to lose 10% of his body weight.   10%

5. Total pounds of fat loss needed to reach ideal weight. Ten percent
   times 185 or 18.5 pounds of fat.   18.5

6. Ideal weight with 14.9% fat (high end of recommended ideal body
   fat for college men) is 167 (185 minus 18 = 167)   167

Fat as a Percentage of Body Weight Based on the Sum of Four Skinfolds, Age, and Sex

SKINFOLDS (MM)	PERCENT OF FAT, MALES (AGE IN YEARS)				PERCENT OF FAT, FEMALES (AGE IN YEARS)			
	17–29	30–39	40–49	50+	16–29	30–39	40–49	50+
15	4.8	—	—	—	10.5	—	—	—
20	8.1	12.2	12.2	12.6	14.1	17.0	19.8	21.4
25	10.5	14.2	15.0	15.6	16.8	19.4	22.2	24.0
30	12.9	16.2	17.7	18.6	19.5	21.8	24.5	26.6
35	14.7	17.7	19.6	20.8	21.5	23.7	26.4	28.5
40	16.4	19.2	21.4	22.9	23.4	25.5	28.2	30.3
45	17.7	20.4	23.0	24.7	25.0	26.9	29.6	31.9
50	19.0	21.5	24.6	26.5	26.5	28.2	31.0	33.4
55	20.1	22.5	25.9	27.9	27.8	29.4	32.1	34.6
60	21.2	23.5	27.1	29.2	29.1	30.6	33.2	35.7
65	22.2	24.3	28.2	30.4	30.2	31.6	34.1	36.7
70	23.1	25.1	29.3	31.6	31.2	32.5	35.0	37.7
75	24.0	25.9	30.3	32.7	32.2	33.4	35.9	38.7
80	24.8	26.6	31.2	33.8	33.1	34.3	36.7	39.6
85	25.5	27.2	32.1	34.8	34.0	35.1	37.5	40.4
90	26.2	27.8	33.0	35.8	34.8	35.8	38.3	41.2
95	26.9	28.4	33.7	36.6	35.6	36.5	39.0	41.9
100	27.6	29.0	34.4	37.4	36.4	37.2	39.7	42.6
105	28.2	29.6	35.1	38.2	37.1	37.9	40.4	43.3
110	28.8	30.1	35.8	39.0	37.8	38.6	41.0	43.9
115	29.4	30.6	36.4	39.7	38.4	39.1	41.5	44.5
120	30.0	31.1	37.0	40.4	39.0	39.6	42.0	45.1
125	30.5	31.5	37.6	41.1	39.6	40.1	42.5	45.7
130	31.0	31.9	38.2	41.8	40.2	40.6	43.0	46.2
135	31.5	32.3	38.7	42.4	40.8	41.1	43.5	46.7
140	32.0	32.7	39.2	43.0	41.3	41.6	44.0	47.2
145	32.5	33.1	39.7	43.6	41.8	42.1	44.5	47.7
150	32.9	33.5	40.2	44.1	42.3	42.6	45.0	48.2
155	33.3	33.9	40.7	44.6	42.8	43.1	45.4	48.7
160	33.7	34.3	41.2	45.1	43.3	43.6	45.8	49.2
165	34.1	34.6	41.6	45.6	43.7	44.0	46.2	49.6
170	34.5	34.8	42.0	46.1	44.1	44.4	46.6	50.0
175	34.9	—	—	—	—	44.8	47.0	50.4
180	35.3	—	—	—	—	45.2	47.4	50.8
185	35.6	—	—	—	—	45.6	47.8	51.2
190	35.9	—	—	—	—	45.9	48.2	51.6
195	—	—	—	—	—	46.2	48.5	52.0
200	—	—	—	—	—	46.5	48.8	52.4
205	—	—	—	—	—	—	49.1	52.7
210	—	—	—	—	—	—	49.4	53.0

In two-thirds of the instances the error was within ± 3.5% of the body-weight as fat for the women and ± 5% for the men.

Source: J.V.G.A. Dumin and J. Womersley, "Body Fat Assessed from Total Body Density and Its Estimation from Skinfold Thickness." *British Journal of Nutrition* (published by Cambridge University Press, Cambridge) 32 (1974): 95. Reprinted with the permission of Cambridge University Press.

Lab Activity 9.2

Determining Your Caloric Needs

INSTRUCTIONS: *Complete each of the following steps carefully to identify how many calories you need daily to attain and maintain your ideal weight as determined in Lab Activity 9.1: Determining Your Percent of Body Fat.*

1. Rate your level of physical activity from the list below by honestly estimating your activity level.

ACTIVITY PATTERN	CALORIES NEEDED PER LB
Very inactive (sedentary, never exercise)	13
Slightly inactive (occasional physical activity)	14
Moderately active (fairly active on the job; engage in aerobic exercise twice weekly)	15
Relatively active (almost always on the go; engage in aerobic exercise three to four times a week)	16
Frequent strenuous activity (daily aerobic exercise for one hour or more)	17

2. Multiply your rating (calories per pound) times your actual weight. A sedentary 18- to 21-year-old female who weighs 130 pounds, for example, would need 1690 calories per day ($130 \times 13 = 1690$). In theory, if she is consistently eating more than 1690 calories daily, she is gaining weight.

3. Multiply your physical activity rating times your ideal weight from Lab Activity 9.1: Determining Your Percent of Body Fat. This figure is the number of calories needed per day to maintain your ideal weight. The ideal weight in the example in Lab Activity 9.1: Determining Your Percent of Body Fat is 167 pounds. Since John is sedentary, he needs only 13 calories per pound and 2171 calories daily to maintain this weight ($167 \times 13 = 2171$).

Once you find your ideal weight, you can eventually reach that weight by consuming only the number of calories necessary to maintain that weight. This is a common, sound approach to weight and fat loss and is used in some clinics in the United States. Weight loss that occurs slowly and safely is much more likely to be maintained in the future.

10

STRESS MANAGEMENT AND PHYSICAL FITNESS

Chapter Objectives

By the end of this chapter, you should be able to:

1. Define stress, stressor, and stress reactivity.

2. List sources of stress and differentiate between distress and eustress.

3. Describe the bodily changes that occur when a person experiences stress.

4. Manage stress by using coping mechanisms at various levels of the stress response.

5. Use time management techniques to free up time for regular exercise.

6. Detail the role of exercise in the management of stress.

EMILIO'S WIFE DIED last year, and he grieved long and hard for her. He felt that her death was unfair (she was such a kind person), and a sense of helplessness crept over him. Loneliness became part of his days, and tears became the companions of his late evening hours. There were those who were not even surprised at Emilio's own death just one year after his wife's. They officially called it a heart attack, but his friends know he died of a broken heart.

You probably know some Emilio's—people who have died or become ill from severe stress with seemingly little physically wrong with them. That is what stress can do. You will soon learn how stress can actually change your body to make you susceptible to illness and disease or other negative influences. Contrary to what some people might tell you, it is not all in your mind. And you will learn how you can prevent these negative consequences from occurring, including the role of exercise in that process.

STRESS-RELATED CONCEPTS

Even the experts do not agree on the definition of **stress**. Some define it as the stimulus that causes a physical reaction (such as being afraid to take a test), while others view it as the reaction itself (for example, increases in blood pressure, heart rate, and perspiration). For our purposes in this text, we define stress as a combination of the cause (**stressor**) and the physical reaction (**stress reactivity**). The significance of these definitions is not merely academic. It is important to consider a stressor as having the potential to result in stress reactivity but not necessarily to do so.

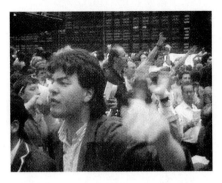

A demanding, fast-paced job can cause a great deal of stress if you let it. (Photo Courtesy of Cable News Network.)

Common Stressors

There are biological stressors (toxins, heat, cold), sociological stressors (unemployment), philosophical stressors (deciding on a purpose in life), and psychological stressors (threats to self-esteem, depression). Each has the potential to result in a stress reaction.

We all encounter stressors in our daily lives. You may have stressors associated with school (getting good grades, exams, or having teachers think well of you), with work (too much to do in a given amount of time, not really understanding what is expected of you, or fear of a company reorganization), with family (still being treated as a child when you are an adult, arguing often, lack of trust), or with your social life (making friends, telephoning for dates). Even scheduling exercise into your already busy day may be a stressor.

Stress Reactivity

When a stressor leads to a stress response, several changes occur in the body. The heart beats faster, muscles tense, breathing becomes rapid and shallow, perspiration appears under the arms and on the forehead, and blood pressure increases. These and other changes prepare the body to respond to the threat (stressor) by either fighting it off or running away. That is why stress reactivity is sometimes called the **fight-or-flight response**. Although many people consider the fight-or-flight response harmful, it is only bad for you if it is inappropriate to fight or run away, that is, when it is inappropriate to do something physical. For instance, if you are required to present a speech in front of your class, you cannot run from the assignment (you will fail the class if you do so) and you cannot strike out at the professor or

your classmates. It is in these situations, when you do not or cannot use your body's preparedness to do something physical, that the stress reaction is unhealthy. Your blood pressure remains elevated, more cholesterol roams about your blood, your heart works harder than normal, and your muscles remain tense. That, in turn, can lead to various illnesses, such as coronary heart disease, stroke, hypertension, and headaches. At this point, pay attention to your body, particularly to your muscle tension. If you think you can drop your shoulders, that means your muscles are unnecessarily raising them. If your forearm muscles can be relaxed, you are unnecessarily tensing them. This wasted muscle tension—since you are not about to do anything physical—is the result of stress and can cause tension headaches, back ache, or neck and shoulder pain. Lab Activity 10.1: Experiencing Stress Reactivity at the end of this chapter provides

Stress The combination of a stressor and stress reactivity.

Stressor A stimulus that has the potential to elicit stress reactivity.

Stress reactivity The physical reaction to a stressor that results in increased muscle tension, heart rate, blood pressure, and so forth.

Fight-or-flight response A physiological reaction to a threatening stressor; another name for stress reactivity.

Psychosomatic Illnesses or diseases that are either worsened or develop in the first place because of the body changes resulting from an interpretation of thoughts.

you with an activity to identify how your heart reacts to stress.

Psychosomatic Disease

When built-up stress products (for example, increased heart rate and blood pressure) are chronic, go unabated, or occur frequently, they can cause illness and disease. These are called **psychosomatic**, from the Greek words *psyche* (the mind) and *soma* (the body). That does not mean these conditions are all in the mind; instead it means that there is a mind-body connection causing the illness. An example is the effect of stress on allergies. Stress results in fewer white blood cells in the immunological system which, in turn, can lead to an allergic reaction (teary eyes, stuffy nose, itchy throat). That is because it is the white blood cells that fight off *allergens* (the substances to which people are allergic); fewer of them will make a person more susceptible to an allergic reaction.

To determine to what degree you experience physical symptoms of stress complete Table 10.1 on page 208. If your score indicates excessive physical stress symptoms, pay particular attention to the stress management techniques described later in this chapter.

A MODEL OF STRESS

Stress can be better understood by considering the model depicted in Figure 10.1 on page 209. The model begins with a *life situation* occurring that is *perceived as distressing*. Once it is perceived this way, *emotional arousal* (anxiety, nervousness, anger) occurs that, in turn, results in *physiological arousal* (increased heart rate, blood pressure, perspiration). That can lead to negative *consequences* such as psychosomatic illness, low grades at school, or arguments with family and friends.

Now let us see how the model operates in a stressful situation. Imagine you are a college senior and that all you need to graduate this semester is to pass a physical fitness class. Imagine further that you fail this class (life situation). You might say to yourself, "This is terrible. I will not be able to start work. I must be a real dummy. What will all my friends and relatives think?" In other words, you view the situation as distressing (perceived as distressing). That can result in fear and insecurity about the future, anger at the physical-fitness instructor, or worry about how

Diversity Issues

Stress and the Family

Stress is often the result of specific life events, such as school, work, or family. Greater sources of stress include loss of job, divorce, physical illness, or death in the family. An increasingly common stressor in the United States is the dual-career family. When both husband and wife work, whether the reasons are financial or career-goal oriented, they face such stress as how best to care for the children, how to find time to get the household chores done, and how to find enough quality time to spend as a family. When family responsibilities conflict with work requirements, such as when a child is sick and a parent needs to stay home, stress can build up.

There are no easy answers for alleviating dual-career family stressors. Sometimes the demands of work and family are severe and they need to be resolved creatively. Outlets for reducing stress include physical activity, relaxation, and time-management techniques. By working a combination of these stress relievers into their schedules, dual-career families can work their way toward a happier, healthier, lower-stress family life. ✦

friends and family members will react (emotional arousal). These emotions can lead to increased heart rate, muscle tension, and the other components of the stress response (physiological arousal). As a result, you can develop a tension headache or an upset stomach (consequences).

It is as though a road winds its way through the towns of Life Situation, Perceived as Stressful, Emotional Arousal, Physiological Arousal, and Consequences. And that means that, as with any road, a roadblock can be set up that interferes with travel. Remember, a stressor only has the potential to lead to stress. A roadblock can prevent that stressor from proceeding to the next "town." That is the very essence of stress management; that is, setting up roadblocks on the stress model to interfere with travel to the next level.

Using the example of failing a physical-fitness class again, imagine that your reaction was, "It's not good that I failed this course, but I still have my health and people who love me. They'll help me get

Table 10.1 ✦ Physical Stress Symptoms Scale

Indicate how often each of the following effects happen to you either when you are experiencing stress or following exposure to a significant stressor. Respond to each item with a number between 0 and 5, using the scale that follows:

0 = Never	2 = Every few months	4 = Once or more each week
1 = Once or twice a year	3 = Every few weeks	5 = Daily

Cardiovascular Symptoms

_____ Heart pounding   _____ Heart racing or beating erratically

_____ Cold, sweaty hands   _____ Headaches (throbbing pain)   Subtotal _____

Respiratory Symptoms

_____ Rapid, erratic, or shallow breathing   _____ Shortness of breath

_____ Asthma attack   _____ Difficulty in speaking because of poor breathing control   Subtotal _____

Gastrointestinal Symptoms

_____ Upset stomach, nausea, or vomiting   _____ Constipation

_____ Diarrhea   _____ Sharp abdominal pains   Subtotal _____

Muscular Symptoms

_____ Headaches (steady pain)   _____ Back or shoulder pains

_____ Muscle tremors or hands shaking   _____ Arthritis   Subtotal _____

Skin Symptoms

_____ Acne   _____ Dandruff

_____ Perspiration   _____ Excessive dryness of skin or hair   Subtotal _____

Immunity Symptoms

_____ Allergy flare-up   _____ Common cold

_____ Influenza   _____ Skin rash   Subtotal _____

Metabolic Symptoms

_____ Increased appetite   _____ Increased craving for tobacco or sweets

_____ Thoughts racing or difficulty sleeping   _____ Feelings of anxiety or nervousness   Subtotal _____

Overall Symptomatic Total (add all seven subtotals) _____

What Does Your Score Mean?

0 to 35   Moderate physical stress symptoms
A score in this range indicates a low level of physical stress manifestations, hence minimal overall probability of encounter with psychosomatic disease in the near future.

36 to 75   Average physical stress symptoms
Most people experience physical stress symptoms within this range. It is representative of an increased predisposition to psychosomatic disease but not an immediate threat to physical health.

76 to 140   Excessive physical stress symptoms
If your score falls in this range, you are experiencing a serious number and frequency of stress symptoms. It is a clear indication that you may be headed toward one or more psychosomatic diseases sometime in the future. You should take deliberate action to reduce your level of stress.

Source: Roger J. Allen and David Hyde, _Investigations in Stress Control._ Minneapolis, MN: Burgess, 1980, pp. 101–105.

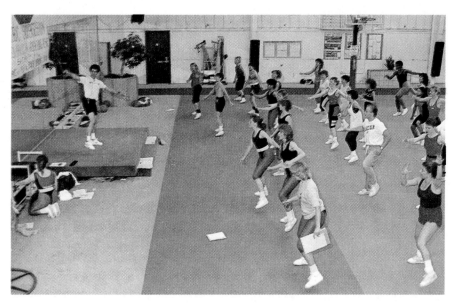

Exercise is particularly useful as a means of managing stress. (Photo Courtesy of the Aspen Hill Club.)

through this." In this case, the life situation is not perceived as distressing. Consider this change in perception a roadblock preventing emotional arousal. Without emotional arousal, there will be no physiological arousal and no negative consequences. In fact, there might even be positive consequences. Maybe failing the course will result in your studying extra hard the next time with the benefit of learning much more about physical fitness and becoming more fit than you would have been otherwise. In that instance, rather than experience distress you have experienced **eustress**. That is stress that results in personal growth and positive outcomes.

Figure 10.1 ✦ A Model of Stress

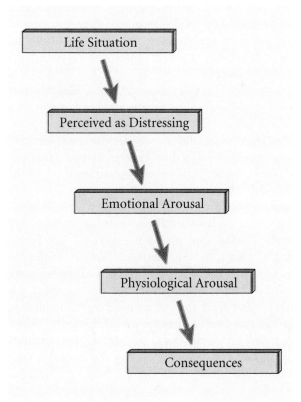

εXERCISE'S UNIQUE CONTRIBUTION TO STRESS MANAGEMENT

Exercise is a unique stress-management intervention since it can be plugged in at many levels on the stress model. It is a life situation intervention when you give up stressful habits (for example, cigarette smoking) because they interfere with your exercising. When you make friends through participating in a training program, you may also be using exercise as a life situation intervention since loneliness and social isolation may be remedied.

Eustress Stress that results in personal growth or development and, therefore, the person experiencing it is better for having been stressed.

Exercise can be a perception intervention as well. The brain produces neurotransmitters (endorphins) during exercise, and their euphoric, analgesic effect serves to relax the brain and the rest of the body. That relaxed state helps us perceive stressors as less stressful.

Exercise is also an emotional arousal intervention. During exercise, we focus on what we are doing and away from our problems and stressors. It can therefore be relaxing to engage in physical activity. Furthermore, numerous research studies have found that exercise enhances well being. It reduces feelings of depression and anxiety while increasing the sense of physical competence. The result is a higher level of self-esteem. And exercise can use up the built-up stress by-products and the body's preparedness to do something physical. Consequently, it can also be a physiological arousal intervention.

It is because of its unique ability to be plugged into all the different levels of the stress model that exercise is particularly useful as a means of managing stress. Be careful, however, to exercise in ways recommended in this book rather than inappropriately. Whereas exercise is an excellent stress-management coping mechanism, if it is done incorrectly, it can result in injury or discomfort. In that case, it will be a stressor rather than a stress reliever. And if exercise in itself is not your cup of tea but you participate anyway because you know it is good for you, you can still make it more pleasant. Exercise with a friend. Listen to music while you are exercising. Engage in physical activity out of doors in a pleasant setting, listening to the birds chirp and the wind rustling through the leaves. These and other accommodations can make your exercise more pleasing and, therefore, make you more likely to maintain your program.

Selective awareness A means of managing stress by consciously focusing on the positive aspects of a situation or person.

Progressive relaxation A relaxation technique in which you contract, then relax, muscle groups throughout the body.

Autogenic training A relaxation technique in which you imagine your arms and legs are heavy, warm, and tingly.

Body scanning A relaxation technique in which you identify a part of your body that feels relaxed and transport that feeling to another part of your body.

MANAGING STRESS

To manage stress you need to set up roadblocks at each level of the stress model.

The Life Situation Level

At the life situation level, you can make a list of all your stressors, routine ones that occur regularly and unusual ones that are often unanticipated. Then go through the list trying to eliminate as many of them as you can. For example, if you jog every day but find jogging stressful, try a different aerobic exercise or vary exercises from day to day. If you commute on a crowded highway and often become distressed about the traffic and construction slowdowns, try taking a different route. If you often argue with a friend and the associated stress interferes with your work, see the friend less often or not at all. There are probably many stressors that you tolerate by habit but that can be eliminated, thereby decreasing the stress in your life.

The Perception Level

You can perceive or interpret stressors that cannot be eliminated as less distressing. One way to do that is called **selective awareness**. In every situation there is some good and some bad. Choosing to focus on the good, while not denying the bad, will result in a more satisfying and less distressing life. For example, rather than focusing on the displeasure of standing in line at the checkout counter, you choose to focus on the pleasure of being able to do nothing when your day is usually so hectic.

Consider the story about a female college student who wrote her parents that she was in a hospital after having fallen out of her third-floor dormitory window. Luckily, she landed in some shrubs and was only temporarily paralyzed on her right side (that explained why her handwriting was so unclear). In the hospital, she met a janitor, fell in love with him, and now they are planning to elope. The reason for eloping is that he is of a different religion, culture, and ethnic background and she suspected her family might object to the marriage. She is confident, though, that the marriage will work since her lover learned from his first marriage not to abuse his spouse and since the jail term he served reinforced that lesson. She went on to say in the letter, "Mom and Dad, I really am not in a hospital, have not fallen out of any window, and have not met someone with whom I am planning on eloping. However, I did fail chemistry and wanted you to be able to put that in its proper perspective." Now that is selective awareness.

The Emotional Arousal Level

An excellent way to control your emotional responses to stress is to engage regularly in some form of relaxation. Some of the more effective ways of relaxing are described in this section.

There is no research to allow us to diagnose which relaxation technique is best for you. The only way to determine that is to try several and evaluate their ability to make you feel relaxed. To help you do that we have provided a relaxation technique rating scale (Table 10.2 on page 212). Use it after you try each of the relaxation techniques.

Progressive Relaxation With **progressive relaxation**, you first tense a muscle group for 10 seconds, all the while paying attention to the sensations that are created. Then relax that muscle, paying attention to that sensation. The idea is to learn what muscular tension feels like so you will be more likely to recognize it when you are experiencing it and to be familiar with muscular relaxation so that, when you are tense, you can relax those muscles. It is called *progressive* because you progress from one muscle group to another throughout the body.

Autogenic Training **Autogenic training** involves imagining your arms and legs are heavy, warm, and tingly. When you are able to imagine that, you are increasing the blood flow to those areas. This precipitates the relaxation response. After the body is relaxed, think of relaxing images (a day at the beach, a park full of trees and green lawn, a calm lake on a sunny day) to relax the mind.

Body Scanning Even when you are tense, there is some part of your body that is relaxed. It may be your thigh or your chest or your hand. The relaxation technique called **body scanning** requires you to search for a relaxed body part and transport that feeling to the tenser parts of your body. That can be done by imagining the relaxed part as a fiery, hot ball that you roll to the tenser parts of your body. The more you practice this technique, the more effective you will become with it. This is true with all relaxation techniques.

Biofeedback This technique involves the use of an instrument to mirror what is going on in the body

Fitness Heroes

Mike Utley was a young, successful, professional football player. During a game, he was hit by another player, broke his neck, and was completely paralyzed. He and his wife were devastated when doctors predicted that he would never walk again. Mike, however, predicted otherwise.

Determined to walk as well as he used to, Mike struggled through years in therapy. After extensive sessions came a breakthrough—Mike was able to wiggle his toe. Last year, without any help, he stood for the first time on his own with only a walker and steel braces.

Every day is full of challenges for Mike Utley. Although he is walking, he still requires regular therapy to help him learn to control his muscle functions. Things that he took for granted before, such as walking to the refrigerator to get a drink, are much more challenging than they used to be, but he doesn't let it stop him.

Mike's mental and physical strength gave him the ability to fight and to overcome. He is a true fitness hero. ✦

and to report the results back to the individual. Biofeedback instrumentation can measure and *feed back* to the person numerous physiological parameters: temperature, blood pressure, heart rate, perspiration, breathing rate, muscle tension, brain waves, and many others. One interesting aspect of biofeedback is that individuals can control these previously thought-to-be involuntary responses once the measure has been reported back to them. The physiological parameters already enumerated in this paragraph can be increased or decreased with biofeedback training. Since the body and the mind are connected, changes in either can effect changes in the other. Consequently, when a person is taught to decrease heart rate and muscle tension, for example, the psychological states of anxiety and nervousness may also be decreased.

Lab Activity 10.2: Measuring the Effects of Meditation teaches meditation, which is another effective relaxation technique. Complete this lab activity at the end of the chapter to determine the effectiveness of meditation for you.

Table 10.2 ✦ The Relaxation Technique Rating Scale

To determine which is most effective for you, try each relaxation technique presented in this chapter and evaluate it by answering these questions, using this scale:

1 = Very true

2 = Somewhat true

3 = I'm not sure

4 = Somewhat untrue

5 = Very untrue

1. It felt good.

2. It was easy to fit into my schedule.

3. It made me feel relaxed.

4. I handled my daily chores better than I usually do.

5. It was an easy technique to learn.

6. I was able to shut out my surroundings while I was practicing this technique.

7. I did not feel tired after practicing this technique.

8. My fingers and toes felt warmer after trying this relaxation technique.

9. Any stress symptoms I had (headache, tense muscles, anxiety) before doing this relaxation technique disappeared by the time I was done.

10. Each time I concluded this technique, my pulse rate was much lower than it was when I began.

Now sum up the values you responded with for a total score. Compare the scores of all the relaxation techniques you try. The lower the score, the more appropriate a particular relaxation technique is for you.

Source: Jerrold S. Greenberg, *Comprehensive Stress Management,* 4th Edition. Dubuque, IA: Wm. C. Brown, 1993, p. 183.

The Physiological Arousal Level

This is the point at which your body is already prepared to do something physical. To manage stress at this level requires engaging in some physical activity, which can range from the obvious to the obscure. Running around the block as fast as you can will use the stress by-products and do wonders for your disposition. Dribbling a basketball up and down the court mimicking several fast breaks, serving 30 tennis balls as

hard as you can, biking as fast as you can, or swimming several laps at breakneck speed, as well as other tiring exercises, can also relieve stress. Still you need not engage in formal sports activities to relieve stress at this level on the model. You can simply punch your mattress or pillow as hard and as long as you can. You will not hurt them nor yourself, but you will feel better.

> **Type A behavior pattern** A constellation of behaviors that makes individuals susceptible to coronary heart disease.
>
> **Type B behavior pattern** A combination of behaviors that seem to protect people from contracting coronary heart disease, i.e., lack of hostility, anger, aggression; cooperativeness; focusing on one task at a time.

TYPES A AND B BEHAVIOR PATTERNS AND THE EXERCISER

Researchers have discovered a **behavior pattern (Type A)** related to the subsequent development of coronary heart disease. Type A people are aggressive and competitive, never seem to have enough time, do two or more things at once (this is called being *polyphasic*), are impatient, and become angry easily. **Type B behavior pattern** seems to be protective of the development of coronary heart disease. Type B

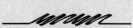

Myth and Fact Sheet

Myth	Fact
1. Stressful events of necessity cause stress and a stress reaction.	1. Stressful events only have the potential to cause a stress reaction. They need not do so if they are interpreted as nonstressful.
2. There is really nothing that can be done about stress. It is just a normal part of living.	2. There are many ways to manage stress so it does not make you ill or interfere with the satisfaction you derive from living.
3. Exercise is stressful because of the toll it takes physically.	3. Exercise is an excellent way of managing stress since it responds to every level of the stress model.
4. You should try to eliminate all stress from your life.	4. There is an optimal level of stress that results in joy and stimulation and encourages your best performance. Therefore, you need some stress to make life worth living.

people exhibit no free-floating hostility, always seem to have enough time to get things done and if they do not do so they are not worried, are more cooperative than competitive, and are concerned with quality rather than quantity (it is not how fast they run but whether they enjoy their run).

Recent research has clarified the relationship between Type A and coronary heart disease. It appears that the hostility is the trait of major concern. People who tend to become angry easily are more apt to develop coronary heart disease than are others.

Our friend Jorge, mentioned on page 41, characterizes the Type A exerciser. If you remember, on a sunny, windless day, Jorge was playing tennis when he hit one too many backhands that went awry. Losing control, he threw his racket over the fence, over several trees, and into the creek alongside the court. As the racket floated downstream never to be seen again, Jorge was at a loss about what to berate more severely, his tennis skills or his temper. This aggressiveness and hostility are classical characteristics of Type A behavior.

Type A exercisers are aggressive (they may smack their golf clubs into the ground when they hit a shot off target), hostile (they may accuse their opponents of cheating), competitive (losing may be more than they can bear), and evaluate themselves by numbers (how many matches they won rather than whether they played well or had fun participating). If you see yourself as a Type A, think about a change. Use the behavior change techniques and strategies presented in chapter 3 to become more Type B. You may be healthier, and you will probably be happier.

TIME MANAGEMENT: FREEING UP TIME TO EXERCISE

To manage stress, you need to set aside time. To exercise regularly, you also need to set aside time. Since stress can capture your attention, energy, and time, it can interfere with your exercise regimen. After all, stress can be a threat to your physical self or to your self-concept. Who can blame you for postponing or canceling exercise to manage that threat? This section shows you how to organize your time better so there is plenty of time for exercise, managing stress, and the myriad of other things you need, and choose, to do.

To be serious about using time-management strategies you need to realize that:

1. Time is one of your most precious possessions.

2. Time spent is gone forever.

3. You cannot save time. Time moves continually and it is used, one way or another. If you waste time, there is no bank where you can withdraw the time you previously saved to replace the time wasted.

4. To come to terms with your mortality is to realize that your time is limited. None of us will live forever, and none of us will be able to do everything we would like to do.

You can *invest* time to free up (not to save) more time than that you originally invested. Then you will have sufficient time to use the stress-management techniques presented in this chapter and plenty of time to participate in a regular exercise program. The techniques we will now describe will help you to do that. As you read the following suggestions for better managing your limited time, try to make direct application of these techniques to your situation. Most of these techniques you will want to incorporate into your lifestyle; others you will decide are not worth the effort or the time.

Assessing How You Spend Time

As a first step, analyze how you spend your time now. To do this, divide your day into 15-minute segments as shown in Table 10.3. Record what you are doing every 15 minutes. Review this time diary and total the time spent on each activity throughout the day. For example, you might find you spent three hours socializing, four hours eating meals, three hours watching television, one hour doing homework, two hours shopping, two hours listening to music, six hours sleeping, and three hours on the telephone as shown on the example in Table 10.4 on page 216. Evaluate your use of time as shown in Table 10.4, and note in the *adjustment* column that, even while study time by an hour, the adjustment would free up 6.5 hours a day. That would leave plenty of time to exercise. A good way to actually make the changes you desire is to draw up a contract with yourself that includes a reward for being successful. Refer to chapter 3 for the most effective way to develop such a contract.

Table 10.3 ✦ Daily Activity Record

Time (AM)	Activity	Time (PM)	Activity
12:00		12:00	
12:15		12:15	
12:30		12:30	
12:45		12:45	
1:00		1:00	
1:15		1:15	
1:30		1:30	
1:45		1:45	
2:00		2:00	
2:15		2:15	
2:30		2:30	
2:45		2:45	
3:00		3:00	
3:15		3:15	
3:30		3:30	
3:45		3:45	
4:00		4:00	
4:15		4:15	

Table 10.3 ✦ Daily Activity Record *(continued)*

Time (AM)	Activity	Time (PM)	Activity
4:30		4:30	
4:45		4:45	
5:00		5:00	
5:15		5:15	
5:30		5:30	
5:45		5:45	
6:00		6:00	
6:15		6:15	
6:30		6:30	
6:45		6:45	
7:00		7:00	
7:15		7:15	
7:30		7:30	
7:45		7:45	
8:00		8:00	
8:15		8:15	
8:30		8:30	
8:45		8:45	
9:00		9:00	
9:15		9:15	
9:30		9:30	
9:45		9:45	
10:00		10:00	
10:15		10:15	
10:30		10:30	
10:45		10:45	
11:00		11:00	
11:15		11:15	
11:30		11:30	
11:45		11:45	

Table 10.4 ✦ Summary of Daily Activities

ACTIVITY NEEDED	TOTAL TIME SPENT ON ACTIVITY	ADJUSTMENT
Socializing	3 hours	1 hour less
Eating meals	4	1 hour less
Watching television	3	1.5 hours less
Doing homework	1	1 hour more
Shopping	2	1 hour less
Listening to music	2	1 hour less
Sleeping	6	None
On telephone	3	2 hours less

Prioritizing

One important technique for managing time is to prioritize your activities. Not all of them are of equal importance. You need to focus on those activities of major importance to you, and only devote time to other activities after the major ones are completed. One of the major activities for which you should prioritize your time is exercise.

To prioritize your activities, develop A, B, C lists. On the A list (Table 10.5) place those activities that *must* get done, that are so important that not to do them would be very undesirable. For example, if a

Table 10.5 ✦ A. List of Activities for Today

LIST ONLY THOSE ACTIVITIES ON WHICH YOU MUST SPEND TIME TODAY.

1. _____
2. _____
3. _____
4. _____
5. _____
6. _____
7. _____
8. _____
9. _____
10. _____

Table 10.6 ✦ B. List of Activities for Today

LIST THOSE ACTIVITIES ON WHICH YOU WOULD LIKE TO SPEND TIME TODAY BUT THAT COULD WAIT UNTIL TOMORROW.

1. _____
2. _____
3. _____
4. _____
5. _____
6. _____
7. _____
8. _____
9. _____
10. _____

term paper is due tomorrow and you have not typed it yet, that gets on your A list.

On the B list (Table 10.6) are those activities you would like to do today and need to get done. If they don't get done today, however, it would not be too terrible. For example, if you have not spoken to a

Table 10.7 ✦ C. List of Activities for Today

LIST THOSE ACTIVITIES TO WHICH YOU WILL DEVOTE TIME TODAY ONLY IF AND AFTER YOU HAVE COMPLETED ALL A AND B ACTIVITIES.

1. _____
2. _____
3. _____
4. _____
5. _____
6. _____
7. _____
8. _____
9. _____
10. _____

close friend and have been meaning to telephone, you might put that on your B list. Your intent is to call today, but if you don't get around to it, you can always call tomorrow or the next day.

On the C list (Table 10.7) are those activities you would like to do if you get all the A- and B-list activities done. If the C-list activities never get done, that is no problem. For example, if a department store has a sale and you would like to go browse, put that on your C list. If you do all of the As and Bs, you can go browse.

In addition, make a list of things not to do. For example, if you tend to waste your time watching television, you might want to include that on your not-to-do list (Table 10.8). In that way, you will have a reminder not to watch television today. Other time wasters should be placed on this list as well.

Other Ways to Free Up Time for Exercise

There are numerous other time-management strategies you can use to make time for exercise.

Say No Because of guilt, concern for what others might think, or a real desire to engage in an activity, we often have a hard time saying no. A, B, C lists and prioritizing your activities will help identify how much time remains for other activities and make saying no easier.

Table 10.8 ✦ Not-to-Do List of Activities for Today

LIST THOSE ACTIVITIES ON WHICH YOU WILL AVOID SPENDING TIME TODAY.

1. _____
2. _____
3. _____
4. _____
5. _____
6. _____
7. _____
8. _____
9. _____
10. _____

Delegate to Others When it is possible, get others to do things that need to be done but that do not need your personal attention. Conversely, avoid taking on chores that others try to delegate to you. This does not mean that you use other people to do work you should be doing or that you do not help out others when they ask. What it means is that you should be more discriminating regarding delegation of activities. Another way of stating this is not to hesitate to seek help when you are short on time and overloaded. Help others when they really need it and when you have the time available to do so.

Give Tasks the Once-Over Many of us will open our mail, read through it, and set it aside to act on it later. This is a waste of time. If we pick it up later, we have to familiarize ourselves with it once again. As much as possible, look things over only once.

Use the Circular File How many times do you receive junk mail that is obvious from its envelope and in spite of knowing what is enclosed in the envelope and that you will eventually throw it all out anyhow, you probably still take the time to open it and read the junk inside. You would be better off bypassing the opening and reading part, and going directly to the throwing out part. That would free up time for more important activities, such as exercise.

Limit Interruptions Throughout the day you will be interrupted. Recognizing this fact, you should actually schedule in times for interruptions. That is, don't make your schedule so tight that interruptions will throw you into a tizzy. On the other hand, try to keep these interruptions to a minimum. There are several ways you can accomplish this. You can accept phone calls only between certain hours. You can also arrange to have someone take messages so you can call back later, or you can use an answering machine. Do the same with visitors. Anyone who visits should be asked to return at a more convenient time, or you can schedule a visit with them for later. If you are serious about making better use of your time, you will adopt some of these means of limiting interruptions.

Recognize the Need to Invest Time The bottom line of time management is that you need to invest time initially in order to free it up later. We often hear people say, "I don't have the time to organize myself the way you suggest. That would put me further in the hole." This is an interesting paradox. If you are so pressed for time that you believe you do not even have sufficient time to get yourself organized, that in

Behavioral Change and Motivational Strategies

There are many things that might interfere with your ability to manage stress. Here are some barriers (roadblocks) and strategies for overcoming them.

Roadblock	Behavioral Change Strategy
You may have a lot to do with little time to get it all done. Term papers are due, midterm or final exams are approaching, you are invited to a party, you are expected to attend a dinner celebrating your sister's birthday, your team is scheduled for an intramural game, and your professor is holding a study session.	When responsibilities are lumped together, they often appear overwhelming. Use the behavior change strategy of *divide and conquer*. Buy a large calendar, and schedule the semester's activities by writing on the calendar when you will perform them, when you will do library research for term papers, when you will begin studying for exams, and when you will read which chapters in which textbooks. Do not forget to include nonacademic activities as well. For example, write your intramural team's schedule and times of parties or dinners to attend on the calendar. You will soon realize that you have plenty of time. You just need to get organized. That realization will go a long way in relieving unnecessary stress.
You are not accomplishing your fitness objectives and because of that you feel distressed. You are not running as fast as you would like to run, nor are you lifting the amount of weight you would like to lift, doing the number of repetitions you would like to do, losing the amount of weight you would like to lose, or participating in aerobic dance classes.	Use *goal setting* strategies outlined in chapter 3. Set realistic fitness goals; give yourself enough time to achieve them; and make your workout fun. If you are distressed because your goals seem elusive, perhaps they are. Maybe they are too difficult to achieve or too difficult to achieve in the amount of time you have allotted. If you are injuring yourself regularly, perhaps your fitness program is too difficult or too intense. Use *gradual programming* and *tailoring* to devise a program specific to you and to the level of fitness you presently possess.
You try to relax but you cannot. Your thoughts seem nonstop. Your body becomes fidgety. You are anxious to move on to do something that needs doing. Finding the time to engage in a relaxation technique is impossible. You are just too busy.	Use *material reinforcement* to encourage the regular practice of relaxation. Every time you set aside time to relax, reward yourself with something tangible. You might put aside a certain amount of money or buy a healthy snack. Another behavior change technique that could help is *boasting*. Be proud of taking time to relax and share that feeling of pride with friends. That will make you feel good and more likely to engage in that relaxation technique again.
	You will also need to assess periodically your relaxation method. Use Table 10.2 to help you perform this assessment. You will find that some relaxation techniques are more effective for you than others, so you will learn which ones to use regularly.
List roadblocks interfering with your ability to manage stress.	Cite behavior-change strategies that can help you overcome the roadblocks you just listed. If you need to, refer back to chapter 3 for behavioral-change and motivational strategies.
1. _____	1. _____
2. _____	2. _____
3. _____	3. _____

itself tells you that you are in need of applying time-management strategies. The investment in time devoted to organizing yourself will pay dividends by allowing you to achieve more of what is really impor-tant to you. After all, what is more important than your health and wellness? And, what better way is there to achieve health and wellness than freeing up time for regular exercise?

SUMMARY

Stress-Related Concepts

Stress can be defined as a combination of the cause (stressor) and the physical reaction (stress reactivity). A stressor has the potential to result in stress reactiv-ity, but does not necessarily do so. Whether it does depends on how the stressor is perceived or inter-preted. Stressors can take a variety of forms: biologi-cal (toxins, heat, cold), sociological (unemployment), philosophical (deciding on a purpose in life), or psy-chological (threats to self-esteem or depression).

When a stressor leads to a stress response, sever-al changes occur in the body. The heart beats faster, muscles tense, breathing becomes rapid and shallow, perspiration appears under the arms and on the fore-head, and blood pressure increases. These and other changes make up the fight-or-flight response.

When built-up stress products (for example, in-creased heart rate and blood pressure) are chronic, go unabated, or occur frequently, they can cause illness and disease. These are called *psychosomatic.* That means these conditions consist of a mind-body inter-action that causes the illness or makes an existing dis-ease worse.

A Model of Stress

A model to better understand stress and its effects begins with a life situation occurring that is perceived as distressing. Once the situation is perceived this way, emotional arousal occurs (anxiety, nervousness, anger), which in turn results in physiological arousal (increased heart rate, blood pressure, muscle tension, perspiration). This can lead to negative consequences such as psychosomatic illness, low grades at school, or arguments with family and friends. The essence of stress management is to set up roadblocks on the stress model to interfere with travel to the next level.

The goal, however, is not to eliminate all stress. Certainly, some stress (distress) is harmful. On the other hand, some stress is useful since it encourages peak performance, or eustress.

Exercise's Unique Contribution to Stress Management

Exercise is a unique stress-management interven-tion since it can be plugged in at many levels on the stress model. It is a life situation intervention when you give up stressful habits because they interfere with exercising. It is a perception intervention when your brain produces neurotransmitters during exer-cise that make you feel relaxed. It is an emotional arousal intervention when you focus on the physical activity and ignore problems and stressors. And it is a physiological arousal intervention when you use the built-up stress by-products by doing something physical.

Managing Stress

Managing stress involves interventions at each of the levels of the stress model. At the life situation level, you can assess routine stressors and eliminate them. At the perception level, you can use selective awareness. At the emotional arousal level, you can do progressive relaxation, autogenic training, body scan-ning, biofeedback training, and meditation, and at the physiological level, you can exercise regularly.

Types A and B Behavior Patterns and the Exerciser

People who are aggressive, competitive, never seem to have enough time, do two or more things at once, are impatient, and become angered easily exhibit Type A behavior patterns. Type As are prone to coronary heart disease, with the most harmful characteristic being free-floating hostility. Type B people, who exhibit no free-floating hostility, always seem to have enough time to get things done, are more cooperative than competitive, and are concerned with quality rather than quantity, seem to be protected from de-veloping coronary heart disease.

Time Management: Freeing Up Time to Exercise

Time can not be saved, but you can free up time by being more organized. Some effective time-management strategies include assessing how you spend time so you can make sensible adjustments, prioritizing your activities, learning to say no so you do not take on too many responsibilities, delegating tasks to others, looking things over only once, avoiding spending time on junk mail, and limiting interruptions. Time invested in applying time-management strategies will pay off in terms of freeing up time for such important activities as regular exercise.

Lab Activity 10.1

Experiencing Stress Reactivity

INSTRUCTIONS: *While seated in a comfortable position, determine how fast your heart beats at rest using one of these methods. (Use a watch that has a second hand.)*

1. Place the first two fingers (pointer and middle finger) of one hand on the underside of your other wrist, on the thumb side. Feel for your pulse and count the number of pulses for 30 seconds.

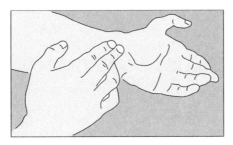

2. Place the first two fingers of one hand on your lower neck, just above the collar bone; move your fingers toward your shoulder until you find your pulse. Count the pulse for 30 seconds.

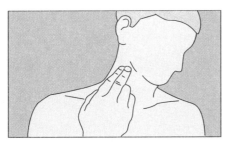

3. Place the first two fingers of one hand in front of your ear; move your fingers until you find a pulse. Count the pulse for 30 seconds.

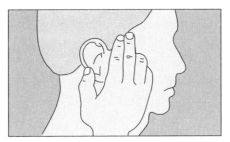

Multiply your 30-second pulse count by two to determine how many times your heart beats each minute while you are at rest. Now close your eyes and think of either someone you really dislike or some situation you experienced that really frightened you. If you are recalling a person, think of how that person looks and smells and what he or she does to incur your dislike. Really feel the dislike, do not just think about it. If you recall a frightening situation, try to place yourself back in that situation. Sense the fright, be scared, vividly recall the situation in all its detail. Think of the person or situation for one minute and then count your pulse rate for 30 seconds, as you did earlier. Multiply the rate by two and compare your first total with the second.

Most people find that their heart rates increase when they are experiencing stressful memories. This increase occurs despite a lack of any physical activity; the very thoughts increase heart rate. This demonstrates two things: the nature of stressors and the nature of stress reactivity.

Source: Jerrold S. Greenberg, *Comprehensive Stress Management,* 4th Edition. Dubuque, IA: Wm. C. Brown, 1993, p. 11.

Lab Activity 10.2

Measuring the Effects of Meditation

INSTRUCTIONS: *Learning how to meditate is easy. Just close your eyes and repeat the word* calm *or* one *or some other relaxing word in your mind every time you exhale. Make sure not to eat anything or ingest a stimulant beforehand. Stimulants such as caffeine or nicotine will interfere with your ability to relax. Do this for 20 minutes but recognize that no one can stay focused on a word for that long. As soon as you realize your mind has wandered, just return to repeating the relaxing word as you did before.*

To measure whether meditation has a relaxing effect on you, follow these instructions:

1. Using one of the techniques presented in Lab Activity 10.1: Experiencing Stress Reactivity, determine your resting pulse rate per minute. Place that number in the space marked "Pulse Rate before Meditating."

2. After determining how fast your heart beats at rest, meditate for 20 minutes. Be sure not to set an alarm clock since it will speed up your heart rate when it goes off. Merely look at your watch when you think 20 minutes has passed.

3. After meditating, determine your pulse rate per minute again. Place that number in the space marked "Pulse Rate after Meditating."

Pulse Rate before Meditating _____

Pulse Rate after Meditating _____

Difference in Pulse Rate _____

Most people find their heart rate decreases after meditating (or engaging in any other relaxation technique). That finding should not be unexpected since we know that one of the effects of relaxation is to slow down the heart.

11

How Chemicals Affect Physical Fitness

Chapter Objectives

By the end of this chapter, you should be able to:

1. Differentiate between drug use, misuse, and abuse and give examples of each.

2. Describe the prevalence of alcohol on college campuses and make suggestions for drinking responsibly.

3. Cite methods taken by colleges to control alcohol on their campuses.

4. Describe the prevalence of tobacco use and its effects on the body.

5. Describe strategies to quit smoking and/or to make smoking less harmful.

6. List drugs used to enhance athletic performance and discuss their safety and effectiveness.

The Thomas and the Lopez families both experienced a very difficult year. Glenn Thomas was diagnosed with angina (pain in the chest due to constricted coronary arteries) and started taking nitroglycerin pills periodically. His wife, Barbara, contracted a sinus infection in February and was prescribed antibiotics. In May her gynecologist recommended she begin regular doses of estrogen to replace her body's decreased production of estrogen caused by menopause. Their son, Clark, was diagnosed with Attention Deficit Disorder and his pediatrician put him on the drug Ritalin.

The Lopezes were no more fortunate. Felipe decided that he needed assistance to stop smoking and was encouraged by his doctor to wear a nicotine patch. Flore Lopez was diagnosed with high blood pressure and instructed to take hypertension medication daily. And Melinda, the Lopez's teenage daughter, was found to be anemic and began taking an iron supplement each day.

More than ever before, drugs—prescription and nonprescription drugs—are available to treat medical and psychological conditions, thereby improving the quality of our lives. Without these drugs, the Thomases and the Lopezes would not feel as well each day and would probably either live shorter lives and/or have their activities limited.

You, too, are a drug user; we all are. In fact, America is a drug-taking society. And, in many respects, it is fortunate that we are. Think about the important drugs we use:

1. Vaccines that provide protection from diseases that can wipe out whole societies.

2. Antibiotics that control previously fatal bacterial diseases.

3. Oral contraceptives that help some people plan families, and that have a profound, though controversial, effect on our society.

4. Tranquilizers that allow people with mental illness to function.

For all the good that has come from drugs, many people believe that U.S. society has become too reliant on medication and mood-altering substances. Too often the remedy for anxiety is a tranquilizer, the response to a headache is an aspirin or some other painkiller, the answer to a problem is alcohol, and social occasions are more stimulating with cocaine.

DRUG USE, MISUSE, AND ABUSE

You will soon see that differentiating between drug use, misuse, and abuse is not as easy as it at first appears. Start this section by listing the last ten times you can remember taking a drug.

Drug Use

Your list probably includes an occasion when you were ill and took either a drug prescribed by your physician or one available over the counter. Perhaps you had a strained muscle from exercising and took aspirin or ibuprofen to control the inflammation and pain. If you used this drug properly, it probably

---

Drug use The proper use of a drug.

Drug misuse The inappropriate use of a legal drug.

Drug abuse The use of an illegal drug or the use of a legal drug for purposes other than those it was intended for.

Cirrhosis A scarring of cells of the liver that is associated with the excessive use of alcohol.

---

helped you overcome your illness. In fact, this drug might have been so important to your health that if you had not used it, you may have gotten even more ill. For example, if you contract pneumonia and do not take the antibiotic prescribed for you, you might die. This is **drug use**; that is, when drugs are used as they are recommended to be used and for the purposes for which they were recommended.

Drug Misuse

Unfortunately, some people ruin a good thing. They take too many aspirin tablets in too short a period of time, or ingest ibuprofen without drinking enough fluids. The result could be intestinal problems such as bleeding stomach caused by damage to stomach tissue. When a legal drug is used inappropriately, it is **drug misuse**.

Drug Abuse

When an illegal drug is used or when a legal drug is used for purposes other than for what it was intended, that is **drug abuse**. Typical drugs of abuse include marijuana, cocaine, heroin, anabolic steroids, and amphetamines. These drugs are often taken for the euphoria they produce rather than for any medical or physiological reason. Legal drugs that are sometimes abused include Demerol (meperidine), Dilaudid (hydromorphine), and Darvon (propoxyphene). These drugs are prescription pain relievers that are sometimes sold illicitly for their narcotic effects.

Drugs That Are Difficult to Categorize

Although the differentiation between drug use, misuse, and abuse may at first appear clear, there are a number of drugs and drug usages that are difficult to categorize. For example, how would you classify the use of tobacco products? They are legal but cause the body harm. What about the use of alcoholic beverages? In this case, the amount of drug used (the dosage) might dictate its categorization. And, in which category would you place the use of over-the-counter diet remedies? They, too, can be taken in excessive amounts or in place of changes in eating and exercise habits.

Space dictates we limit our discussion of drugs and fitness, and the effects of drugs on health and wellness. Consequently, we have chosen to discuss only the more prevalent drugs or those with direct application to physical fitness.

ALCOHOL

Studies indicate that 64 percent of young adults aged 18 to 25 are current consumers of alcohol, and in general almost half of men (46 percent) and a quarter of women (25 percent) are heavy drinkers who average four or more drinks daily (National Center for Health Statistics, pp. 104 and 108). Drinking starts even earlier. Thirty-one percent of high school seniors report that most or all of their friends get drunk at least once a week. This situation is probably not dissimilar to what occurs on college campuses throughout the United States (see Table 11.1). Alcohol is the drug of choice on college campuses and leads to too many accidents, fights, suspensions and expulsions from school, injuries, and even death. All of this occurs in spite of the legal drinking age in many states having been returned to 21 in recent years.

People drink for many reasons: to relax, to be sociable, to have something to do with their hands during social occasions, and to decrease inhibitions and become less shy. When drinking is limited, alcohol-related problems usually do not occur. When too much alcohol is ingested in too short a period of time, is taken with other drugs or medications, or is combined with events requiring coordination and speedy reflexes (such as driving an automobile), however, serious consequences can result.

Alcohol's Effects

Alcohol affects the body in many different ways. It results in blood vessels in the head dilating, which can lead to headaches. It also increases heart rate and blood pressure while at the same time constricting (narrowing) the blood vessels supplying the heart. And when the liver is subjected to excessive doses of alcohol over a period of time, it too can be damaged. **Cirrhosis** of the liver is a condition to which alcoholics are prone; it is irreversible and sometimes leads to death. Malnutrition, cancer (of the liver,

---

Table 11.1 ✦ Facts and Figures on College Students and Alcohol

The U.S. Department of Health and Human Services reports these statistics pertaining to college students and alcohol:

- Of the current student body in the United States, between two and three percent will eventually die from alcohol-related causes, about the same number that will get advanced degrees, masters and doctorate degrees combined.

- For the over 12 million college students in the United States, the annual consumption of alcoholic beverages totals well over 430 million gallons. To visualize this, imagine an Olympic-sized swimming pool filled with beer, wine, and distilled spirits. In a single year, the student body of each college in the country drinks the equivalent of one pool.

- Over one-half of all college students participate in drinking games that involve the consumption of extremely high quantities of alcohol. The average amount consumed in these games is between six and ten drinks in a short period of time.

- Approximately 35 percent of all college newspaper advertising revenue comes from alcohol advertisements.

- Fraternity members drink more frequently and more heavily than other college students.

- Depending on the particular study, between 53 and 84 percent of college students get drunk at least once a year. Between 26 and 48 percent get drunk once a month.

- College administrators believe alcohol is a factor in 34 percent of all academic problems and in 25 percent of dropouts.

- Almost half of college athletes who drink admit that their use of alcohol has had a harmful or slightly harmful effect on their athletic performance.

Source: U.S. Department of Health and Human Services, *Prevention Resource Guide: College Youth.* Washington, DC: DHHS Publication No. (ADM) 91-1803, 1991.

Diversity Issues

Alcohol

Alcohol use has its own cultural, ethnic, and gender differences. For instance, women drink less than men, have relatively low rates of heavy drinking, and have fewer alcohol-related problems.

African-American men are less likely to drink than are white men, and, of the drinkers, white men are more likely to be heavy drinkers. However, African-American men are more likely to experience health problems and symptoms of alcohol dependence than are their white counterparts. Nearly half of African-American women are abstainers, compared to one-third of white women.

Drinking rates among Hispanics differ considerably depending on gender and country of origin. Therefore, studies that group all members of Hispanic societies together have limitations. Some studies indicate that more than 70 percent of Hispanic women drink either less than once a month or not at all, whereas the same percentage of Hispanic men are drinkers. More than half of male Hispanics in Spain report drinking nearly every day. The cultural mores in Spain value drinking as a relaxant as well as a stimulant.

Asian Americans have the lowest level of alcohol consumption and alcohol-related problems of all ethnic groups in the United States. The moral and cultural standards of Asian populations suggest that drinking and becoming inebriated are not acceptable behaviors. ✦

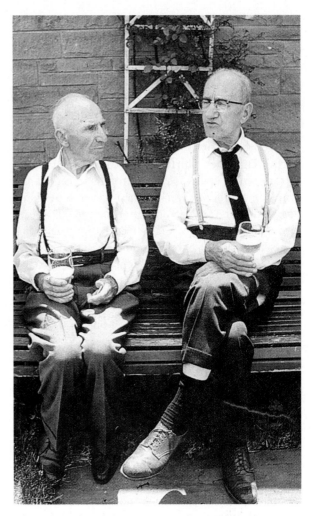

Although it is a social custom for friends to share a drink together, too much alcohol can lead to dependence and a range of illnesses. (Photo Courtesy of the National Cancer Institute.)

esophagus, nasopharynx, and larynx), endocrine and reproductive problems, neurological disorders, and mental illness are but a few other potential effects of the abuse of alcohol.

How to Take Control of Your Drinking

As you can see in Table 11.2, alcohol can significantly impair your physical functioning. To be physically fit, be healthy, and possess a high level of wellness all require either abstaining from ingesting alcohol or drinking responsibly. That means limiting the amount of alcohol ingested to no more than one drink containing no more than 0.6 fluid ounces of alcohol per hour (the amount your liver can metabolize in an hour), drinking only when it is appropriate and never when you are driving, and refraining from drinking when you need good judgment.

And yet, saying no to alcohol is often easier said than done. Imagine that your friends drink alcohol every time you socialize. Either they go to a bar near campus, bring in beer and sit around and drink, or attend a party where alcohol is available. If you do not drink, they will think you are strange. You fear they might not want anything more to do with you. What can you do?

You can adopt any of the following strategies:

1. Take one drink and nurse it for a long time to limit the amount of alcohol you ingest.

Table 11.2 ✦ Effects of Blood-Alcohol Level (BAL) on Functioning

BAL	EFFECTS OF ALCOHOL ON FUNCTIONING
Less than .03	Reflexes, sensory function generally intact, but subtle changes can be detected with sensitive tests.
.03–.05	Greater impairment of judgment, reflexes, and coordination; alterations of sensory perception; changes are enough to alter driving skills but not enough to be illegal in the United States; occurs after consuming the equivalent of 2 oz of 86-proof spirits, 8 oz of wine, or two 12-oz beers.
.05–.15	Judgment, reflexes, and coordination usually impaired measurably; blood levels above .1 are sufficient for a charge of legally impaired driving; the equivalent of six oz of 86-proof spirits, drunk quickly, is enough to produce a blood level of .15.
.15–.40	Moderate to severe intoxication with deteriorating judgment, reflexes, and coordination; aggressive behavior often develops, followed by progression to lethargy, sedation.
.40–.60	Severe intoxication; individual usually sleeps and arousal is difficult; blood levels of approximately .5 or more are liable to produce coma and death.

Source: From *The Nurse, Pharmacology, and Drug Therapy,* Second Edition, by Marshal Shlafer. Copyright (©) 1993 by Addison-Wesley Publishing Company. Reprinted by permission.

2. Tell your friends you are taking medication that prohibits you from drinking.

3. Invite someone else to join you who also does not want to drink. With company it will be easier to withstand peer group pressure.

4. Practice refusal skills in which you assertively tell your friends that you prefer not to drink. Do so without turning them off by not being judgmental. For example, you might say, "You can drink if you like but I would prefer not to." You might have to say this several times for your friends to believe you mean it, but once they do, they will usually accept your decision.

If you do decide to drink, however, follow these guidelines:

1. Drink in moderation.

2. Never drink on an empty stomach. Food in your stomach will slow down the absorption of the alcohol.

3. Never drink when you are taking medication.

4. Never ingest alcohol in combination with other drugs.

5. Drink slowly.

6. Dilute your drinks with water or a mixer.

7. Do not drink and eat salty or spicy foods at the same time. The salts and spices will make you thirsty, and you will drink more.

Too many people have a problem with alcohol. To determine whether you have a problem with alcohol, complete Lab Activity 11.1: Signs of Alcoholism at the end of this chapter.

Alcohol on College Campuses

A number of strategies have been developed in response to the problems created by alcohol on college campuses. These include, but are not limited to, the following:

1. Some universities have offered dry bars. That is, bars that only serve nonalcoholic beverages. Then students can gather and meet as they do at alcoholic bars but with neither the pressure nor the opportunity to ingest alcohol. An example is the University of Maryland's Dry Dock.

2. Some universities have offered hangover-free Friday mornings that include music and dancing.

3. A national organization has formed to educate students about how to drink responsibly,

how to help friends who have been drinking from experiencing problems (such as driving drunk), and how to control their own drinking. This organization, funded by the alcohol industry, is called BACCHUS (Boost Alcohol Consciousness Concerning the Health of University Students) and is now present on many campuses across the United States.

4. College theater groups have presented skits educating students regarding responsible use of alcohol. An example is the Wellesley College's Alcohol Information Theater (Project WAIT).

5. Sporting and other events on campuses that once boasted of having kegs of beer are refraining from the alcohol connection. An example is George Washington University where they used to have a "Miller's Rocks the Block" party with free beer, T-shirts, and hats distributed. Now, although the beer distributors are still present on the George Washington campus, they no longer provide beer; instead, they sponsor a superdance for Muscular Dystrophy.

6. On some campuses, college administrators have prohibited beer kegs at parties and re-

Table 11.3 ✦ Alcohol-Related Groups, Organizations, and Programs for College Students

Al-ANON Family Groups, Inc.
World Service Office
P.O. Box 862, Midtown Station
New York, NY 10159
212-254-7230
1-800-344-2666

Alcohol Policies Project Center for Science in the Public Interest
1875 Connecticut Avenue, NW, #300
Washington, DC 20009
202-332-9110

Alcoholics Anonymous (AA)
World Service, Inc.
468 Park Avenue, South
New York, NY 10016
212-686-1100

American College Health Association
15879 Crabbs Branch Way
Rockville, MD 20855
301-963-1100

American College Personnel Association
Central Michigan University
Mt. Pleasant, MI 48859
517-774-3381

American Council on Education
One Dupont Circle
Washington, DC 20036
202-466-5030

Campuses Without Drugs, Inc.
National Office
2530 Holly Drive
Pittsburgh, PA 15235
412-731-8019

Center for Science in the Public Interest
1875 Connecticut Avenue, NW, #300
Washington, DC 20009
202-332-9110

The Coalition of (Campus) Drug and Alcohol Educators
250 Arapahoe, Suite 301
Boulder, CO 80302
303-443-5696

Commission on Alcohol and Other Drugs of the American College Personnel Association
Central Michigan University
Mt. Pleasant, MI 48859
517-774-3381

Health Promotion Resources
509 University Avenue
St. Paul, MN 55103
1-800-782-1878

Integrated Substance Abuse Consultants (INSAC)
P.O. Box 7505
Arlington, VA 22205
703-237-3840

Nar Anon Hotline
800-780-3951

National Association of Student Personnel Administrators
One Dupont Circle, Suite 330
Washington, DC 20036
202-293-9161

The Marin Institute for the Prevention of Alcohol and Other Drug Problems
24 Belvedere Street
San Rafael, CA 94901
415-456-5692

National Interfraternity Conference
3901 West 86th Street
Suite 390
Indianapolis, IN 46268
317-872-1112

National Organization of Student Assistance Programs and Professionals (NOSAPP)
250 Arapahoe, Suite 301
Boulder, CO 80302
800-972-4636

Network of Colleges and Universities Committed to the Elimination of Drug and Alcohol Abuse
Office of Educational Research and Improvement
U.S. Department of Education
555 New Jersey Avenue, SW
Washington, DC 20208-5644
202-357-6265

Peterson's Drug and Alcohol Programs and Policies
Dept. 9377
P.O. Box 2123
Princeton, NJ 08543
800-338-3282

quire that food and soft drinks be served where beer is available. Such a policy was begun at Roanoke College in Virginia.

7. Universities such as William and Mary College, the University of Virginia, James Madison University, and Louisiana State University have instituted dry fraternity and sorority rushes.

8. At the University of Maryland, campus-area alcohol retailers have begun a program entitled SUDS (Students Understanding Drinking Sensibly). They distribute SUDS T-shirts and buttons, train local bartenders, and arrange for local police officers to have breathalyzers available for those drinkers who voluntarily choose to have their blood-alcohol levels tested.

What is your campus doing to respond to both the pressure to drink and the problems resulting from the consumption of alcohol? If you decide to become proactive, you can obtain assistance from the organizations listed in Table 11.3.

TOBACCO

Another too prevalent drug is tobacco and its products. These include cigarettes, cigars, pipes, and chewing tobacco. The U.S. government estimates that tobacco use is responsible for one of every six deaths in the United States and is the most preventable cause of death and disease in our society. Tobacco use is the major risk factor for heart and blood diseases; chronic bronchitis and emphysema; cancers of the lung, larynx, pharynx, oral cavity, esophagus, pancreas, and bladder; and other problems such as respiratory infections and stomach ulcers. Cigarette smoking accounts for approximately 390,000 deaths each year including 21 percent of coronary disease deaths, 87 percent of lung cancer deaths, and 30 percent of all cancer deaths. Smokers of more than two packs of cigarettes a day are 15 to 25 times more likely to die of lung cancer than people who never smoked (U. S. Department of Health and Human Services, p. 137).

Smoking Rates

It is estimated that by the late 1990s smoking rates for women will exceed those for men. Presently, 32 percent of men and 27 percent of women aged 20 and older smoke cigarettes. Overall, 29 percent of the people in the United States smoke (U. S. Department of Health and Human Services, p. 140). Most people

Diversity Issues

Smoking

The United States Department of Health and Human Services recognized cultural, gender, and ethnic differences related to cigarette smoking. These differences were translated into Year 2000 National Health Objectives. Several are described below.

Gender
Presently 32 percent of men and 27 percent of women smoke. One Year 2000 health objective speaks to decreasing the overall rate of smoking among people aged 20 and older to no more than 15 percent. Among *pregnant women,* the objective is to decrease smoking from the present 25 percent to 10 percent. Among *women of reproductive age,* the objective is to decrease smoking from the present 29 percent to 12 percent. And, among *women who use oral contraceptives,* the objective is to decrease smoking from the present 36 percent to 10 percent.

Other Variables
In addition, the national health objectives are directed toward decreasing cigarette smoking among other groups.

1. People with a high school education or younger than 20; from 34 percent to 20 percent.
2. Blue-collar workers aged 20 and older; from 36 percent to 20 percent.
3. Military personnel; from 42 percent to 20 percent.
4. African-Americans aged 20 and older; from 34 percent to 18 percent.
5. Hispanics aged 20 and older; from 33 percent to 18 percent.
6. Native Americans/Alaska Natives; from 42 to 70 percent to 20 percent.
7. Southeast Asian men; from 55 percent to 20 percent.
8. Lower economic status youth; from 40 percent to 18 percent. ✦

start smoking regularly when they are young, before the age of 20. If that same percentage of the 70 million children in the United States start smoking and continue smoking cigarettes as adults, at least 5 million of them will die of smoking-related diseases.

Smokeless Tobacco

Smokeless tobacco includes primarily moist or dry snuff and chewing tobacco. It is used by almost seven percent of males aged 12 through 17 and nine percent of males aged 18 through 24 (U. S. Department of Health and Human Services, p. 147). Smokeless tobacco users are quite susceptible to oral cancer, with long-term snuff users being 50 times more likely to develop oral cancer than nonusers. Adolescent males make up the great majority of new users of smokeless tobacco (only one percent of females use it). They may see their favorite athlete (usually a baseball player) chew tobacco and emulate that behavior.

Tobacco's Effects on the Body

Tobacco effects the body in many ways. The nicotine in tobacco is a central nervous system stimulant and therefore increases the heart rate. Tobacco use also constricts blood vessels, increases blood pressure, destroys air sacs in the lungs, and increases the production of hydrochloric acid in the stomach. The result is shortness of breath; upset stomach; cold and clammy fingers and toes; the development of heart disease, hypertension, stroke, emphysema, and/or digestive disorders; and lung and other cancers.

Why People Use Tobacco Products

Before reading further, complete Lab Activity 11.2: Why Do You Smoke? at the end of this chapter. If you are not a smoker, complete the Lab Activity by guessing how most smokers would respond to the statements presented.

The purpose of tobacco advertising is to sell tobacco products. And they do a pretty good job of it as the statistics presented above prove. In our search to be desirable, envied, "cool," and admired we are taught to emulate the people depicted in the tobacco product ads. They are handsome and pretty, they are smiling and obviously happy, and they appear wealthy enough to have fine furniture and expensive clothing.

There are other reasons people use tobacco products. They provide something to do with the hands. Best friends or parents may smoke, so their behavior is copied. It is *anti-authority* (schools and workplaces disallow it and parents often object) and, therefore, "cool" to do. It relieves boredom and is psychologically relaxing for some people, in spite of it being a central nervous system stimulant. It substitutes for food and can be used to control weight.

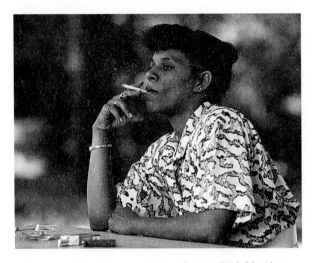

Tobacco use contributes to heart disease, high blood pressure, cancer, emphysema, and numerous other illnesses, and is one of the largest causes of disease in the United States. (Photo Courtesy of the National Cancer Institute.)

How to Quit

Researchers have found that the best way to quit smoking is simply to quit. That might sound simplistic but what usually happens is that smokers try to quit when they are not really committed to doing so. Eventually they get to the point where they are well motivated and during that next attempt are successful. That is why it is difficult to cite any one program that is better than another. The key ingredient in any program is the motivation and seriousness of the smoker wishing to quit.

Imagine you smoke cigarettes and cannot seem to quit. They relax you after dinner and give you something to do with your hands during social occasions. You have tried to quit many times without any success. Do not give up. There are strategies you can employ that are effective.

You can write a *contract* using the form in chapter 3 with the goal being to decrease the number of cigarettes you smoke progressively over several weeks until you quit altogether. The contract can be witnessed by a friend or relative who will check on your progress at predetermined intervals.

You can also use *chaining*. In this case you want to increase the links in the chain leading to smoking. For example, you can take your pack of cigarettes and place it in a sweat sock. Then wrap the sock with masking tape and place it in a locked draw as far away from where you usually smoke as possible (perhaps upstairs if you tend to smoke downstairs). Next, take the key to the drawer and place that in the other sock, wrap it with masking tape, and deposit it in a drawer far away from the drawer in which the pack of cigarettes is located. Now to smoke, you have to go through a bunch of inconveniences. Compare this to just reaching into your pocket or pocketbook and lighting up almost without thinking.

Here are some other suggestions that can help motivated smokers stop smoking or at least lessen the harm they expose themselves to:

- Smoke only one cigarette per hour and eventually taper down.
- Smoke exactly half as many cigarettes each week as you did the week before.
- Inhale less and with less vigor, avoiding deep inhalation.
- Smoke each cigarette only halfway.
- Remove the cigarette from your mouth between puffs.
- Smoke slowly.
- Smoke brands with low tar and nicotine content.
- Place unlighted cigarettes in your mouth when you have the urge to smoke.
- Switch to a brand you dislike.
- Put something else in your mouth when you want a cigarette (for example, chewing gum, fruit, hard candy).
- Exercise regularly so you do not smoke out of boredom.
- Develop the sense of wanting to do well by your body.
- Spend time in places where smoking is prohibited.
- Brush your teeth directly after every meal.
- Alter your behavior pattern. For example, avoid friends who smoke for several weeks after quitting and substitute another activity for smoking after dinner.
- Remind yourself frequently why you quit smoking.

Anabolic steroids Drugs that are derivatives of the male sex hormone testosterone; sometimes used illegally by those desiring to increase their body size, speed, or strength.

- Use the other behavior change techniques discussed in chapter 3 to quit smoking.

DRUG-TAKING TO ENHANCE ATHLETIC PERFORMANCE

Athletes are competitive by nature. They try hard to beat someone else at their sport or, competing against themselves, strive to do better than they have ever done before. It stands to reason they would want whatever edge they can get. This desire to perform at their best has led some athletes to a search for drugs that can enhance performance. Among these drugs are anabolic steroids, caffeine, amphetamines, and cocaine.

Anabolic Steroids

So you want to be strong? So you want to run faster than you ever thought you could? Well, forget about all the work of weight training or exercise that makes you perspire. Try steroids. In today's quick-weight-loss, quick-fitness, quick-everything society why not engage in quick bulking up? As we shall soon see, the answer to that question is No. The use of anabolic steroids is quite dangerous.

Anabolic steroids made the news when Olympic world-record-holder Ben Johnson was disqualified from receiving a gold medal for winning the 100-meter sprint at the 1988 Olympic Games. When he was routinely tested just after the race, Johnson tested positive for a steroid. The death of former professional football player Lyle Alzado of cancer, which was attributed to anabolic steroid use in an attempt to gain strength, also fueled the publicity about these drugs.

Anabolic steroids are derivatives of the male sex hormone testosterone. They are prescribed as treat-

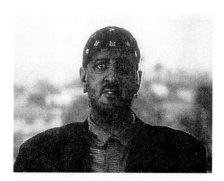

Lyle Alzado blamed his years of steroid use for his brain cancer, which eventually caused his death. (Photo Courtesy of Cable News Network.)

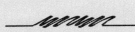

Myth and Fact Sheet

Myth	Fact
1. Beer will not get you as drunk as hard liquor will.	1. It is the alcohol that is responsible for inebriation. You can ingest just as much alcohol from beer as you can from other sources.
2. Drinking alcohol is relaxing.	2. A small amount of alcohol initially acts as a stimulant. Larger amounts depress the central nervous system. The feeling of relaxation, however, is because the brain is deadened. The price paid is that other bodily functions are depressed as well, such as the ability to think well or be coordinated. The result can be accidents or poor decisions that result in injury or ill health.
3. Anabolic steroids can make you a better athlete.	3. There is no scientific evidence that using steroids will in any way increase athletic performance.
4. Being physically fit and possessing a high level of wellness means never using drugs.	4. We all use drugs. We take prescribed antibiotics, we buy over-the-counter cold remedies, and we ingest aspirin or ibuprofen when our muscles ache. The key is to use safe drugs safely, as they were intended to be used.

ment for anemia and growth problems and as an aid in recovery from surgery. A black market has developed, however, and steroids are illegally used to increase body weight and muscle mass, gain power, and increase strength.

Steroids can be taken in pill form or injected directly into the blood stream. It is not unusual for steroid users to take more than one steroid at a time, believing that by doing so the effect will be hastened or enhanced. This is called *stacking*.

Steroid users place themselves at risk for liver cancer, high blood pressure, heart disease, sterility, and increased hostility. In men steroid use can lead to atrophied testicles, prostate cancer, and breast growth. In women it can result in menstrual irregularities, a deepening of the voice, decreased breast size, baldness, and facial hair growth. In both men and women, anabolic steroid use can lead to clogging of the arteries, eating compulsions, and increased aggressiveness.

The *Physician's Desk Reference* (p. 2122) states that "anabolic steroids have not been shown to enhance athletic ability." And the American College of Sports Medicine (ACSM) states that although steroids can increase body weight and muscular strength, they do not increase aerobic power or the capacity for exercise. The ACSM goes on to say that anabolic steroid use is contrary to the rules and eth-

ical principles of athletic competition, and that they deplore its use by athletes. And yet, almost five percent of high school seniors, not to mention other students and athletes, use anabolic steroids illegally.

Suppose, in the gym in which you work out, there are many men and women your age who look fantastic. The men are chiseled. Their muscles are round and hard, and they do not have a inch of fat on them—or so it seems. And the women are curved to perfection. They have muscles in all the right places and are round where they should be round. Upon inquiring, you learn they take steroid drugs. Without the drugs, you are told, they would not look so good. You would love to look like they do and are tempted to try these drugs. How can you overcome this temptation?

You can always use *selective awareness*. Instead of focusing on how good you could look if you took steroids, concentrate on their potential effect on your liver, your sexual organs (atrophied or shrunken testicles if you are a male and menstrual irregularities if you are a female), and the threat they pose to your life. Imagine you could be the most chiseled corpse ever, without any life to enjoy the perfect body.

You could also use *covert modeling*. After watching someone weight train who looks good and does not take steroids, close your eyes and imagine you are doing just what you observed the other person doing.

Smell the smells, hear the noise, see the sights, and so forth. Make it vivid. Refer back to chapter 3 for other ways to take charge of your behavior.

Caffeine

Caffeine is a stimulant drug that appears in coffee, tea, chocolate, and soft drinks. Caffeine can activate the brain, thereby decreasing drowsiness and fatigue. It also increases heart and breathing rates. In addition, caffeine serves as a stimulant for skeletal muscles and enables the body to use fatty acids for energy better. The result is an increase in physical work output. That is why caffeine has been suggested as an aid to physical fitness and athletic activities.

Caffeine consumption as an adjunct to physical activity, however, is not recommended because caffeine can have serious side effects. Depending on the dosage, caffeine can result in irregular heart beat, hyperactivity, headache, insomnia, an increase in low-density lipoprotein (LDL) which is associated with coronary heart disease, and low birth weight when consumed by pregnant women.

Amphetamines

Amphetamines are central nervous system stimulant drugs. They result in increased heart rate, blood pressure, rate of breathing, and blood sugar and in high arousal levels. It is this psychological arousal effect, along with the physiological arousal effects, that disguises muscle fatigue so greater work output can occur.

Amphetamines should not be used to increase work output for several reasons. First, there is no evidence to show that their use enhances athletic performance. In fact, they may even interfere with athletic performance by increasing hyperactivity when more controlled physical responses are needed. Second, amphetamine users often become dependent on these drugs and to come down from an amphetamine high resort to taking barbiturates. This yo-yo drugging effect can be quite dangerous. Not enough people know that barbiturates are extremely addictive and that withdrawing from them without medical supervision can be deadly.

Cocaine

Cocaine is another drug people take to improve physical performance or for "recreational" reasons. Cocaine can be snorted through the nose, smoked as crack, or injected. It, too, can increase work output by

Fitness Heroes

John Lucas was a star basketball player at the University of Maryland. He was a first player draft pick in the NBA, leading him down the path to stardom and money. But the good life got the best of him; John got caught up in drugs and became addicted to cocaine. His habit cost him his wife, his children, and a promising professional basketball career.

John's fighting spirit was the only thing that rehabilitated him. It took several years, but John turned his life around. He fought hard to reestablish his career, and he became the head coach of the San Antonio Spurs in 1993. He was so successful that he was even mentioned as a candidate for coach of the year.

While he spent a good deal of time turning his own life around, John was also concerned about the effects of drug abuse on his fellow athletes. He recently opened a drug-treatment center so that he could help other drug-dependent athletes recover. ✦

the nature of its stimulating effect on the central nervous system. It also produces a euphoria that disguises fatigue.

Aside from cocaine being illegal, however, it can result in dire consequences. It can cause tremors and rapid heart beat, raise blood pressure dangerously high to the point of threatening stroke, lower the effectiveness of the immune system thus subjecting its users to various illnesses, and decrease appetite resulting in malnutrition. In addition, it can cause acute anxiety, confusion, and depression. In a few cases, *cocaine psychosis* has occurred in heavy users, leading to delusions and violence.

Caffeine A stimulant drug present in coffee, tea, and colas and other soft drinks that have not been decaffeinated.

Amphetamines Drugs that stimulate the central nervous system, increasing heart rate, blood pressure, and other body processes.

Cocaine A drug that stimulates the central nervous system and that can cause tremors, rapid heart beat, and harmful psychological effects.

Behavioral Change and Motivational Strategies

There are many things that might interfere with your healthy use of chemical substances. Here are some barriers (roadblocks) and strategies for overcoming them.

Roadblock	Behavioral Change Strategy
You want to quit smoking but you are afraid you will gain weight. Your looks are important to you. Therefore, you decide not to stop smoking in order to look better.	The U.S. Public Health Service reports that 60 percent of women and 47 percent of men say they continue to smoke because they are afraid of gaining weight. And yet most smokers do not gain weight when they quit. In fact, only one-third gain weight, another one-third stay the same weight, and the rest actually lose weight. Even when weight gain does occur, it is usually minimal and certainly worth the health benefits of not smoking.
Weight gain is only one of the excuses smokers use for not quitting. Others include, "The air is polluted anyway, I might as well smoke," and "It's too late to quit, I've been smoking too long."	Knowledge can go a long way in dispelling these myths. The truth is that the U. S. Public Health Service advises that even in heavily polluted urban areas, the concentration of pollutants in the air are tiny in comparison with the concentrations of them in cigarette smoke. Regarding smoking for a long time, it is never too late to prevent a serious disease. After you quit, your chances of dying from smoke-related diseases gradually decreases until they are close to those of people who have never smoked.
You have an important examination next Tuesday so you plan to stay up all Monday night studying. Around 1:00 AM. Tuesday morning, however, you start feeling drowsy so you think about drinking a large amount of caffeine to keep going. You realize, though, that a large amount of caffeine can make your heart beat irregularly, give you a headache, and increase the LDL in your blood.	Of course, the best strategy is to plan to study for several nights rather than pulling an all-nighter. But, given you did not follow this advice, you can use selective awareness to focus on the benefits you will derive from getting some sleep. It will make your learning more efficient since you will not be drugged, it will be healthier, and you will be more alert during the examination. A few hours of sleep can do wonders for your performance. You can also focus on the negative aspects of ingesting a lot of caffeine. After all, who wants to subject themselves to heart problems? A bad grade on an examination is better than a bad electrocardiogram (ECG).
List roadblocks interfering with your using chemicals appropriately.	Now cite behavior-change strategies that can help you overcome the roadblocks you just listed. If you need to, refer back to chapter 3 for behavioral-change and motivational strategies.
1. _____	1. _____
2. _____	2. _____
3. _____	3. _____

SUMMARY

Drug Use, Misuse, and Abuse

When drugs are used as they are recommended and for the purposes for which they were recommended, that is drug use. When a legal drug is used inappropriately, that is drug misuse. When an illegal drug is used or a legal drug is used for purposes other than those for which it was intended, that is drug abuse.

Alcohol

Alcohol is the most prevalent drug on college campuses. It is so widely used that it is estimated that between 2 and 3 percent of the current college student body will eventually die from alcohol-related causes. Between 53 and 84 percent of college students get drunk at least once a year, and between 26 and 48 percent get drunk once a month.

Alcohol dilates blood vessels in the head thus causing headaches; narrows the blood vessels supplying the heart; damages cells in the liver; often leads to malnutrition, endocrine, and reproductive system problems; and can cause cancer in several body sites.

Drinking responsibly means not getting inebriated by limiting the amount of alcohol ingested to no more than one average-sized drink (.6 fluid ounces) an hour, drinking only when appropriate, never drinking and driving, and refraining from drinking when good judgment is needed. To control drinking drink in moderation, never drink on an empty stomach, never drink when taking medication, never ingest alcohol in combination with other drugs, drink slowly, dilute drinks, and do not eat salty or spicy foods when drinking.

Tobacco

Tobacco use is the most preventable cause of death in the United States. It is the major risk factor for heart and blood diseases; chronic bronchitis and emphysema; cancers of the lung, larynx, pharynx, oral cavity, esophagus, pancreas, and bladder; and other problems such as respiratory infections and stomach ulcers.

Tobacco use constricts blood vessels, increases blood pressure, destroys air sacs in the lungs, and increases the production of hydrochloric acid in the stomach. The results are shortness of breath; upset stomach; cold and clammy fingers and toes; the development of heart disease, hypertension, stroke, emphysema, and digestive disorders; and lung and other cancers.

To quit, or cut down on, smoking, smoke only one cigarette an hour, smoke only half the cigarette, inhale less, smoke slowly, smoke brands you dislike, place unlighted cigarettes in your mouth when you get the urge, exercise regularly as a divergence, and spend time in places where smoking is prohibited.

Drug-Taking to Enhance Athletic Performance

Among the drugs taken in an attempt to improve on athletic performance are anabolic steroids, caffeine, amphetamines, and cocaine. None of these are effective in this regard and all of these drugs present a serious threat to health.

Anabolic steroids subject the user to liver cancer, high blood pressure, heart disease, sterility, and increased hostility. In men it can lead to atrophied testicles, prostate cancer, and breast growth. In women it can result in menstrual irregularities, a deepening of the voice, decreased breast size, baldness, and facial hair growth. In both men and women, anabolic steroid use can lead to clogging of the arteries, eating compulsions, and increased aggressiveness.

Caffeine is a stimulant. It increases heart and breathing rates, enables skeletal muscles to use fatty acids for energy more efficiently, and decreases fatigue and drowsiness. Caffeine, however, can have serious side effects depending on the amount ingested. It can result in irregular heart beats, hyperactivity, headache, insomnia, an increase in LDL which is associated with coronary disease, and low birth weight when it is consumed by pregnant women.

Amphetamines and cocaine are also stimulants. They can create feelings of psychological and physiological arousal. However, they are drugs on which people can become dependent, and they can cause serious cardiac problems that can even result in death.

REFERENCES

National Center for Health Statistics. *Health, United States, 1992.* Hyattsville, MD: U.S. Public Health Service, 1993.

U. S. Department of Health and Human Services. *Healthy People: National Health Promotion and Disease Prevention Objectives.* Washington, DC: U. S. Government Printing Office, 1991, Pub. No. (PHS) 91-50212.

Physicians' Desk Reference, 48th Edition. Montvale, NJ: Medical Economics Data Production Company, 1994.

Lab Activity 11.1

Signs of Alcoholism

INSTRUCTIONS: *Answer each of the questions below. Then read the interpretation section to find out what your score indicates about you and symptoms of alcoholism.*

Yes	No	
_____	_____	Do you ever drink too heavily when you are disappointed, under pressure, or have had a quarrel with someone?
_____	_____	Have you ever been unable to remember part of the previous evening even though your friends say you did not pass out?
_____	_____	Has a family member or close friend ever expressed concern, or complained, about your drinking?
_____	_____	Do you often want to continue drinking after your friends say they have had enough?
_____	_____	When you are sober, do you sometimes regret things you did or said while you were drinking?
_____	_____	Are you having financial, work, or school and/or family problems as a result of your drinking?
_____	_____	Has a physician ever advised you to cut down on drinking?
_____	_____	Do you eat very little or irregularly at times when you are drinking?
_____	_____	Have you recently noticed that you cannot drink as much as you used to?
_____	_____	Have any of your blood relatives ever had a problem with alcohol?

Interpretation: Any "yes" indicates you may be at greater-than-average risk for alcoholism. More than one "yes" may indicate the presence of an alcohol-related problem or alcoholism, and the need for consultation with an alcoholism professional. To find out more, contact the National Council on Alcoholism and Drug Dependence in your area.

Source: These questions have been excerpted from "What Are the Signs of Alcoholism? The NCAAD Self Test," published by the National Council on Alcoholism and Drug Dependence, Inc. For a copy of this brochure, please send $.50 to NCAAD, 12 West 21 St., New York, NY, 10010.

Lab Activity 11.2

Why Do You Smoke?

INSTRUCTIONS: *Here are some statements made by people to describe what they get out of smoking cigarettes. If you are a smoker, how often do you feel this way when smoking cigarettes? If you are not a smoker, how often do you think smokers feel this way when they smoke? Perhaps responding to these questions, even if you do not smoke cigarettes, will help you better understand why other people smoke. Circle one number for each statement.* **Important: Answer all statements.**

		Always	Frequently	Occasionally	Seldom	Never
A.	I smoke cigarettes in order to keep myself from slowing down.	5	4	3	2	1
B.	Handling a cigarette is part of the enjoyment of smoking it.	5	4	3	2	1
C.	Smoking cigarettes is pleasant and relaxing.	5	4	3	2	1
D.	I light up a cigarette when I feel angry about something.	5	4	3	2	1
E.	When I have run out of cigarettes, I find it almost unbearable until I can get them.	5	4	3	2	1
F.	I smoke cigarettes automatically without even being aware of it.	5	4	3	2	1
G.	I smoke cigarettes to stimulate me, to perk myself up.	5	4	3	2	1
H.	Part of the enjoyment of smoking a cigarette comes from the steps I take to light it up.	5	4	3	2	1
I.	I find cigarettes pleasurable.	5	4	3	2	1
J.	When I feel uncomfortable or upset about something, I light up a cigarette.	5	4	3	2	1
K.	I am very much aware of the fact when I am not smoking a cigarette.	5	4	3	2	1
L.	I light a cigarette without realizing I still have one burning in the ashtray.	5	4	3	2	1
M.	I smoke cigarettes to give me a "lift."	5	4	3	2	1
N.	When I smoke a cigarette, part of the enjoyment is watching the smoke as I exhale it.	5	4	3	2	1

	Always	Frequently	Occasionally	Seldom	Never
0. I want a cigarette most when I am comfortable and relaxed.	5	4	3	2	1
P. When I feel "blue" or want to take my mind off cares and worries, I smoke cigarettes.	5	4	3	2	1
Q. I get a real gnawing hunger for a cigarette when I haven't smoked for a while.	5	4	3	2	1
R. I've found a cigarette in my mouth and didn't remember putting it there.	5	4	3	2	1

◆ Scoring

1. Enter the numbers you have circled in the test questions in the spaces below, putting the number you have circled for question A over line A, for question B over line B, and so on.
2. Add the three scores on each line to get your totals. For example, the sum of your scores over lines A, G, and M gives you your score on *Stimulation*; lines B, H, and N give the score on *Handling*, etc.

Totals

$$\frac{\quad}{A} + \frac{\quad}{G} + \frac{\quad}{M} = \frac{\quad}{\text{Stimulation}}$$ 11 or above suggests you are stimulated by the cigarette to get going and keep going. To stop smoking, try a brisk walk or exercise when the smoking urge is present.

$$\frac{\quad}{B} + \frac{\quad}{H} + \frac{\quad}{N} = \frac{\quad}{\text{Handling}}$$ 11 or above suggests satisfaction from handling the cigarette. Substituting a pencil or paper clip or doodling may aid in breaking the habit.

$$\frac{\quad}{C} + \frac{\quad}{I} + \frac{\quad}{O} = \frac{\quad}{\text{Pleasurable relaxation}}$$ 11 or above suggests you receive pleasure from smoking. For this type of smoker, substitution of other pleasant habits (eating, drinking, social activities, exercise) may aid in eliminating smoking.

$$\frac{\quad}{D} + \frac{\quad}{J} + \frac{\quad}{P} = \frac{\quad}{\text{Crutch: tension reduction}}$$ 11 or above suggests you use cigarettes to handle moments of stress or discomfort. Substitution of social activities, eating, drinking, or handling other objects may aid in stopping.

$$\frac{\quad}{E} + \frac{\quad}{K} + \frac{\quad}{Q} = \frac{\quad}{\text{Craving: psychological addiction}}$$ 11 or above suggests an almost continuous psychological craving for a cigarette. "Cold turkey" may be your best method of breaking the smoking habit.

$$\frac{\quad}{F} + \frac{\quad}{L} + \frac{\quad}{R} = \frac{\quad}{\text{Habit}}$$ 11 or above suggests you smoke out of mere habit and may acquire little satisfaction from the process. Gradually reducing the number of cigarettes smoked may be effective in helping you to stop.

Scores can vary from 3 to 15. Any score of 11 or above is *high*; any score of 7 and below is *low*.

Source: National Clearinghouse for Smoking and Health (USPHS).

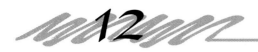

$\mathcal{E}$XPLORING $\mathcal{E}$XERCISE $\mathcal{I}$NJURIES

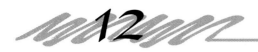

$\mathcal{C}$hapter $\mathcal{O}$bjectives

By the end of this chapter, you should be able to:

1. Design a 10-point injury-prevention plan for someone who is about to begin a new exercise program.

2. Describe the body's response to soft-tissue injury and the three stages of healing.

3. Discuss the correct use of cold, heat, and massage in the emergency treatment of exercise injuries.

4. Demonstrate the correct technique of RICE therapy in the treatment of an ankle sprain and other soft-tissue injuries.

5. Describe the proper use of common over-the-counter and prescription drugs for the treatment of soft-tissue injuries.

6. Describe the proper emergency treatment for at least 25 common exercise injuries.

$\mathcal{M}$OST OF LEE'S friends exercise regularly. Some jog, cycle, and swim; others engage in aerobic exercise classes, or play sports such as tennis, racketball, basketball, soccer, and touch football. At some time or other, it seems as if every one of them has experienced an injury of some sort. Sprained ankles, torn Achilles tendons, sore knees and backs, inflamed shoulders and elbows are just a few of the complaints Lee hears. Lee feels good most of the time although her weight is creeping upward, and she is generally tired by late afternoon. If it were not for the risk of injury, Lee would join her friends in an aerobic activity she enjoys.

This chapter presents a program designed to keep Lee injury-free while she receives the full benefits of an exercise program of her choice. Although there are no guarantees, the information in this chapter can significantly reduce Lee's risk of injury.

Entering into a fitness program involves a slight risk of injury or illness during the first month or so. Later a key benefit of improved conditioning is the reduction in the incidence and severity of serious exercise-, job-, and home-related injuries. The danger of injury increases considerably, however, when you fail to follow simple rules of training. For the *weekend athlete*, exercise can even be fatal. This chapter is designed to help you avoid common hazards and to make exercise a safe, enjoyable experience. It includes ten steps for injury prevention for your body; discusses how tissue responds to injury; describes the proper use of cold, heat and massage; provides basic treatment procedures for common injuries and illnesses; and discusses the special injury-proofing problems of women.

PROTECTING YOUR BODY FROM INJURY AND ILLNESS

Common sense and the application of some basic conditioning concepts can eliminate the majority of risks in most exercise programs. The ten-point injury-prevention program that follows is designed to help minimize your risk of injury and initiate a sound, safe fitness program.

Analyze Your Medical History before You Begin

If you are over 40 years of age, have been inactive for more than two to three years regardless of age, or are in a high-risk group (obese, hypertense, diabetic, or have high blood lipids), a thorough physical examination is recommended. A qualified fitness instructor can also check your heart rate and blood pressure during exercise on a stationary bicycle to secure valuable information about how you will respond to a program. Although the chances of a serious problem are slight for young people, even they are better safe than sorry.

Improve Your General Conditioning Level

It is important to be extra careful in the first month of a new exercise program when you are particularly vulnerable to muscle, joint, **ligament**, tendon, **cartilage**, and other **soft-tissue** injuries. Injuries of all types are also more likely to occur when you are generally fatigued since blood supply to muscles is re-

duced, muscle fibers are somewhat devitalized and easily torn, and joint stability and muscle groups are weakened. A state of general fatigue is common during the early stages of an exercise program. Strengthening the injury-prone areas such as the ankle, wrist, knee, shoulders, lower back, and neck (see chapter 6) before beginning a new program will help reduce the incidence of fatigue-related injuries.

Warm Up Properly before Each Workout

At the beginning of every exercise session, it is important to raise your body temperature one to two degrees to prepare muscles, ligaments, and tendons for vigorous movement. A fast walk, a slow jog, or a mild form of exercise specific to your workout activity for four to five minutes to elevate core temperature, followed by several minutes of stretching will help prevent common muscle pulls, strains, sprains, and lower back discomfort and reduce muscle soreness that may occur 8 to 24 hours later (chapter 7).

Cool Down at the End of Each Exercise Session

The cooldown is a key phase of the fitness workout that should be enjoyed rather than avoided. Experienced joggers or runners, for example, complete the final half- to one mile at a slow, easy pace rather than with a kick or sprint. The final three to five minutes of any workout should also include several minutes of stretching as the body cools and slowly returns to a near resting state (see chapter 4). The cooldown will reduce the incidence of injury during this fatigued state of your workout and decrease muscle soreness the next day.

Progress Slowly

It is wise to add only small increments to your workout each exercise session. Too much, too soon is a common cause of muscular injuries. Plan your program over a three- to six-month period to maximize enjoyment and minimize pain and the risk of injury.

Table 12.1 classifies runners, a group who typically tend to add extra mileage too soon, according to mileage and pace and identifies the injuries common to each group. Within each category, injuries are often the result of excessive mileage, intensive workouts, and a rapid increase in distance over a short time period. Compounding the problem is running surface (a soft, level surface is preferred); running up

Table 12.1 ✦ Classification of Runners and Potential Injuries

CLASSIFICATION	MILEAGE	POTENTIAL INJURIES
Jogger or Novice Runner	3–20 miles per week at 9–12 minutes per mile	Shin splints, chondromalacia (runner's knee), soreness, hamstring strains, and low back pain
Sports Runner	20–40 miles per week, participant in fun runs and races of 3–6 miles	Achilles tendonitis, stress fractures
Long Distance Runner	40–70 miles per week at 7–8 minutes per mile; may compete in 10,000 meters (6.2 miles) or marathons (26.2 miles)	More serious injuries to thigh, calf, and back; sciatica and tendon pulls
Elite Marathoner	70–200 miles per week at 5–7 minutes per mile	Stress fractures, acute muscle strain in the back, sciatica

© Copyright 1980, Ciba-Geigy Corporation. Reprinted with permission from *Clinical Symposia* by David M. Brody, MD, illustrated by Frank H. Netter, MD.

and down curbs, which increases shock to the legs, feet, and back; sloping or banked roads, which force the foot on the higher part of the slope to twist inward excessively; overstressing tendons and ligaments; or uphill (strains the Achilles tendon and lower-back muscles) and downhill (force to the heel is increased) running. Complete Lab Activity 12.1: Evaluating Your Potential for Foot and Leg Injuries at the end of this chapter.

Your workout should also avoid increasing your heart rate to more than 60 percent of your maximum the first two to four weeks. After this acclimation period you can train at higher heart rates more safely.

Alternate Light and Heavy Workout Days

Many people make the mistake of trying to exercise hard every day. The body then does not have adequate time to repair or rebuild, and the full benefit of your workout may not be realized. In addition, injuries, boredom, and peaking out early are much more likely to occur. The chance of an exercise-related injury can be reduced by alternating light and heavy workout days each week.

Avoid the Weekend Athlete Approach to Fitness

One sure way to guarantee numerous injuries and illnesses is to exercise vigorously only on weekends. The older weekend athlete is particularly susceptible to heart attack, while individuals of all ages increase their chances of soft-tissue injuries to muscles, tendons, and ligaments.

In the early spring of each year and during the first major snowfall, approximately 25 to 50 men die of heart attacks. The early spring victims are generally middle-aged men who recently purchased a pair of $200.00 running shoes and decided to get in shape in just one workout. The five-mile run usually attempted is often the first time this person has exercised in the past year. Or the snow shoveling after the first major snowfall is the first exposure to exercise since the previous winter. For these individuals, who may have underlying disease, the result is often fatal. These deaths can probably be prevented by a few months of walking as a means of preconditioning.

Death occasionally occurs following unaccustomed exertion in cold weather even though an autopsy reveals no signs of a heart attack. While this condition is rare, it is a possibility when men and women try to do it all in one weekend workout. Cold air constricts the blood vessels of the skin and increases blood pressure slightly. Vigorous exercise also increases blood pressure, heart rate, and the oxygen needs of the heart dramatically. Without proper warmup and with the presence of hidden signs of heart disease, a heart attack may occur.

Ligament Fibrous bands or folds that support organs, hold bones together, or attach muscles to bones.

Cartilage Fibrous connective tissue between the surfaces of movable and immovable joints.

Soft tissue Tissue other than bone.

If the weekend is the only time you can exercise, avoid long bouts in hot or cold weather and strenuous exercise (jogging, running, racketball, handball, tennis, basketball, soccer, rugby, and so on) unless you take frequent breaks. Consider supplementing your weekend routine with one other workout during the week. After one month, try increasing to two workouts during the week in addition to one on weekends. If you choose an aerobic activity and progress slowly for several months, you can minimize the risk of serious illness or injury. With a total of three workouts weekly, you have the foundation for a good conditioning program.

Pay Close Attention to Your Body Signals

Pain and other distress signals during exercise should not be ignored. Although some breathing discomfort and breathlessness is common and minor pain may be present in joints or muscles, severe, persistent, and particularly sharp pain is a warning sign to stop exercising. Also stop exercising immediately if you notice any abnormal heart action (pulse irregularity, fluttering, palpitations in the chest or throat, rapid heart beats); pain or pressure in the middle of the chest, teeth, jaw, neck, or arm; dizziness; lightheadedness; cold sweat; or confusion.

After each workout, let your body analyze the severity of your exercise session. The workout was probably too light if you did not sweat, and it was too heavy if you were still breathless 10 minutes after you stopped exercising, your pulse rate was above 120 beats per minute 5 minutes after stopping, prolonged fatigue remained for more than 24 hours, nausea or vomiting occurred, or sleep was interrupted. To remedy these symptoms in the future, exercise less vigorously and lengthen your cooldown period.

Exercise may also be inadvisable for some individuals afflicted with certain medical conditions. Study Table 12.2 to identify the adjustments that should be made when you are ill, injured, or suffering from a medical condition that requires modifications. When you are obviously ill or not up to par, avoid exercise, rest a few days, and return to a lower level or an easier workout.

Master the Proper Form in Your Activity

For all activities, correct form improves efficiency and reduces the risk of injury. Proper running form, for example, is important to most fitness programs. Joggers should avoid running on the toes, which produces soreness in the calf muscles. The heel should strike the ground first before rolling the weight along

Table 12.2 ✦ Disqualifying Conditions for Sports Participation

CONDITIONS	COLLISION[a]	CONTACT[b]	NONCONTACT[c]	OTHERS[d]
General health				
Acute infections	×	×	×	×
Respiratory, genitourinary, infectious mononucleosis, hepatitis, active rheumatic fever, active tuberculosis				
Obvious physical immaturity in comparison with other competitors	×	×		
Hemorrhagic disease	×	×	×	
Hemophilia, purpura, and other serious bleeding tendencies				
Diabetes, inadequately controlled	×	×	×	×
Diabetes, controlled	e	e	e	e
Jaundice	×	×	×	×
Eyes				
Absence or loss of function of one eye	×	×		
Respiratory				
Tuberculosis (active or symptomatic)	×	×	×	×
Severe pulmonary insufficiency	×	×	×	×

Table 12.2 ✦ Disqualifying Conditions for Sports Participation *(continued)*

CONDITIONS	COLLISION[a]	CONTACT[b]	NONCONTACT[c]	OTHERS[d]
Cardiovascular				
Mitral stenosis, aortic stenosis, aortic insufficiency, coarctation of aorta, cyanotic heart disease, recent carditis of any etiology	×	×	×	×
Hypertension on organic basis	×	×	×	×
Previous heart surgery for congenital or acquired heart disease	f	f	f	f
Liver, enlarged	×	×		
Skin				
Boils, impetigo, and herpes simplex gladiatorum	×	×		
Spleen, enlarged	×	×		
Hernia				
Inguinal or femoral hernia	×	×	×	
Musculoskeletal				
Symptomatic abnormalities or inflammations	×	×	×	×
Functional inadequacy of the musculoskeletal system, congenital or acquired, incompatible with the contact or skill demands of the sport	×	×	×	
Neurological				
History of symptoms of previous serious head trauma or repeated concussions	×			
Controlled convulsive disorder	g	g	g	g
Convulsive disorder not moderately well controlled by medication	×			
Previous surgery on head	×	×		
Renal				
Absence of one kidney	×	×		
Renal disease	×	×	×	×
Genitalia				
Absence of one testicle	h	h	h	h
Undescended testicle	h	h	h	h

[a]Football, rugby, hockey, lacrosse, and so forth.

[b]Baseball, soccer, basketball, wrestling, and so forth.

[c]Cross country, track, tennis, crew, swimming, and so forth.

[d]Bowling, golf, archery, field events, and so forth.

[e]No exclusions.

[f]Each individual should be judged on an individual basis in conjunction with his or her cardiologist and surgeon.

[g]Each patient should be judged on an individual basis. All things being equal, it is probably better to encourage a young boy or girl to participate in a noncontact sport rather than a contact sport. However, if a patient has a desire to play a contact sport and this is deemed a major ameliorating factor in his or her adjustment to school, associates, and the seizure disorder, serious consideration should be given to letting him or her participate if the seizures are moderately well controlled or the patient is under good medical management.

[h]The Committee approves the concept of contact sports participation for youths with only one testicle or with an undescended testicle(s), except in specific instances such as an inguinal canal undescended testicle(s), following appropriate medical evaluation to rule out unusual injury risk. However, the athlete, parents, and school authorities should be fully informed that participation in contact sports with only one testicle carries a slight injury risk to the remaining healthy testicle. Fertility may be adversely affected following an injury. But the chances of an injury to a descended testicle are rare, and the injury risk can be further substantially minimized with an athletic supporter and protective device.

Source: Daniel D. Arnheim, *Modern Principles of Athletic Training.* St. Louis: Times Mirror/Mosby College Publishing, 1989, pp. 51–52.

Fitness Heroes

The Los Angeles Dodgers' manager Tommy Lasorda is strict about stretching. The 66-year-old spends his days hurling pitch after pitch at his players, all the while maintaining a regular stretching and strengthening routine for his team. Lasorda, team physicians, and team trainers created the regular stretching and strengthening routine to keep the Dodgers healthy and injury-free. The program has substantially reduced the number of injuries sustained by members of his team.

At first, the players were annoyed because missing a stretching routine was a big demerit for any team member. Once they started participating, though, they realized the benefits quickly. Relief pitcher Jim Gott, who frequently suffered from elbow and shoulder injuries, has recovered fully in response to the strengthening routine and has not had an injury since.

Lasorda and his trainers feel that the days of players getting by on talent alone are over. Regular stretching and strengthening not only lengthens the baseball careers of the team members but also helps the Dodgers to avoid the wrath of Tommy Lasorda! ◆

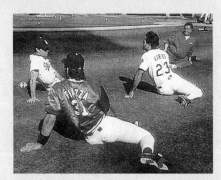

Under the management of Tommy Lasorda, the Dodgers are required to stretch before each practice and each game. The team has considerably reduced its injury rate. (Photo Courtesy of Cable News Network.)

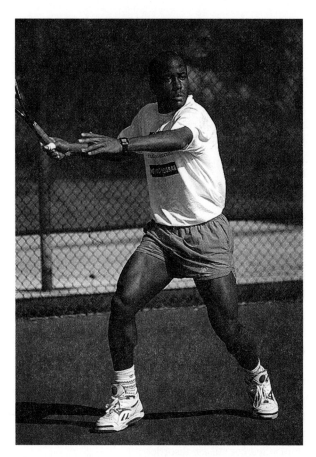

Mastering the proper form improves efficiency and reduces the risk of injury. Tennis players are especially susceptible to elbow, shoulder, wrist, and lower back problems. (Photo Courtesy of the United States Handball Association.)

and wrist inflammation and lower-back problems) from faulty stroke mechanics such as elbow-led ground strokes, bent-elbow hits, muscles not firming at impact, and so on. A few professional lessons in your sport can help to reduce the risk of these types of injuries.

Dress Properly for the Weather

Weather extremes can also cause health problems during exercise. Consider the suggestions in Table 12.3 to reduce the risk of overheating on hot, humid days or overexposure on cold days. It is also helpful to become familiar with the early symptoms and emergency treatment for heat- and cold-related injuries such as heat exhaustion, heat stroke, **hypothermia,** and **frostbite** (see Table 12.4 on pages 253–261.).

If you are a runner, plan your jogging course to avoid being too far out on either a hot or cold day

the bottom of the foot to the toes for the pushoff. A number of other running form problems often produce mild muscle or joint strain.

Participants in racket sports are also susceptible to numerous form-related injuries (elbow, shoulder,

Table 12.3 ✦ Preventive Techniques on Hot and Cold Days

HOT, HUMID WEATHER	COLD WEATHER
1. Listen to weather reports and avoid vigorous exercise if the temperature is above 90° and the humidity is above 70 percent. Make hot days your light workout.	1. Listen to weather reports noting temperature and wind-chill factor. Unless the equivalent temperature is in the "little danger" area, avoid outside exercise.
2. Avoid adding to normal salt intake. Do not use salt tablets. Increase consumption of fruits and vegetables.	2. Eat well during cold months: the body needs more calories in cold weather.
3. Avoid lengthy warm-up periods.	3. Warm up carefully until sweating is evident.
4. Wear light-colored, porous, loose clothing to promote evaporation. Remove special equipment, such as football gear, every hour for 15 minutes.	4. Use two or three layers of clothing rather than one heavy warm-up suit.
5. Avoid wearing a hat (except for an open visor with brim) since considerable heat loss occurs through the head.	5. Protect the head (warm hat), ears, fingers, toes, nose, and genitals. A hat should cover the ears and face. Fur-lined supporters for men can also prevent frostbite to sensitive parts.
6. Never use rubberized suits that hold the sweat in and increase fluid and salt/potassium loss.	6. Never use rubberized, air-tight suits that keep the sweat in. When the body cools, the sweat starts to freeze.
7. Wet clothing increases salt and sweat loss. Replace whenever possible.	7. Keep clothing dry, changing wet items as soon as possible.
8. Slowly increase the length of your workout by 5 to 10 minutes daily for nine days to acclimate to the heat.	8. Slowly increase the length of your workout by 5 to 10 minutes daily for nine days to acclimate to the cold.
9. Drink cold water (40°F) before (10–20 ounces 15 minutes prior to exercise), during, and after exercise. Hydrate before the workout with two or three glasses of water.	9. Drink cold water freely before, during, and after exercise. Let thirst be your guide.

should symptoms of heat exhaustion or overexposure to cold occur. If you run against the wind in cold weather on the way out, on the way back, when you are likely to be sweating much more, you will be running with the wind. Running into a head wind with wet clothes will draw heat away from your body.

Both weather extremes can be dangerous. Heat stroke (when core temperature may rise to 105 or 106 degrees Fahrenheit) symptoms are difficult to reverse unless immediate, rapid cooling takes place. On the other hand, a one-degree drop in core temperature will produce pain. Should body temperature drop to 94 degrees, shivering ceases and rigidity sets in; at 75 degrees death usually occurs from heart failure.

Properly fitted shoes, appropriate equipment, avoidance of gimmicky exercise devices, and acceptable equipment for contact sports are also important for injury prevention and need special attention. A good quality shoe is your best protection against injury to the feet, ankles, knees, hips, and lower back.

TISSUE RESPONSE TO INJURY

The actual healing process is unique to each individual and to different types of tissue. Age, nutrition, and the proper use of treatment techniques also effect the way tissue responds to the injury and the healing process. An understanding of how soft tissue

Hypothermia Subnormal body temperature.
Frostbite Destruction of tissue by freezing.

Diversity Issues

Injury Prevention

During and after adolescence, boys are encouraged to begin strength-training programs that help add muscle mass and improve strength, endurance, and physical appearance. This training also helps boys avoid exercise injuries by strengthening soft tissue and making the body less susceptible to bruises and muscle pulls. Unfortunately, girls are not encouraged at an early age to weight train, and weight rooms in most public schools in the United States are still male dominated and not well suited for women. Strength training, particularly with free weights, is still considered a male activity that has not been fully accepted as an appropriate training method for women.

With the advent of aerobics and the increasing number of women frequenting gyms, however, more women are beginning to see the benefits of weight training. Whether they train on Nautilus machines or with free weights, they are realizing that strengthening the muscles increases overall body strength, increases basal metabolism, and generally improves the body's appearance. Sometimes, however, women who have never trained with weights tend to overdo their first time around. Lifting too much weight with too many repetitions leads to muscle pulls and soft-tissue injuries, and the pain associated with these injuries can be very discouraging.

Weight-training injuries for both women and men can be avoided by following a few simple suggestions. The proper lifting techniques described in chapter 6 for each exercise should be carefully mastered. A first attempt at weight training requires light-to-moderate weights and a relatively high number of repetitions. This approach will slowly prepare the muscles and other soft tissue for heavier weight and fewer repetitions in the future. Training with a partner who acts as a spotter, or protector, is a necessary precaution, particularly when using free weights. A safe, injury-free weight-training program is attainable for all. ✦

responds (heals) to **acute** and **chronic** injuries will help you understand emergency treatment techniques and reinforce the correct use of heat, cold, and massage as treatment modalities.

Musculoskeletal injuries incurred through sports or exercise fall into three phases: acute, repair and regeneration, and remodeling.

Acute Phase

The acute phase of inflammation (the first 3 or 4 days after an injury) occurs as the body initially reacts to an injury with redness, heat, swelling, pain, and loss of function or movement. During this period, pressure on nerve endings or **ischemia** may produce considerable pain. Some tissue death also takes place from the initial trauma or the lack of oxygen following the trauma. Acute inflammation is actually a protective mechanism designed to keep the problem local and remove some of the injurious agents so healing and repair can begin. Almost immediately after the injury occurs, blood flow to that area is decreased for a period from several seconds to as long as ten minutes and coagulation begins to seal the broken blood vessels. Numerous other vascular and cellular events occur to prepare the site for the next phase.

Repair and Regeneration Phase

For a period of from 48 to 72 hours after the injury to about six weeks, healing begins when cellular debris, erythrocytes, and the fibrin clot are being removed. Although some scar tissue will form following soft-tissue injuries, a desirable goal is to treat the injury properly to produce as little of such tissue as possible since scar tissue is less viable than normal tissue. Primary healing occurs with little scar tissue formation in injuries where the edges are held closely together. When a gaping lesion and large tissue loss is present, considerable scar tissue forms during the healing process to replace lost tissue and bridge the gap.

Remodeling Phase

In this phase, which overlaps the repair and regeneration phase, scar tissue continues to increase and become stronger for three to six weeks following an injury. The actual strength of scar tissue increases for three months to a year. The complete remodeling of ligamentous tissue generally requires a year.

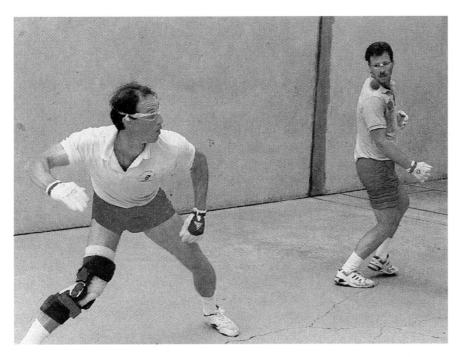

Always wear appropriate protective equipment. Eye guards should be worn while playing handball, raquetball, and squash in order to prevent serious eye injuries. (Photo Courtesy of the United States Handball Association.)

GENERAL TREATMENT MODALITIES

Cryotherapy

The application of cold (cryotherapy) to the skin for 20 minutes or less at a minimum temperature of 50 degrees Fahrenheit causes the constriction of vessels and reduces the flow of blood to the injured area. When cold is applied for longer than 20 minutes, an intermittent period of **vasodilation** occurs for 4 to 6 minutes. This prevents tissue damage from too much exposure to cold. At this point, cold is no longer effective. It also reduces muscle spasm, swelling, and pain; slows metabolic rate; and increases **collagen** inelasticity and joint stiffness. Cold is somewhat more penetrating than heat, and the effects last longer.

Cold applications should be used immediately after an injury and continued for several days until swelling subsides. Cold can be applied intermittently for 20 minutes every 1-1/2 waking hours in combination with compression, elevation, and rest (see RICE later in this chapter). The longer the cold is applied, the deeper the cooling. *Ice massage* can be used on a small body area by freezing water in a plastic-foam cup to form a cylinder of ice. After removing one or two inches of the plastic-foam at the top of the cup, the cup portion can be used as a handle, and the ice can be rubbed over the skin in overlapping circles for 5 to 10 minutes to produce cold, burning, aching, and numbness in the area. *Ice packs* can be made by placing flaked or crushed ice in a wet towel or self-sealing plastic bag. Unless ice massage is being used, ice should not come in direct contact with the skin.

Acute Disease or pain characterized by sudden onset and a short, severe course.

Chronic Disease or pain of slow onset and long duration.

Ischemia A condition of localized diminished blood supply.

Vasodilation Increase or opening of the blood vessels.

Collagen The connective tissue portion of the true skin and of other organs.

Thermotherapy

In general, proper **thermotherapy** to an injured area raises skin temperature and increases the amount of blood flow to the area. Heat can also be used to relieve joint stiffness, pain, muscle spasm, and inflammation, and to increase the extensibility of collagen tissues. Temperatures should not exceed 116 degrees Fahrenheit and a treatment session should never exceed 30 minutes. Additional cautions in the use of heat include:

1. Never apply heat immediately after an injury.
2. Never use heat when there is loss of sensation or decreased arterial circulation.
3. Never apply heat directly to the eyes, genitals, or the abdomen of a pregnant woman.
4. Never fall asleep while applying heat or apply heat over Ben Gay® or other topical heat ointment.

Heat can be safely applied through the use of moist heat and commercial packs as well as whirlpool and paraffin baths. You can use moist heat at home by soaking a towel in hot water and allowing it to drain for several seconds before applying to an injured area, which is already covered by four to six layers of toweling. The moist towel should not directly contact the skin.

Electrotherapy

The use of **electrotherapy** as a form of heat should be performed only by a physician, physical therapist, or licensed athletic trainer.

Massage

The use of massage to manipulate soft tissue is a helpful adjunct to heat and cold. Stroking, kneading, friction, percussion, and rapid shaking are some of the more common techniques used to increase heat, improve blood flow to the injured area, remove metabolites such as lactic acid, overcome edema, improve circulation and the venous return of blood to the heart, and aid relaxation.

Thermotherapy The application of heat.

Electrotherapy The use of electricity (infrared radiation therapy, shortwave and microwave diathermics, and ultrasound therapy) in the treatment of disease or injury.

PREVENTION AND EMERGENCY TREATMENT OF COMMON EXERCISE INJURIES AND ILLNESSES

Additional common injuries, illnesses, and problems associated with exercise are discussed in Table 12.4 which serves as a guide for diagnosis, prevention, emergency treatment, and determination of the need for a physician. If in doubt, consult a physician immediately or transport the injured person to a hospital emergency room.

RICE

Emergency home treatment for most muscle, ligament, and tendon strains, sprains, suspected fractures, bruises, and joint inflammations involve four simple actions known as the RICE approach.

Rest To prevent additional damage to injured tissue, stop exercising and immobilize the injured area immediately. If the lower extremities are effected, use crutches to move about.

Ice To decrease blood flow to the injured area and decrease swelling, apply ice (crushed in a towel or ice pack) directly to the skin immediately for 15 to 20 minutes. Use cold applications intermittently for 1 to 72 hours.

Compression To limit swelling and decrease likelihood of hemorrhage and hematoma formation, wrap a towel or bandage firmly around the ice and injured area. An elastic wrap soaked in water and frozen in a refrigerator can be used to apply both compression and cold.

Elevation To help drain excess fluid through gravity, improve the venous return of blood to the heart, and reduce internal bleeding and swelling, raise the injured limb above heart level.

Home treatment should begin as soon as possible. The procedure should be: (1) Evaluate the injured area. (2) Apply ice for 20 minutes. (3) Compress the ice firmly against the injury. (4) Replace the ice pack with a compress wrap and pad. (5) Rest the injured area. (6) Reapply ice in 1 to 1½ hours. (7) Remove the elastic wrap and elevate the area before you go to bed. (8) Begin ice therapy immediately on rising in the morning. On the fourth or fifth day, discontinue cold treatments, and begin to apply moist heat or dry heat or use a whirlpool twice daily for 15

(text continues on page 261)

Table 12.4 ✦ Prevention and Emergency Treatment of Common Exercise Injuries

Injury	General comments	Prevention and treatment	Need for a physician
Extremities			
Ankle	Most injuries involve inversion sprains (outer edge of foot turns inward). Ankles are not strong enough for most sports, and are poorly supported by muscles and ligaments that often stretch and tear from high-speed direction changes, cutting, and contact.	Improved support muscle strength offers some protection, along with preventive taping (inversion sprains only). RICE therapy is the preferred treatment. Use crutches for two or three days if pain is severe.	If swelling or pain remains for three days; If ligament or tendon damage is present; If pain prevents walking; If symptoms of fracture exist.
Bruise (charley horse)	A charley horse is nothing more than a thigh contusion from a direct blow to a relaxed thigh muscle (the tissue is compressed against the bone). Bruises to other areas occur in similar fashion.	Prevention involves use of proper equipment in contact sports. RICE therapy is the preferred emergency and home treatment. Replace ice with heat on the third or fourth day.	If pain and discoloration do not disappear with rest, treatment, and mild exercise.
Elbow (tennis and pitcher's)	The movement causing the condition is a forceful extension of the forearm and a twisting motion (serve in tennis, curve in baseball). The more you play and the older you are, the more likely you are to be afflicted. Pain is present over the outer (lateral epicondyle) or inner (medial epicondyle) elbow and radiates down the arm. Pain is produced by tears, inflammation and scar tissue at the attachment of the extensor muscles to the bony prominence of the elbow.	Prevention centers around use of warmup, correction of poor stroke mechanics, avoiding use of wet tennis balls and heavy, inflexible rackets, and reducing the frequency of curve ball pitches (should be greatly restricted in little league baseball with growing youngsters).	If condition remains more than two or three weeks; If pain makes exercise impossible; If severe swelling is present.
Fractures	A fracture should be suspected in most injuries where pain and swelling exist over a bone.	Apply ice packs, protect and rest the injured part for 72 hours. In severe cases, splint the bone where the victim lies and transport to emergency room.	If limb is cold, blue, or numb; If pelvis or thigh are involved; If limb is crooked or deformed; If shock symptoms are present; If rapid, severe swelling occurs.
Hamstring strains	The large muscle group in the back of the upper leg is commonly strained during vigorous exercise. Pain is severe and prohibits further activity. In a few days, discoloration may appear.	Prevention includes proper stretching before exercise. proper diet, improved flexibility, and care in running around wet areas. For treatment use RICE therapy followed by heat application in three to four days.	If severe discoloration occurs; If pain and discomfort remain after 10 to 15 days of treatment.

Table 12.4 ✦ Prevention and Emergency Treatment of Common Exercise Injuries *(continued)*

INJURY	GENERAL COMMENTS	PREVENTION AND TREATMENT	NEED FOR A PHYSICIAN
Knee	The knee is a vulnerable joint that depends on ligaments, cartilage, and muscles for support. *Chondromalacia* of the patella, or roughing of the undersurface of the kneecap, is the most common injury; kneecap pain and grating symptoms are evident. A tear of the cartilage is the second most common injury. Pain is evident along the inner or outer part of the knee joint along with swelling. *Ligament* tears are less common but occur from a blow to the leg. Swelling and knee instability result.	Prevention involves flexibility and strength. Exercises should stretch and strengthen the hamstrings, quadriceps, and Achilles tendon. Chondromalacia is treated through use of arch supports, or by bulking up the inner part of the heel of the shoe. Aspirin and quadriceps exercises also help. Serious knee injury (cartilage and ligament damage) requires an examination by an orthopedic surgeon. Use of the arthroscope to examine and insert small tools through puncture wounds offers effective treatment and rapid recovery.	If swelling and pain persist more than three to five days; If ligament or cartilage damage is suspected; If chondromalacia is suspected.
Shin splints	A shin splint is merely an inflammation of the anterior and posterior tendons of the large bone in the lower leg. It is an overuse syndrome developing in poorly conditioned individuals in the beginning of their training program. Hard surfaces add to the problem.	Avoid hard surfaces, too much mileage, doing too much too soon, using improperly fitted shoes, and running on banked tracks or road shoulders. RICE therapy is recommended for two to four days, followed by taping and heat therapy, and stretching exercises.	If condition remains more than two to three weeks; If condition reoccurs after reconvening your exercise routine.
Tendonitis	The location of the pain and swelling of the tendon varies in different sports. With considerable running, the Achilles tendon is affected. In those involving repeated movement of the upper arms (swimming, baseball), it is the shoulder tendon. When a snapping or rotation of the elbow is involved (tennis/ handball), it is the elbow tendon.	For both prevention and treatment, stretch the involved tendon (daily and exercise lightly until pain disappears. RICE therapy is helpful in the early stages for three to four days. See *Elbow* this table. Pain may disappear during a workout, only to return and grow worse later.	If pain and inflammation continue after two to three weeks of treatment.
Varicose veins	Varicose veins are nothing more than abnormally lengthened, dilated veins. Surrounding muscles support deep veins, whereas superficial veins get little support. In some individuals, vein valves that prevent blood from backing up become defective, enlarged, and lose their elasticity. The condition is uncommon in young people.	Prevention and treatment for those with symptoms or a family history include bed rest and leg elevation, avoiding long periods of standing, use of elastic bandages and support stockings, surgery for severe cases, and removal of intraabdominal pressure (obesity, tumor, or tight girdles).	If pain is severe enough to make walking difficult; If cosmetic problem is bothersome.

Table 12.4 ✦ Prevention and Emergency Treatment of Common Exercise Injuries *(continued)*

INJURY	GENERAL COMMENTS	PREVENTION AND TREATMENT	NEED FOR A PHYSICIAN
Feet and Hands			
Athlete's foot	Athlete's foot is caused by a fungus, and is accompanied by a bacterial infection. Itching, redness, and a rash on the soles, toes, or between the toes is common.	Prevention and treatment are similar; wash between the toes with soap and water, dry thoroughly, use medication containing Tinactin twice daily, and place fungistatic foot powder in shoes and sneakers.	If treatment does not relieve symptoms in two to three weeks.
Blisters	Blisters are produced by friction causing the top skin layer to separate from the second layer. Blisters can become severely inflamed or infected unless properly treated. A porous inner sole can be purchased that almost completely eliminates getting blisters on the feet.	Use clean socks, comfortably fitting shoes, and Vaseline to reduce friction. Avoid breaking open blisters (skin acts as a sterile bandage). If the blister breaks, trim off all loose skin and apply antibiotic salve. Avoid use of tincture of benzoin, and of powder that increases friction, since this is more likely to cause blisters than prevent them.	If inflammation and soreness develop; If redness occurs in the involved limb; If pain or sensitivity occurs under the arms or in the groin area.
Bunions	Bunions are merely growths on the head of the first or fifth toe that produce inflammation (swelling, redness, and pain).	Bunions can be prevented by using properly fitted shoes.	If symptoms of infection occur.
Corns	Hard corns may result from poorly fitted shoes. Inflammation and thickening of soft tissue (top of toes) occur. Soft corns are often caused by excessive foot perspiration and narrow shoes. The corn forms between the fourth and fifth toe in most cases.	Prevention and treatment involves use of properly fitted shoes, soaking feet daily in warm water to soften the area, and protecting the area with a small felt or sponge rubber doughnut. Trim and file corns to reduce pressure.	If a change of shoes and treatment does not improve the condition.
Heel bruise	The most common cause of heel pain is plantar fascitis—inflammation of the broad band of fibrous tissue that runs from the base of the toes back to the heel and inserts on the inner aspect of the heel. Mild tears and severe bruises are also common.	Prevention involves proper stretching and use of a plastic heel cup. Aspirin should be used to reduce inflammation (two tablets, four times daily); rest is indicated for five to seven days.	If pain persists for more than five to seven days after rest and treatment.
Ingrown toenails	The edge of the toenail grows into the soft tissue, producing inflammation and infection.	Prevention and treatment involves proper nail trimming, soaking the toe in hot water two to three times daily, and inserting a small piece of cotton under the nail edge to lift it from the soft tissue.	If infection occurs.

Table 12.4 ✦ Prevention and Emergency Treatment of Common Exercise Injuries *(continued)*

INJURY	GENERAL COMMENTS	PREVENTION AND TREATMENT	NEED FOR A PHYSICIAN
Stress fracture	A stress fracture is a small crack in a bone's surface, generally a foot, leg, or hand. Unexplained pain may exist over one of the small bones in the hand or foot. X-ray will not reveal small cracks until the bone heals and a callus (scar tissue) forms.	Prevention involves not running too many miles, not increasing mileage too fast, running on soft surfaces, and taking care to progress slowly in your fitness program. Treatment requires rest and proper equipment (especially footwear).	If unexplained pain exists in the lower back, hip, ankle, wrist, hands, or feet.
Head and Neck			
Cauliflower ear	A deformed painful outer ear is common in wrestling, rugby, and football from friction, hard blows, and wrenching in a headlock position. With poor circulation to the ear, fluid is absorbed slowly, and the ear remains swollen, sensitive, and discolored.	Use protective ear guards, apply Vaseline to reduce friction, and apply ice as soon as a sore spot develops. Once a deformed ear develops, only a plastic surgeon can return the ear to normal appearance.	If symptoms of infection develop; If cosmetic surgery is desired.
Concussion	Any injury to the head producing dizziness or temporary unconsciousness should be considered serious.	Apply ice to the area. Observe the patient for 72 hours for alertness, unequal pupil size (although about one person in four has unequal pupil size all the time), and vomiting. Pressure inside skull may develop in 72 hours.	If unconsciousness occurred; If bleeding occurs from ears, eyes, or mouth; If there is unequal pupil size, lethargy, fever, vomiting, convulsions, speech difficulty, stiff neck, or limb weakness.
Dental injuries	Common in basketball and contact sports from elbow contact.	Chipped tooth—avoid hot and cold drinks. Swelling due to abscess—apply ice pack. Excessive bleeding of socket—place gauze over socket and bite down. Toothache—aspirin and ice packs.	If tooth is chipped, abscess is present, or bleeding of socket or toothache is present.
Eye (object in eye, contusion from a ball or elbow)	Eye injuries are more common in racket sports and handball from ball contact, and in contact sports from elbow contact. In racket sports, the ball may ricochet off the top of the racket into the eye, or the victim may turn to see where his or her partner is hitting the ball in doubles play.	Protective eye guards should be used in racketball and handball. Never turn your head in doubles play. Avoid rubbing—you could scratch the cornea. Close both eyes to allow tears to wash away a foreign body. Grasp the lashes of the upper lid and draw out and down over the lower lid. If it feels like an object is in the eye but none can be seen, cornea scrape probably occurred, and will heal in 24 to 48 hours. To remove object, moisten corner of handkerchief and touch object lightly.	If object is on the eye itself; If object remains after washing; If object could have penetrated the globe of the eye; If blood is visible in eye; If vision is impaired; If pain is present after 48 hours.

Table 12.4 ✦ Prevention and Emergency Treatment of Common Exercise Injuries *(continued)*

INJURY	GENERAL COMMENTS	PREVENTION AND TREATMENT	NEED FOR A PHYSICIAN
Nasal fracture	The blow may come from the side or front. The side hit causes more deformity. Hemorrhage is profuse (mucous lining is cut), and swelling is immediate.	Prevention involves use of a face guard in football. Bleeding should be controlled immediately (see *Nosebleed*).	If bleeding continues; If deformity and considerable swelling are present.
Extremities			
Neck	Neck injuries are more common in contact sports, and require immediate and careful attention. Assume a vertebrae is involved, and avoid movement of any kind until a physician or rescue squad arrives.	Neck flexibility exercises should be a part of your warmup routine. Neck strengthening exercises are a necessity for contact sport participants.	If any injury to the neck occurs.
Nosebleed	Nosebleed may occur even from mild contact to the nose.	Do not lie down when bleeding starts. Squeeze the nose between the thumb and forefinger just below the hard portion for 5 to 10 minutes while seated with the head tilted back. Avoid blowing the nose or placing cold compresses on the bridge of the nose.	If bleeding occurs frequently and is associated with a cold; If victim has a history of high blood pressure; If emergency treatment fails to stop the bleeding.
Torso			
Back	The first 7 vertebrae control the head, neck, and upper back. The next 12 provide attachments for the ribs. The 5 lumbar vertebrae of the lower back support the weight of the upper half of the body. It is this area that plagues millions of Americans.	Avoid exercise motions that arch the back. Back pain may be caused by muscular and ligamentous sprains, mechanical instability, arthritis, and ruptured discs. Most problems will improve with rest, heat, pain medication, and an exercise program.	If pain, weakness, or numbness in legs is present; If pain remains after rest and heat therapy; If aching sensation occurs in buttocks, or further down the leg.
Chest pain	Chest pain provides a heart attack scare to everyone over age 30. Actually, pain could be in the chest wall (muscle, rib, ligament, or rib cartilage), the lungs or outside covering, or the gullet, diaphragm, skin, or other organs in the upper part of the diaphragm. Sharp pain that lasts a few seconds, pain at the end of a deep breath, or one that worsens with a deep breath, pain upon pressing a finger on the spot of discomfort, and painful burning when the stomach is empty are all symptoms that are probably not associated with a heart attack.	Any of the symptoms to the right require immediate hospitalization and physician care.	If any of the following symptoms are present: mild to intense pain with a feeling of pressure, or squeezing on the chest; pain beneath the breastbone; accompanying pain in the jaw, or down the inner side of either arm; accompanying nausea, sweating, dizziness, or shortness of breath; or pulse irregularity.

Table 12.4 ✦ Prevention and Emergency Treatment of Common Exercise Injuries *(continued)*

INJURY	GENERAL COMMENTS	PREVENTION AND TREATMENT	NEED FOR A PHYSICIAN
Groin strain	The groin muscles (area between the thigh and abdominal region) are easily torn from running, jumping, and twisting. It is a difficult injury to prevent and cure. Pain, weakness, and internal bleeding may occur.	Prevention involves proper stretching prior to exercise. R-I-C-E therapy is suggested for treatment.	If symptoms remain after several weeks of rest and mild exercise.
Hernia	The protrusion of viscera (body organs) through a portion of the abdominal wall is referred to as a hernia. Hernias associated with exercise and sports generally occur in the groin area.	Prevention involves attention to proper form in weight lifting and weight training, and care in lifting heavy objects.	If a protrusion is located that protrudes further with coughing.
Hip pointer	A hard blow to the iliac crest or hip produces what is commonly called a hip pointer. The injury is severely handicapping, and produces both pain and spasm.	Prevention involves the use of protective hip pads in contact sports. R-I-C-E therapy is suggested for treatment.	If symptoms of a fracture are present.
Jock itch	Jock itch is acquired by contact and is associated with bacteria, fungi, molds, and ringworm.	Prevention and treatment involve practicing proper hygiene (showering in warm water, use of antiseptic soap, powder, and proper drying); drinking enough water; regularly changing underwear, supporter, and shorts; disinfecting locker benches, mats, and other equipment; and avoiding long periods of sitting in warm, moist areas.	If condition persists for more than 10 days.
Wind knocked out	With a hard blow to the right place, such as a relaxed midsection, breathing is temporarily hampered. Although you will have trouble convincing the victim, breathing will return. The blow has only increased abdominal pressure, produced pain, and interfered with the diaphragmatic cycle reflex due to nerve paralysis or muscle spasm.	The victim should be told to try to breath slowly through the nose (no easy task for someone who is gasping, dizzy, and 100 percent convinced death is only seconds away). Clothing is loosened at the neck and waist, and ice is applied to the abdomen.	If breathing is still not normal in one or two minutes; If breathing stops (start CPR); If pain persists in the midsection.

Shoulder

INJURY	GENERAL COMMENTS	PREVENTION AND TREATMENT	NEED FOR A PHYSICIAN
Tendonitis	Tendonitis is common in tennis and baseball. Soreness results on the front of the shoulder when elevating the arm from the side.	Ice and aspirin are used. Prevention and treatment involves flexibility and weight-training exercises. Flexibility movements concentrate on back stretching while weight-training choices are lateral lifts, military, and bench presses.	If soreness remains for 7 to 10 days.

Table 12.4   ✦   Prevention and Emergency Treatment of Common Exercise Injuries *(continued)*

INJURY	GENERAL COMMENTS	PREVENTION AND TREATMENT	NEED FOR A PHYSICIAN
Thorax			
Rib fracture and bruises	Fractures may occur from direct contact or, uncommonly, from muscular contraction. A direct blow may displace the bone and produce jagged edges that cut the tissue of the lungs, producing bleeding or lung collapse.	The type of contact helps reveal rib fracture. Pain when breathing and palpitation are also signs. RICE therapy should be initiated immediately.	If pain is present when breathing after a direct blow to the thorax; If fracture is suspected.
Miscellaneous Injuries and Illnesses			
Abrasions	Superficial skin layers are scraped off. Injury imposes no serious problem if cleaned properly.	Clean with soap and warm water. Use a bandage if the wound oozes blood. Remove loose skin flaps with sterile scissors if dirty; allow to remain if clean.	If all dirt and foreign matter cannot be removed; If infection develops.
Common cold	Handshaking with an infected person or breathing in particles after a sneeze are two ways of transmitting a cold virus. Contributing factors may be low resistance, improper nutrition, tension, bacteria entering the respiratory tract, and remaining indoors in winter months, which increases the likelihood of close contact with a contagious person.	A cold will typically last about seven days. There is no known protection or cure. Antihistamines, decongestants, and cold tablets are of little value. Aspirin (for those over 16 years of age) or acetaminophen (for those under 16), combined with rest and plenty of fluids are sound advice. Exercise only lightly and include one or two days of rest.	If fever or sore throat lasts more than a week; If pain is present in one or both ears.
Fainting and dizziness	Lack of blood flow to the brain commonly occurs with increasing age, and may result in temporary loss of vision or lightheadedness.	Place the victim in a lying position with the feet elevated. If it is not possible to lie down, an alternative position is a sitting posture with the head lowered between the legs.	If loss of consciousness occurs; If dizziness occurs frequently.
Frostbite	Frostbite, a destruction of tissue by freezing, is more likely to occur on small parts of the nose, cheeks, ears, fingers, and toes.	Thaw rapidly in a warm water bath. Avoid rubbing areas with snow. Water should be comfortable to a normal, unfrozen hand (not over 104°F). When a flush reaches the fingers, remove the frostbitten part from the water immediately. For an ear or nose, use cloths soaked in warm water.	Always see a doctor.

Table 12.4 ✦ Prevention and Emergency Treatment of Common Exercise Injuries *(continued)*

Injury	General comments	Prevention and treatment	Need for a physician
Heat exhaustion/ heat stroke	The body loses heat to the environment and maintains normal temperature by: *Evaporation*—sweat evaporates into the atmosphere. *Radiation*—With body temperature higher than air temperature, heat loss occurs. *Convection*—As body heat loss occurs, air is warmed. This warmed air rises and cooler air moves in to take its place, cooling the body. *Conduction*—Heat moves from deeper body organs to skin through blood vessels. The skin acts as a radiation surface for heat loss to the air.	Symptoms of heat exhaustion include nausea, chills, cramps, and rapid pulse. Treatment requires immediate cooling with ice packs to the head, torso, and joints, and maintaining proper water and electrolyte balance.	If rapid improvement is not evident; If multiple cramps occur; If core temperature does not immediately return to normal.
Hypothermia	With extremely cold temperatures and high wind chill, core body temperature may drop below normal levels.	Prevention involves following the steps outlined in the section "Dressing Properly for the Weather" in chapter 9. Treatment calls for warming with blankets, heating pads, replacing wet clothing, and administering warm drinks.	If core temperature drops below 94°.
Infected wounds	Bacterial infection in the bloodstream (septicemia).	Keep area clean, changing the bandage and soaking and cleaning in warm water twice daily. Up to 10 to 12 days may be needed for normal healing.	If fever is above 100°; If thick pus and swelling occur the second day.
Minor cuts	Minor cuts can develop into serious problems if mistreated or neglected. Avoid use of antiseptics that may destroy tissue and actually retard healing.	Clean the wound with soap and water or hydrogen peroxide, removing all dirt and foreign matter. Use a butterfly bandage or steri-strip to bring the edges of the wound tightly together without trapping the fat or rolling the skin beneath.	If cut occurs to face or trunk; If deep cut involves tendons, nerves, vessels, or ligaments; If blood is pumping from a wound; If tingling or limb weakness occurs; If cut cannot be pulled together without trapping the fat; If direct pressure fails to stop the bleeding.

Table 12.4 ✦ Prevention and Emergency Treatment of Common Exercise Injuries *(continued)*

INJURY	GENERAL COMMENTS	PREVENTION AND TREATMENT	NEED FOR A PHYSICIAN
Muscle soreness	You may experience two different types of soreness: general soreness that appears immediately after your exercise session and disappears in 3 to 4 hours, or localized soreness appearing 8 to 24 hours after exercise. The older you are, the longer the period between exercise and soreness.	You can help prevent soreness by warming up properly, avoiding bouncing-type stretching, or flexibility, exercises and progressing slowly in your program. Doing too much too soon is a common cause. You can expect to have some soreness after your first few workouts, especially if you have been inactive. Don't stop exercising, it will only reoccur later.	If muscle soreness persists after the second week.
Muscle cramps	Muscular cramps commonly occur in three areas: back of lower leg (calf), back of upper leg (hamstring group), and front of upper leg (quadriceps group). Cramps may be related to fatigue, tightness of the muscles, or fluid, salt, and potassium imbalance.	Stretch before you exercise and drink water freely. If cramp occurs, stretch area carefully.	If multiple cramps occur If symptoms of heat exhaustion are present.

to 20 minutes. Depending on the severity of the injury and amount of swelling and pain, mild exercise can resume in four or five days. Another acronym to remind you of the proper procedure in treating minor injuries is PRICE; the "P" is a reminder to see a physician.

There is considerable misinformation available concerning proper home emergency treatment. Unfortunately, incorrect treatment can worsen the injury or actually produce serious side effects that may require surgery later.

Shock

Many injuries such as fractures, concussions, profuse bleeding, heart attack, back and neck damage, and severe joint trauma can produce shock. Shock is one of the body's strongest natural reactions to disease and injury. It slows blood flow acting as a natural tourniquet, reduces pain, and decreases the body's agony in serious injury. All three types of shock can kill: *traumatic* (injury or loss of blood), *septic* (infection-induced), and *cardiogenic* (from a heart attack). Shock is much easier to prevent than it is to treat. You

should assume that shock is present with the above injuries and illnesses, splint broken bones, handle the victim with care, stop the bleeding, and keep the victim warm at all times.

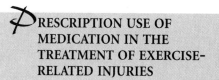

PRESCRIPTION USE OF MEDICATION IN THE TREATMENT OF EXERCISE-RELATED INJURIES

Numerous prescription and nonprescription (over-the-counter) drugs are available to combat infection, treat fungi, control pain and bleeding, and reduce inflammation. It is wise, however, to consult your physician before using any medication. It is also important to update your home medicine cabinet to make certain you are stocking the basics for common illnesses and injuries. Take a moment to analyze your home pharmacy by completing Lab Activity 12.2: Evaluating Your Home Medicine Cabinet at the end of this chapter. Then compare your findings to the recommended home pharmacy in Table 12.5 on page 263.

Myth and Fact Sheet

Myth	Fact
1. When an injury occurs to most body parts, heat should be applied.	1. Injuries to soft tissue should be treated with RICE therapy, which requires ice, not heat. Heat should be avoided for two to three days until swelling begins to subside. Early use of heat in any form increases swelling, delays healing, and can result in serious tissue changes that may require surgery to correct.
2. Ice should be applied directly to the skin for one hour.	2. The maximum amount of time ice should be applied is 20 minutes. Longer periods can actually bring about tissue damage. And it should not come in contact with the skin unless an ice massage is being used.
3. Individuals who have a heart murmur should not exercise.	3. A heart murmur is an abnormal sound caused by turbulent blood flow. The difficulty may be an impaired valve that fails to close completely or valve orifices that are narrowed and slow the flow of blood. A greater-than-normal load is placed on the heart, heart walls may increase in size, and tension increases inside the walls. The heart is less efficient and, in a sense, has to regurgitate blood twice. In what is termed a functional murmur, no structural defect is evident to account for the abnormal sounds. Although individuals with functional murmurs can generally exercise safely, it is important to consult your physician before starting an exercise program.
4. Individuals who have the wind knocked out of them are in danger of dying.	4. The temporary inability to breathe following a blow to a relaxed midsection will slowly subside until breathing is restored. Meanwhile, you will gasp for breath, possibly suffer dizziness, nausea, weakness, or even collapse. A hard blow to the solar plexus increases intra-abdominal pressure, causes pain, and interferes with the diaphragmatic cycle reflex due to nerve paralysis or muscle spasm. Breathing is only temporarily affected by a blow that momentarily paralyzes the nerve control of the diaphragm. Loosen clothing at the neck and waist; apply ice to the abdomen; and breathe slowly through the nose.
5. A popping or snapping sound in the knee is a sign of serious trouble.	5. The sound generally comes from a tendon flipping over bony fulcrums and may be quite natural in some athletes who just never really noticed the sound before. Joint mice or the presence of some loose cartilage or other tissue may also produce a clicking sound as the knee flexes and extends. Bone, tendon, ligament, or cartilage damage may not be indicated unless other symptoms are present such as inflammation, swelling, fluid, and knee locking.

Infection can often be prevented by including at least one antiseptic and one wound protectant in your home medicine kit. Your physician may also prescribe an antibiotic, either a topical dressing or a systemic medication.

Pain may be controlled through the skin by applying a topical anesthesia to inhibit pain sensations through quick evaporation and cooling or by counterirritating the skin so you are no longer aware of the pain. Liniments, analgesic balms, heat, and cold

Table 12.5 ✦ Your Home Pharmacy

MEDICAL CONCERN	MEDICATION
Allergy	**Antihistamines***
Cold and coughs	Cold tablets and cough drops
Constipation	**Milk of magnesia**
Diarrhea	Antidiarrheal, paregoric
Eye irritations	Eye drops
Exercise injury problems (inflammation)	See your physician; **aspirin,** NSAID medication
Exercise injury problems (pain)	**Acetaminophen, aspirin** and use of heat and cold
Pain and fever (children)	Children's aspirin, acetaminophen, liquid acetaminophen, aspirin, rectal suppositories
Fungus	**Antifungal preparations**
Sunburn (preventive)	**Sunblock**
Sprains	**Elastic bandages**
Stomach, upset	Antacid (nonabsorbable)
Wounds (general)	**Adhesive tape, bandages, sodium bicarbonate (soaking agent)**
Wounds (antiseptics)	**Ethyl alcohol (60–90%),** isopropyl alcohol
Wounds (protectant)	Topical antibiotics

*Items in bold print are basic requirements; other preparations are also useful and should be considered.

are examples of **counterirritants**. Some central nervous system drugs such as acetaminophen (Tylenol®) and aspirin reduce pain by acting on the nerves that carry the pain impulse to the brain.

Inflammation to soft tissue can be reduced through the use of one of several drugs. Aspirin is effective for conditions such as tendonitis, bursitis, chondromalacia, and tendosynovitis. Some enzymes can help treat swollen joints, reduce inflammation, edema, pain, swelling, and redness. NSAIDs (nonsteroid-antiflammatory drugs) are also quite effective in eliminating inflammation. A physician's prescription and guidance is needed, however, since side effects may occur and dangers exist with long-term use.

NUTRITION AND HEALING

Individuals who do not eat correctly and have poor nutritional status do not heal as rapidly as normal. Although the recommended daily allowances (RDAs) (see chapter 8) for protein and for some vitamins and minerals increase during periods of recovery from illness and injury, a sufficient safety margin exists in the RDA to promote normal healing and recovery, providing you are consuming adequate fluids and calories.

> **Counterirritants** Medication, heat, cold, electricity, and so forth used to eliminate pain and inflammation.

Behavioral Change and Motivational Strategies

There are many things that might interfere with the use of some practices known to prevent exercise-related injuries. Here are some of these barriers (roadblocks) and strategies for overcoming them.

Roadblock	Behavioral Change Strategy
Although you are aware of the value of proper warmup before exercise, you just never seem to do it. It seems so natural to change into your workout clothing and immediately start the three-mile jog or the tennis match. Yet you have noticed a tightness in the calf muscles after exercise for a week or so now.	Most people are impatient and want to get right into exercise, without wasting time. It is kind of a mind set that is difficult to overcome. One approach may be to avoid viewing warmup as a separate component of your program. Continue what you are doing but divide the run into three continuous segments: (1) Begin jogging immediately but very slowly for the first mile, progressing from a quarter-mile walk to a slow jog. (2) Stop and stretch for at least five minutes, emphasizing calf and Achilles tendon exercises (see chapter 7). (3) Complete the remaining two miles of your run. Other forms of exercise can also be planned that permit considerably less effort in the initial 5 to 10 minutes to build in a warmup period.
You are totally exhausted at the end of your workout and feel nauseated, uncomfortable, and have some muscle soreness.	Most individuals develop the habit of saving the most vigorous part of their workout routine for the final 5 to 10 minutes, before stopping and standing around to talk or sitting down to relax. Failure to use a cooldown period produces the roadblock symptoms. You can avoid this problem by adding one more segment to the three-mile run. Segment three should involve the most vigorous portion of the workout for about 1.5 miles or 10 to 20 minutes followed by a fourth segment involving a half-mile slow jog or walk and a brief stretching period to taper off at the end of your workout.
List roadblocks interfering with your approach to exercise injury prevention.	Now, cite the behavioral-change strategies that can help you overcome the roadblocks you listed. If you need to, refer back to chapter 3 for behavioral-change and motivational strategies.

1. _____

2. _____

3. _____

1. _____

2. _____

3. _____

SUMMARY

Protecting Your Body from Injury and Illness

Many exercise-related injuries are preventable. You can significantly reduce your risk of injury and illness by using a preconditioning period before beginning your exercise program, warming up and cooling down properly, analyzing your medical history, progressing slowly in the early stages of your program, monitoring body signals, dressing properly for the activity, and mastering proper form.

Tissue Response to Injury

The healing process is unique to each individual. Factors such as age, nutrition, treatment, and type and severity of the injury play major roles. In the acute stage immediately following an injury, the body attempts to keep things localized to prevent further damage and aid the healing process that will occur over the next five to six weeks. Complete regeneration and repair, however, may require up to one year.

General Treatment Modalities

The immediate and continued use of cold applications over the first several days after a soft-tissue injury should be followed by heat therapy during the repair and remodeling stage of healing. Numerous techniques to apply heat and cold can be safely used.

Prevention and Emergency Treatment of Common Exercise Injuries and Illnesses

Proper home emergency treatment for a soft-tissue injury to an extremity requires the use of RICE. Certain symptoms suggest the need for immediate care by a physician. If you are in doubt, take the injured person to an emergency room or physician as soon as possible.

Some injuries involving fractures, concussions, bleeding, heart attack, and severe joint trauma can produce shock. Since shock is considerably easier to prevent than it is to treat, precautions should be taken with all patients when dealing with these types of injuries.

Prescription Use of Medication in the Treatment of Exercise-Related Injuries

The home medicine cabinet should contain the basic items necessary for the emergency treatment of common exercise injuries. Over-the-counter medication to treat inflammation, fungi, pain, fever, wounds, and basic problems such as allergy, colds, constipation, diarrhea, and eye irritations should be readily available.

Nutrition and Healing

Sound nutrition is important during recovery from both injury and illness. Nutritional needs increase somewhat during the recovery period, and it is important to continue to eat well, avoid skipping meals, drink plenty of water and other fluids, and consider the use of a multiple vitamin and mineral supplement.

Lab Activity 12.1

Evaluating Your Potential for Foot and Leg Injuries

INSTRUCTIONS: *Injuries to the feet and legs are common in most sports and activities. If you continue the same activity long enough, overuse injuries are almost certain. There are also certain aspects in the makeup of the lower extremities that may require some adjustment to prevent injury. To evaluate your potential for lower extremity injury, examine yourself carefully in the following areas:*

1. **Length of both legs below the ankle:** Stand erect, ankles together, and ask a helper to measure the distance from the floor to a spot marked with a magic marker at the bony protrusion of your ankle.

2. **Length of both legs above the ankle:** Sit in a chair with your feet on the floor, heels together, and toes pointed. If a carpenter's level placed on both knees is uneven, your problem is above the ankle.

3. **Morton's toe:** Stand erect without shoes or socks and determine whether your second toe is larger than your great toe.

4. **Excessive pronation:** Examine your running or athletic shoes for excessive wear on the outside back of the shoe heel.

✦ Results

1. Does the length of your legs differ by more than 1/16 of an inch?

2. Is the problem below the ankle or from the ankle to the knee?

3. Is your second metatarsal longer than your great toe?

4. Are your shoes wearing evenly?

5. Are you experiencing pain in the lower back, hip, knee, ankle, or feet during or following exercise?

If you answered "yes" to any of the questions, consult your orthopedic physician for advice on how to prevent a future injury.

Lab Activity 12.2

Evaluating Your Home Medicine Cabinet

INSTRUCTIONS: *It is very important to analyze your home medicine cabinet at least once a year and discard outdated prescriptions and other medicine. Replace used items, discard unnecessary items, place dangerous medicine out of the reach of children, and purchase newly needed products. Since you are beginning a new exercise program, some new items may be needed to prepare you for the treatment of common injuries. Complete the three steps below to evaluate and update your home medicine cabinet.*

1. Prepare a list of all items in your home medicine cabinet and complete the form below.

ITEM	DATE	PURPOSE	EFFECTIVENESS

2. List all unneeded and outdated items that can be discarded.

3. Study Table 12.5 on page 263 to make certain your cabinet contains the bare necessities for treatment of common exercise injuries and ailments. List the items you are missing and may want to consider purchasing.

13

PREVENTING HEART DISEASE AND CANCER

Chapter Objectives

By the end of this chapter, you should be able to:

1. Cite the prevalence and describe the causes of heart disease.
2. Cite the prevalence and describe the causes of cancer.
3. Describe how to prevent or postpone the development of heart disease.
4. Describe how to prevent cancer.
5. Discuss the role of physical fitness in preventing heart disease and cancer.

WHEN FRANK WAS young he assumed he was invulnerable. He knew intellectually that he would someday die; sooner or later everyone does. But that was not a reality Frank had internalized. In fact, he acted as though he was impervious to the effects of his health decisions. He smoked cigarettes; rarely exercised; took on too much work thereby "stressing himself out"; did not eat well by often choosing fatty meals at fast-food restaurants; and spent prolonged periods lounging in the sun.

Frank eventually paid the price for his health-related choices. By the time he reached his fiftieth year, he had a cough diagnosed as lung cancer, and had blocked arteries that threatened a heart attack. Although he had yet to develop skin cancer, his doctor warned him that cancer was possible unless he altered his exposure to the sun's harsh rays. Contributing to his heart condition was the amount of stress to which he subjected himself, the cigarettes he smoked, and his lack of regular exercise. Contributing to the threat of his developing cancer elsewhere than in the lungs was his ingestion of foods high in fat. Frank's early years may have been carefree but his later adult life was fraught with discomfort and fear. He realized he would not live as long as he might have.

Unfortunately, Frank's situation, extreme though it may sound, is not all that unusual.

Too many people have experienced the death of a loved one from either heart disease or cancer. If you have not experienced any of these illnesses yourself, you certainly know others who have—parents, grandparents, relatives, friends. This is not surprising since heart disease and cancer account for 57 percent of all deaths that occur in the United States each year. Throw in stroke, which is also a developmental disease associated with an unhealthy lifestyle, and you have accounted for almost two-thirds of the deaths that occur in this country every year.

In this chapter, we will define heart disease and cancer and discuss what causes them. More importantly, we describe how to prevent their occurrence or at least how to delay their arrival. Much of that latter discussion pertains to lifestyle decisions that include physical fitness and wellness considerations.

Coronary Heart Disease

One of the authors of this book recently moved into a new house—one built from scratch—and has experienced a most frustrating situation. Every few weeks the faucets have to be dismantled to clean out the debris. The builder says this is to be expected in a new

> **Coronary heart disease (CHD)** A condition in which the heart is supplied with insufficient blood due to clogging of coronary arteries.
>
> **Occluded** Clogged arteries that no longer allow the normal amount of blood to pass through them.
>
> **Plaque** A collection of blood fats and other substances that combine to clog blood vessels.
>
> **Atherosclerosis** A condition in which plaque has formed and blocks the passage of blood through a blood vessel.
>
> **Angina pectoris** Chest pain caused by restricted blood flow to the heart.
>
> **Lipoproteins** Fatty particles that can collect on the walls of the blood vessels.
>
> **Triglyceride** The fatty substance in lipoproteins.
>
> **Low-density lipoproteins (LDL)** Fatty particles in the blood that carry cholesterol to cells throughout the body.
>
> **High-density lipoproteins (HDL)** Fatty particles in the blood that pick up unused cholesterol and transport it for processing and elimination from the body.

house, that it is the lead and material from inside the pipes that accumulates and clogs the faucets. No matter whether it is to be expected, every few weeks the screen in the faucets gets clogged and has to be taken out and cleaned.

The situation with the faucets is analogous to that of the body's fluid system, which includes the heart, the blood, and the blood vessels. As the faucets carry water to where it is needed, so do the blood vessels carry blood to where it is needed. As the pumping station somewhere in town pumps the water, so does the heart pump the blood. And as pipes can become clogged with debris, so can your blood vessels.

How the Heart Functions

The heart's main function is to pump blood containing oxygen and nutrients to parts of the body. It also receives blood filled with waste products (such as carbon dioxide) that are to be eliminated from the body. The heart pumps this blood through the circulatory system and into and from the lungs via blood vessels. If these blood vessels become obstructed or if they rupture thereby interfering with the passage of oxygenated blood, the part of the body deprived of blood can die. And if it is the heart's blood supply that is blocked, it too can die. That is what happens when a heart attack occurs. Since the arteries supplying the heart are called the coronary arteries, any problem with them is called either **coronary heart disease (CHD)** or coronary artery disease.

Coronary Heart Disease (CHD)

Some people are born with heart disease. They may have a heart chamber missing or malformed, a valve between the chambers of the heart not opening or closing adequately, or a weak heart that is unable to pump with enough power to expel sufficient amounts of blood throughout the body. Others may have blood vessels that do not work normally because they are malformed. And still others may have heart disease because they have had rheumatic fever (which affects the heart valves), or they may experience an irregular heart beat known as an *arrythmia*.

The most prevalent form of heart disease, however, is CHD. The coronary arteries can become **occluded** when blood fats and other substances collect on their inside walls thereby narrowing the opening through which blood can flow (see Figure 13.1). This collection of blood fats and other substances can also break loose and travel through the arteries until they get caught and block the flow of blood at that point. That is called a *thrombosis*. The clogging mate-

Figure 13.1 ✦ Coronary Artery Blockage

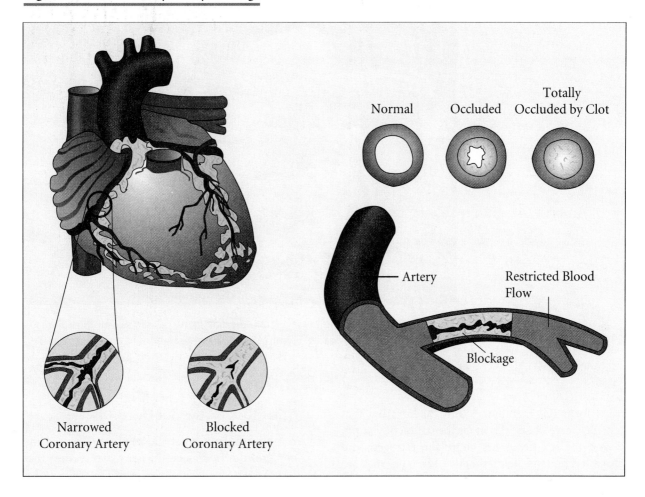

Normal

Occluded

Totally
Occluded by Clot

Artery

Restricted Blood
Flow

Blockage

Narrowed
Coronary Artery

Blocked
Coronary Artery

rial is called **plaque** and the condition is known as **atherosclerosis**. Plaque consists of fatty substances, cholesterol, cellular waste products, calcium, and the clotting material *fibrin*. If blood flow is restricted, a person can become fatigued easily and may feel **angina pectoris** when they are active. If the coronary arteries are so narrowed or blocked that little, if any, blood can pass through, the part of the heart deprived of oxygenated blood can die. And if that part is important or involves a large enough section of the heart, the person to whom this happens can die.

Fat and Cholesterol

Lipoproteins consist of **triglycerides**, a blood protein (to make the fat soluble in the portion of the blood that is water), and cholesterol. Although some people are suspicious of the role of triglycerides in causing CHD, researchers have found no clearcut association between the two. The real culprit in CHD is the cholesterol found in the foods we eat and that is manufactured by the liver. When we eat foods high

in saturated fats, the liver is stimulated to manufacture cholesterol. Add that to the cholesterol in the foods of animal origin that we eat, and the amount in our blood can be excessive. The recommended daily consumption of cholesterol is 300 milligrams. Yet the average person in the United States consumes 1½ to 3 times that amount. The recommended amount of saturated fat to be consumed daily is 10 percent of total calories. Yet the average person in the United States consumes over three times that amount. No wonder heart disease is the leading cause of death in the United States.

Low-Density and High-Density Lipoproteins (LDLs and HDLs)

There are several different kinds of lipoproteins, of which **low-density lipoproteins (LDLs)** and **high-density lipoproteins (HDLs)** have the most significance for CHD. LDLs are produced in the liver and released into the bloodstream where they carry cholesterol to cells throughout the body. Cholesterol

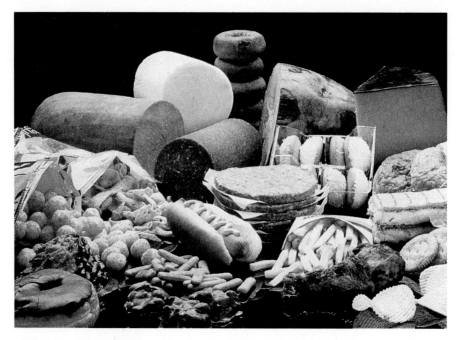

The average American eats too much fat and cholesterol, substances that contribute to both heart disease and cancer. (Photo Courtesy of the National Cancer Institute.)

helps form cell membranes and the covering that protects nerve fibers; aids in the formation of vitamin D and the sex hormones androgen, estrogen, and progesterone; and helps produce bile salts that aid digestion of fats. When LDLs carry more cholesterol than the body requires, however, it can build up on the artery walls.

HDLs are also produced by the liver and released into the bloodstream. Although they also carry cholesterol, HDLs pick up unused cholesterol and return it to the liver where it is used to produce bile salts. In addition, it is thought that HDLs possibly provide a protective layer of grease to help prevent a build-up of substances on artery walls.

When LDL is elevated and HDL is too sparse, there is a likelihood that arteries will be clogged and CHD will be promoted. It is recommended that HDL (the *good* cholesterol) levels exceed 35 for adult men and 45 for adult women and that LDL (the *bad* cholesterol) levels remain less than 165. A total cholesterol/HDL ratio of 5:1 (20 percent of total cholesterol being of the HDL variety) begins to provide some protection from CHD. Physical activity can increase HDL levels in the bloodstream. That is one reason it is recommended as a way of preventing CHD.

To determine if the composition of your blood is healthful, complete Lab Activity 13.1: Is Your Blood in Tune? at the end of this chapter.

Other Risk Factors for Heart Disease

You already know that the foods we eat and the cholesterol our bodies produce are two reasons that blood vessels can become clogged. There are also other causes of clogged coronary arteries and for the development of heart disease.

Hypertension Hypertension is systolic blood pressure in excess of 140 mm Hg or diastolic blood pressure in excess of 90 mm Hg. **Systolic blood pressure** refers to the force of the blood against the arterial blood vessel walls when the left ventricle contracts and blood is pumped out of the heart. **Diastolic blood pressure** represents the force of the blood against the arterial walls when the heart is relaxed. High blood pressure forces the heart to work harder than normal and places the arteries under strain. Eventually, hypertension contributes to heart attacks, strokes, and atherosclerosis. In 90 percent of high blood-pressure *essential hypertension* cases, the causes are unknown. In the remaining 10 percent, it is caused by kidney abnormality, tumor of the adrenal gland, or a congenital defect of the aorta (the main artery leading out of the heart). Regular physical activity and a healthier diet are often recommended for people whose blood pressure is too high. In some cases, medication is needed to reduce blood pressure to healthier levels.

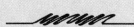

Myth and Fact Sheet

Myth	Fact
1. If CHD runs in your family, there is not much you can do to prevent getting it.	1. CHD is related to a number of factors of which heredity is but one. Other risk factors include smoking, lack of exercise, fatty diets, obesity, and high blood pressure. You can do much to eliminate or diminish the effects of these risk factors.
2. All cholesterol is bad.	2. Cholesterol that accumulates on the walls of the arteries, LDL, is bad for you. HDL, however, helps to carry blood fats out of the body and is therefore helpful.
3. You can recognize if your blood pressure is high but there is little you can do to lower it.	3. High blood pressure occurs without any noticeable symptoms, but with a healthier diet and regular physical activity, blood pressure can be lowered, even without medication.
4. Everything causes cancer.	4. This is just not true. Although cancer can result from toxins, carcinogens in cigarette smoke, chemicals, and viruses, saying that everything causes cancer is just an excuse for ignoring specific causes.
5. Cancer affects all groups of people to the same extent.	5. More African-American men and women than white men and women die of cancer. And white men and women contract skin cancer to a much greater extent than do African-American men and women.

Obesity or Overweight Excess weight places added strain on the heart and increases blood pressure and blood cholesterol. For these reasons, people who have gained more than 20 pounds since they were 18 years old have been found to have doubled their risk of experiencing a heart attack. In addition, obesity is linked to diabetes, and is usually associated with lack of physical activity, thereby further increasing the risk of heart attack.

Stress Excessive stress also increases a person's chances of contracting heart disease. That is because stress results in an increase in cholesterol in the blood, an increase in heart rate, higher blood pressure, and other effects detrimental to normal heart functioning. Stress results in the release of hormones called *catecholamines,* which prepare the body to respond physically to the fight-or-flight response. The heart beats faster, blood pressure increases, and blood glucose and cholesterol levels increase. If stress occurs often, these detrimental effects become chronic and can lead to CHD.

Two researchers (Freidman and Rosenman, 1974) have even found a coronary-prone personality type. They call it Type A behavior pattern, characterized by being focused on time (hurried and time pressured),

competitive, aggressive, hostile, and multiphasic (doing two or more things at a time). The opposite, Type B behavior pattern, seems to protect people from developing CHD. More recent research indicates that hostility is the major ingredient in the Type A behavior pattern. That is, people who are easily angered and who are often hostile are the most susceptible to CHD. Stress also too frequently interferes with people engaging in regular exercise. They become so concerned with managing the source of the stress—whether that be their classes, jobs, or home lives—that they allow too little time, if any, for physical activity.

Hypertension High blood pressure; usually greater than 140 systolic blood pressure and/or greater than 90 diastolic blood pressure.

Systolic blood pressure The force of the blood against the arterial blood-vessel walls when left ventricle contracts and blood is pumped out of the heart.

Diastolic blood pressure The force of the blood against the arterial walls when the heart is relaxed.

𝒟iversity 𝒥ssues

Cardiovascular Disease

In 1987, the death rate from coronary heart disease was 135 per 100,000 for the entire U.S. population. However, the rate was 163 per 100,000 for African Americans. Increasing the level of physical activity and fitness is a major goal for men and women of all ages in the United States today. This need is particularly significant for special populations, such as low-income people, people of various ethnic backgrounds, and people with disabilities.

At one time, mortality from cardiovascular disease among women received little attention. In recent years, however, it has been discovered that the death rates from cardiovascular disease are three to five times higher among African-American women than among white women in every age category past age 18. The prevalence of obesity and high blood pressure is also higher. The prevalence of obesity among all women was 27 percent from the 1976–80 National Health and Nutrition Examination Survey (NHANES II). However, 44 percent of African-American women aged 20 and older were overweight. The prevalence of obesity was 39 percent for Mexican-American women, 34 percent for Cuban women, and 37 percent for Puerto Rican women. The prevalence of obesity ranged from 29 to 75 percent among Native Americans and Native Alaskans in 1975. Furthermore, 50 percent of women with high blood pressure were also obese.

These startling statistics are partially explained by the low level of cardiovascular fitness among women from the different ethnic backgrounds. Many nonwhite women are from the low-income population. Research has shown that less than 7 percent of lower-income people aged 18 and older engage in vigorous physical activity. (*Vigorous activity* is defined as the type of activity that promotes the development of cardiovascular fitness three or more days per week for 20 minutes or more per exercise session.) Furthermore, in 1985, 32 percent of lower-income people reported no leisure-time physical activity. Given the beneficial effects of physical activity on obesity, high blood pressure, and cardiovascular disease, the government is seeking to increase community availability and accessibility of physical fitness facilities. ♦

Sedentary Lifestyle We have just discussed the effect of stress on physical activity. In addition, a sedentary lifestyle does not allow for the production of sufficient HDL, strengthen the heart muscle, or help control mild hypertension. To make matters worse, inactivity is associated with overweight and obesity, two other risk factors for CHD. And, inactivity deprives you of an outlet for the release of built-up stress by-products (for example, cholesterol).

Smoking Tobacco Research has linked smoking with various diseases such as cancer, emphysema, and heart disease. When a person smokes, the blood vessels constrict thereby causing increased blood pressure. In addition, the heart speeds up in response to nicotine, a central nervous system stimulant. Furthermore, cigarettes contain substances that can damage the inside walls of the arteries. Once they have been damaged, it is easier for cholesterol and other substances to adhere to, and accumulate in, the arteries. All of this, coupled with carbon dioxide from cigarette smoke replacing oxygen in the bloodstream, means the heart is overworking and heart disease is more likely.

Family History Not all risk factors are amenable to change. Heredity, for example, is not. Some people are born with a predisposition to heart disease. However, that predisposition only means there is the *potential* to develop CHD. Your lifestyle will influence whether you do and when you do. Some people prefer to use a family history of heart disease as an excuse for behaving in ways that are unhealthy for the heart. That is unfortunate because they might be able to delay or even prevent CHD if they change their behavior.

To determine your risk of acquiring CHD, complete Lab Activity 13.2: Risk Factor Analysis: The Game of HEALTH at the end of this chapter.

How to Prevent Coronary Heart Disease (CHD)

It is possible to manage many of the risk factors for CHD. Hypertension can be controlled by some combination of diet, exercise, or medication. Overweight or obesity can be controlled by diet and exercise. Stress can be managed by a change in lifestyle and engaging regularly in some form of relaxation. Sedentary lifestyles can be remedied by participation in an exercise program. Smoking can be stopped by joining a smoking cessation program or quitting cold turkey. And periodic medical screenings can be useful to analyze blood lipids and evaluate the functioning of the heart. The good news is that you have a great deal of influence over whether you develop CHD. If you are serious about preventing CHD, you can do so.

The Role of Physical Activity

Physical activity is one of the most important components of a CHD-prevention program. That is because it is either directly or indirectly related to so many of the risk factors. Physical activity exercises the heart muscle, encourages the production of HDL, and aids in the control and prevention of mild hypertension. It enhances cardiorespiratory endurance and increases stroke volume of the heart (the amount of blood pumped out of the heart with each contraction). It also is an excellent stress-management technique since it uses the stress by-products that prepare the body to respond physically to a stressor. And physical activity can help you maintain desirable weight and the proper amount of lean body mass.

These effects are somewhat direct and obvious, but there are less direct and less obvious CHD-related benefits of physical activity as well. Engaging in regular exercise will tone your body, provide you with confidence in your ability to perform physically, and make you feel better about yourself. In short, it will improve your self-esteem. The result will be less stress, fewer catecholamines produced, and therefore less potential damage to your heart.

Physical activity also encourages smoking cessation. Smoking is incompatible with aerobic activity since carbon monoxide replaces oxygen in the bloodstream. Furthermore, doing one good thing for your health, such as becoming physically fit, encourages other healthy lifestyle adjustments.

It is for these and other reasons that an effective CHD-prevention program includes a physical activity component. As prestigious an organization as the American Heart Association (AHA) recognizes the importance of physical activity in preventing CHD. In 1992, the Committee on Exercise and Cardiac Rehabilitation of the Council on Clinical Cardiology of the AHA published a position paper entitled "Statement on Exercise: Benefits and Recommendations for Physical Activity Programs for All Americans." That AHA statement serves as a good summary of the role physical activity can play in preventing and treating CHD. In it the AHA states that:

Exercise helps control blood lipid abnormalities, diabetes, and obesity. . . . Inactivity is a risk factor for the development of coronary artery disease. . . . There is also evidence that physical activity probably alleviates symptoms of mild and moderate depression and provides an alternative to alcoholism and drug abuse.

The AHA goes on to suggest specific activities that are most beneficial:

Activities such as walking, hiking, stair-climbing, aerobic exercise, calisthenics, jogging, running, bicycling, rowing, and swimming and sports such as tennis, racquetball [sic], soccer, basketball, and touch football are especially beneficial when performed regularly. Brisk walking is also an excellent choice. . . . The evidence also supports the notion that even low-intensity activities performed daily can have some long-term health benefits and lower the risk of cardiovascular disease. Such activities include walking for pleasure, gardening, yard work, house work, dancing, and prescribed home exercise.

CANCER

Cancer is a disease involving abnormal cell growth. Cells grow wildly, divide rapidly, and assume irregular shapes. Tumors develop and invade nearby normal tissue. These abnormal cells can spread to other parts of the body via the bloodstream and lymphatic system in a process called **metastasis**. The result can be disability and/or death.

Cancer is the second leading cause of death in the United States. Tables 13.1 and 13.2 on page 278 clearly demonstrate that lung cancer is by far the leading cause of death from cancer in both men and women, but that need not be the case. If everyone who now smokes cigarettes quit, the incidence of lung cancer would decline dramatically.

Cancer is really more than one disease. Some cancers are caused by chemicals, others by environmental pollutants, some by radiation from the sun, and still others by viruses. As we have already discussed, cancers also occur in different parts of the body. Even the treatment for different cancers can vary. In some cases, surgery is necessary to remove the cancerous tissue. Sometimes radiation or chemotherapy is required. Often a combination of these three treatments is used.

Metastasis The process in which cancerous cells from one part of the body travel to other parts of the body.

Table 13.1 ✦ Estimated Cancer Incidence in the United States, by Site and Sex

MALES		FEMALES	
New Cases	Type	New Cases	Type
165,000	Prostate	182,000	Breast
100,000	Lung	75,000	Colon and rectum
77,000	Colon and rectum	70,000	Lung
39,000	Bladder	44,500	Uterus
28,500	Lymphoma	22,400	Lymphoma
20,300	Oral	22,000	Ovary
17,000	Melanoma of skin	15,000	Melanoma of skin
16,800	Kidney	14,200	Pancreas
16,700	Leukemia	13,300	Bladder
14,800	Stomach	12,600	Leukemia
13,500	Pancreas	10,400	Kidney
10,000	Larynx	9,500	Oral

Source: American Cancer Society, *Cancer Facts & Figures—1993*. New York: American Cancer Society, 1993, p. 12. Used by permission. © American Cancer Society, Inc.

Causes of Cancer

Cancer develops from a number of different causes. By far the greatest cause of cancer is the use of tobacco. An estimated 75 percent of all lung cancer cases are thought to be caused by smoking cigarettes. Smoking a pipe or cigar or chewing tobacco can cause cancer of the mouth and its parts. The use of tobacco products is associated with cancer of the larynx, pharynx, esophagus, pancreas, and bladder.

High fat diets are associated with cancer of the colon, rectum, prostate, stomach, and breast. Conversely, diets low in fat, but high in fruits and vegetables, seem to offer protection against certain cancers.

Repeated exposure to the sun is also a cause of skin cancer. It is the radiation from the sun that is the culprit here. Particularly vulnerable are people with fair skin who burn easily.

Excessive use of alcohol exposes one to the risk of oral cancer and cancers of the larynx, throat, esopha-

Table 13.2 ✦ Estimated Cancer Deaths in the United States, by Site and Sex

MALES		FEMALES	
Deaths	Type	Deaths	Type
93,000	Lung	56,000	Lung
35,000	Prostate	46,000	Breast
28,800	Colon and rectum	28,200	Colon and rectum
12,000	Pancreas	13,300	Ovary
11,500	Lymphoma	13,000	Pancreas
10,100	Leukemia	10,500	Lymphoma
8,200	Stomach	10,100	Uterus
7,600	Esophagus	8,500	Leukemia
6,800	Liver	5,800	Liver
6,600	Brain	5,500	Brain
6,500	Kidney	5,400	Stomach
6,500	Bladder	4,600	Multiple myeloma

Source: American Cancer Society, *Cancer Facts & Figures—1993*. New York: American Cancer Society, 1993, p. 12. Used by permission. © American Cancer Society, Inc.

gus, and liver, especially when accompanied by the use of smokeless tobacco.

Other causes of cancers include occupational hazards (exposure to toxins or chemicals or other **carcinogens**), viruses, obesity, environmental pollutants (such as those contained in automobile exhaust), and hereditary and genetic factors.

To determine how susceptible you are to contracting cancer, complete Lab Activity 13.3: Determining Your Risk of Acquiring Cancer at the end of this chapter.

Cancer Prevention

Although not all cancers can be prevented, in excess of 80 percent probably can be. If people gave up smoking, ate diets consisting of less fat and more vegetables and fruits, limited the amount of alcohol they ingested, and protected themselves from exposure to the sun, the decrease in the incidence of cancer would be significant. Here are some things you can do to decrease your chances of contracting cancer, or if you do contract it, to detect it early:

- Abstain from using tobacco in any form, including the smokeless variety.
- Eliminate or reduce your consumption of alcohol; drink only in moderation.
- Avoid contact with known carcinogens whenever possible.
- Decrease your exposure to the sun; avoid sunbathing for long periods of time; and use a sunscreen with the appropriate sun protection factor (SPF) for your skin type any time you plan to be in the sun.
- Follow a dietary plan that increases your consumption of vitamins A and C, cruciferous vegetables (for example, cauliflower and broccoli), and fiber. Reduce your consumption of

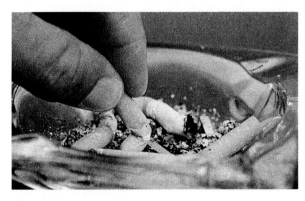

Abstaining from any type of tobacco products greatly reduces the risk of cancer. (Photo Courtesy of the American Heart Association.)

Fitness Heroes

When Rabbi Hirscel Jaffe crossed the finish line of the New York Marathon in 1978, he faced the fight of his life—the fight against cancer. He won the fight and recovered from leukemia. While this was a feat in itself, Rabbi Jaffe decided to share his good fortune and began helping others to overcome adversity as well.

Rabbi Jaffe began counseling cancer patients, became coeditor of *Gates of Healing* (a book distributed to hospital patients everywhere), wrote a highly acclaimed book called *Why Me, Why Anyone?*, and, most recently, developed a videotape titled "Hanging on to Hope." In 1988, he received the American Cancer Society's *Award of Courage* from President Reagan.

Overcoming adversity in Rabbi Jaffe's eyes is about more than physical illness. He visited U.S. hostages in Iran in 1980 to give them comfort and support. In October 1992, he led a unity march in Newburgh, New York, to protest the appearance of the Ku Klux Klan in his town. Over 3,000 people participated.

Those who know him best call him "the running Rabbi" for both his marathon participation and his tireless efforts on behalf of others. Rabbi Jaffe certainly meets our criteria for a fitness hero. ✦

Source: Adapted from "Running for Life," *Alumnus,* Spring 1993, p. 6.

artificial sweeteners, heat-charred food, nitrite-cured or smoked foods, fats, and calories.
- Maintain recommended body weight and fat.
- Memorize the seven warning signs of cancer (see Table 13.3 on page 280) and be alert to these changes if they occur in your body.
- Obtain cancer screenings as recommended (see Table 13.4 on page 281) to identify early signs of cancer.
- Learn how to do breast (females) and testicular (males) self-examinations and do them regularly.

Carcinogens Agents (toxins, chemicals, and so forth) that can cause cancer.

Diversity Issues

Cancer

Ever notice how ads for cigarettes have changed over the years? Well, leaders in the African-American community have! They are appalled at the appeal made to African Americans in particular, and to people of low socioeconomic status and low levels of education in general. The actions of these advertisers and manufacturers of cigarettes are even more distasteful when viewed with the following statistics in mind.

Cancer rates and risk factors—such as cigarette smoking—differ by cultural variables. Whereas the cancer death rate for the general population is 133 per 100,000 people and is 158 per 100,000 people for white men, for African-American men it is 288 per 100,000 people. For white females the cancer death rate is 110 per 100,000 people, whereas for African-American females it is 132 per 100,000 people.

Cigarette smoking is a significant risk factor for cancer. Although 29 percent of people aged 20 and older smoke cigarettes, this differs by gender: 32 percent of men and 27 percent of women smoke. It also differs by other factors. African Americans' and Hispanics' (aged 20 and older) smoking rates are higher than the general population's (34 percent and 33 percent, respectively). Southeast Asian men living in the United States have an even higher smoking rate (55 percent).

Skin cancer rates also differ between different cultural groups. Whereas the rate for whites is 233 per 100,000 people, it is only 3 per 100,000 for African Americans. And, white men experience 1.5 to 3 times the incidence of skin cancer than white women. Recognizing the public's increased awareness of the risk of skin cancer, cosmetic manufacturers have deemphasized suntan lotions and are now pushing sun blockers. Call this good old American ingenuity, or exploitation. In any case, it is a postive change. ♦

- Check for changes in your skin that might indicate skin cancer.
- Report any family history of cancer to your doctor and have that history noted on your medical records.

Table 13.5 on page 282 summarizes the things you can do to prevent developing cancer.

Table 13.3 ♦ The Seven Warning Signs of Cancer

Report any of the following signs of cancer to your doctor:

Change in bowel or bladder habits
A sore that does not heal
Unusual bleeding or discharge
Thickening or lump in breast or elsewhere
Indigestion or difficulty in swallowing
Obvious change in wart or mole
Nagging cough or hoarseness

Source: American Cancer Society, *Cancer Facts & Figures—1993.* New York: American Cancer Society, 1993, p. 12. Used by permission. © American Cancer Society, Inc.

Physical Activity and Cancer Prevention

Physical activity has been found to help prevent the onset of cancer. The exact reason for this is unclear, although several theories have been proposed. For example, some researchers attribute the decreased incidence of cancer among people who are physically active to their being leaner. Excess fat is associated with cancer of the colon, prostate, endometrium, and breast. Whether physical activity has a direct effect on cancer or an indirect effect by reducing body fat is unknown.

The National Cancer Institute also reports that men who exert the energy equivalent of walking 10 or more miles per week have half the risk of developing colon cancer of less active men. One theory explaining this finding is that exercise increases the rate of transit of food through the digestive tract. If there are carcinogens in the fecal stream, the faster they proceed through the system, the less chance there is that they will attach themselves to mucosa lining the tract and develop into cancer.

There is also evidence that women who exercise regularly are less prone to develop cancer of the breast or of the reproductive system. One theory relates a lower rate of these cancers and exercise to the amount of body fat. Fat is needed to make estrogen. This theory hypothesizes that excess fat increases the risk of these cancers because it leads to too much estrogen being produced.

These findings pertain to moderate amounts of exercise. That does not mean that very intense exercise is also protective of cancer. In fact, some researchers believe that very intense exercise is actually detrimental because it suppresses the immune system, resulting in the body being less able to ward off carcinogens. The discovery by researchers that

Table 13.4 ✦ Summary of American Cancer Society Recommendations for the Early Detection of Cancer (for People without Symptoms)

TEST OR PROCEDURE	SEX	AGE	FREQUENCY
Sigmoidoscopy, preferably flexible	M&F	50 and over	Every 3–5 years
Fecal Occult Blood Test	M&F	50 and over	Every year
Digital Rectal* Examination	M&F	40 and over	Every year
Prostate Exam*	M	50 and over	Every year
Pap Test	F	All women who are, or who have been, sexually active, or have reached age 18, should have an annual Pap test and pelvic examination. After a woman has had three or more consecutive satisfactory normal annual examinations, the Pap test may be performed less frequently at the discretion of her physician.	
Pelvic Examination	F	18–40	Every 1–3 years with Pap Test
		Over 40	Every year
Endometrial Tissue Sample	F	At menopause, if at high risk**	At menopause and thereafter the discretion of the physician
Breast Self-Examination	F	20 and over	Every month
Breast Clinical Examination	F	20–40	Every 3 years
		Over 40	Every year
Mammography***	F	40–49	Every 1–2 years
		50 and over	Every year
Health Counseling and Cancer Checkup****	M&F	Over 20	Every 3 years
	M&F	Over 40	Every year

*Annual digital rectal examination and prostate-specific antigen should be performed on men 50 years and older. If either is abnormal, further evaluation should be considered.

**History of infertility, obesity, failure to ovulate, abnormal uterine bleeding, or unopposed estrogen therapy.

***Screening mammography should begin by age 40.

****To include examination for cancer of the thyroid, testicles, ovaries, lymph nodes, oral region, and skin.

Reprinted by permission. © American Cancer Society, Inc.

prostate cancer is more common among male athletes lends credence to this theory.

Early Detection and Diagnosis of Cancer

Many cancers are highly curable if they are detected early. For example, both breast and testicular cancer detected in their earliest stages are well over 90 percent curable. The later the cancer is detected, the less positive is the prognosis. That is why it is so important to detect cancer as early as possible. Obtaining regular medical checkups is one way of assuring that cancers are found in their earliest stages. Medical screenings recommended are listed in Table 13.4. Another method of early detection is by performing regular self-examinations. Two of the most frequently recommended self-examinations are of the breast for women and of the testicles for men. Figures 13.2 on page 283 and 13.3 on page 284 show you how to perform these self-examinations.

Table 13.5   ✦   How to Prevent Cancer

Here are some things you can do to minimize your risk of developing cancer.

Do Not Smoke	Cigarette smoking is responsible for 85 percent of lung cancer cases among men and 75 percent among women—about 83 percent overall. Smoking accounts for about 30 percent of all cancer deaths. Those who smoke two or more packs of cigarettes a day have lung cancer mortality rates 15 to 25 times greater than nonsmokers.
Limit Exposure to Sunlight	Almost all of the more than 600,000 cases of nonmelanoma skin cancer diagnosed each year in the United States are considered to be sun-related. Recent epidemiologic evidence shows that sun exposure is a major factor in the development of melanoma and that the incidence increases for those living near the equator.
Limit Ingestion of Alcohol	Oral cancer and cancers of the larynx, throat, esophagus, and liver occur more frequently among heavy drinkers of alcohol.
Avoid Smokeless Tobacco	Use of chewing tobacco or snuff increases risk of cancer of the mouth, larynx, throat, and esophagus and is highly habit-forming.
Consult with Physician Regarding Estrogen Treatment	For mature women, estrogen treatment to control menopausal symptoms increases risk of endometrial cancer. Use of estrogen by menopausal women needs careful discussion between the woman and her physician.
Limit Exposure to Radiation	Excessive exposure to ionizing radiation can increase cancer risk. Most medical and dental X-rays are adjusted to deliver the lowest dose possible without sacrificing image quality. Excessive radon exposure in homes may increase risk of lung cancer, especially in cigarette smokers. If levels are found to be too high, remedial actions should be taken.
Limit Exposure to Occupational Hazards	Exposure to several different industrial agents (nickel, chromate, asbestos, vinyl chloride, and so forth) increases risk of various cancers. Risk from asbestos is greatly increased when combined with cigarette smoking.
Eat Well	Risk for colon, breast, and uterine cancers increases in obese people. High-fat diets may contribute to the development of cancers of the breast, colon, and prostate. High-fiber foods may help reduce risk of colon cancer. A varied diet containing plenty of vegetables and fruits rich in vitamins A and C may reduce risk for a wide range of cancers. Salt-cured, smoked, and nitrite-cured foods have been linked to esophageal and stomach cancer. The heavy use of alcohol, especially when accompanied by cigarette smoking or chewing tobacco, increases risk of cancers of the mouth, larynx, throat, esophagus, and liver.

Source: American Cancer Society, *Cancer Facts and Figures,* New York: American Cancer Society, 1990, p. 18. Used by permission. © American Cancer Society, Inc.

OTHER DISEASES AND CONDITIONS

Prevention of several other diseases and conditions has also been associated with exercise. Some of these are diabetes, obesity, and hypertension.

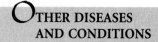

Diabetes

Diabetes is a disease of the pancreas in which an insufficient amount of **insulin** is produced to make use of sugars and other carbohydrates in a normal way. The result is amounts of glucose in the blood, which can lead to a number of other states of ill

health. The sixth leading cause of death in the United States, diabetes contributes to the development of heart disease, stroke, kidney failure, and blindness. Symptoms of diabetes include frequent urination and thirst, extreme hunger, rapid weight loss, blurred vision or a sudden change in visual acuity, tiring easily, and drowsiness. Among the more

> **Insulin** A hormone produced in the pancreas that aids in the digestion of sugars and other carbohydrates.

Figure 13.2   ✦   Breast Self-Examination

Master the following technique and examine your breasts during a bath or shower once per month. Regular examination will soon get you used to the normal feel of your breast. Keep a record of your examination dates and the results. Indicate the type and location of any nodule, changes in the contour of each breast, swelling, dimpling of skin, changes in the nipple, or any discharge. Consult your physician immediately if you notice any of these symptoms.

In the shower. Examine your breasts during your bath or shower since hands glide more easily over wet skin. Hold your fingers flat and move them gently over every part of each breast. Use the right hand to examine the left breast and the left hand for the right breast. Check for any lump, hard knot, or thickening.

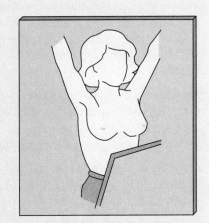

Before a mirror. Inspect your breasts with arms at your sides. Next, raise your arms high overhead. Look for any changes in the contour of each breast: a swelling, dimpling of skin, or changes in the nipple.

Then rest your palms on your hips and press down firmly to flex your chest muscles. Left and right breast will not exactly match—few women's breasts do. Again look for changes and irregularites. Regular inspection shows what is normal for you and will give you confidence in your examination.

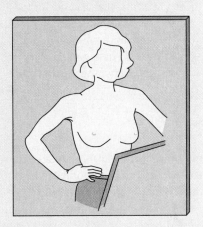

Lying down. To examine your right breast, put a pillow or folded towel under your right shoulder. Place your right hand behind your head: This distributes tissue more evenly on the chest. With the left hand, fingers flat, press gently in small circular motions around an imaginary clockface. Begin at the outermost top of your right breast for 12 o'clock, then move to 1 o'clock and so on around the circle back to 12. (A ridge of firm tissue in the lower curve of each breast is normal).

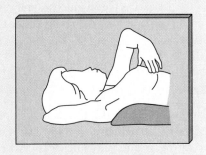

Then move one inch inward toward the nipple and keep circling to examine every part of your breast, including the nipple. This requires at least three more circles. Now slowly repeat the procedure on your left breast with a pillow under your left shoulder and your left hand behind your head. Notice how your breast structure feels.

Finally, squeeze the nipple of each breast gently between thumb and index finger. Any discharge, clear or bloody, should be reported to your doctor immediately.

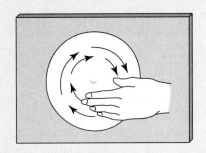

Figure 13.3 ◆ Testicular Self-Examination

Follow the instructions in the diagram carefully and examine your testes immediately after your next hot bath or shower. Heat causes the testicles to descend and the scrotal skin to relax, making it easier to find unusual lumps.

Examine each testicle by placing the index and middle fingers of both hands on the underside of the testicle and the thumbs on the top. Gently roll the testicle between your thumb and fingers, feeling for small lumps.

Changes or anything abnormal will appear at the front or side of your testicle. Did you find any unusual lumps? Are there any unusual signs of any kind? Are there any markings or lumps at any site?

Keep in mind that not all lumps are a sign of testicular cancer. Unusual lumps at any location, however, should be checked by a physician. Early detection greatly increases your chances of a complete cure. Repeat the examination every month and record your findings.

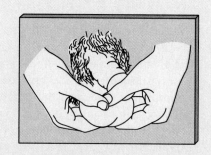

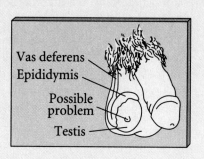

Vas deferens
Epididymis
Possible problem
Testis

than 10 million diabetics in the United States, some need to take insulin into their bodies to help regulate the amount of glucose in their blood. Others, however, can control insulin-insufficiency (sometimes called *glucose intolerance*) by diet and exercise. Exercise uses up the excess blood glucose, and diet can limit the amount of sugar and carbohydrates ingested in the first place.

Obesity

The relationship between leanness and colon and other cancers and that between body fat, the production of estrogen, and subsequently breast cancer were mentioned earlier in this chapter. Obesity, 20 percent or more above recommended weight, is also related to CHD, stroke, hypertension, diabetes, and other conditions. Exercise helps reduce body fat, tone muscles, and decrease body weight. When that occurs, the heart has to pump less forcefully since blood vessels are not occluded, there is less distance the blood has to travel since there is less body to travel through, and there is less blood glucose since it is being used for muscular contractions during physical activity. For these reasons, obesity is best treated by diet control in conjunction with an exercise program.

Hypertension

When blood vessels are partially blocked, the heart has to work harder to pump blood through them. This increased tension of the blood against the walls of the blood vessels is called hypertension, or high blood pressure. Blood pressure is measured as diastolic and systolic blood pressure. The recommended blood pressure reading is 120 systolic/80 diastolic. Usually, readings above 140 systolic and/or 90 diastolic are considered high.

Since high blood pressure creates stress on the walls of the arteries, it can result in the rupture of these blood vessels. When that happens in the brain, a stroke occurs. In addition, high blood pressure can create small tears on the walls of the coronary arteries, making it easier for plaque to attach and accumulate and CHD to develop.

In many cases, hypertensives need medication for the remainder of their lives. In many other cases, however, exercise and diet can help control hypertension. Exercise uses blood fats that might otherwise be available to accumulate on the walls of blood vessels. Exercise also helps the heart become stronger so it can pump blood as required. In addition, physical activity contracts muscles around blood vessels so blood is more efficiently transported through the circulatory system.

Behavioral Change and Motivational Strategies

There are many things that might interfere with your behaving in ways to prevent CHD and cancer. Here are some barriers (roadblocks) and strategies for overcoming them.

Roadblock	Behavioral Change Strategy

Friends or relatives may smoke cigarettes. That means that you may be tempted to do so yourself. Even though we like to think we act independently, other people's behaviors influence us, particularly if we like and respect those people. Furthermore, you do not even have to smoke to be subjected to the harmful effects of tobacco products. All you need do is breathe in second-hand, or sidestream, smoke, which can effect your susceptibility to CHD and cancer.

Two behavior change strategies appropriate here are contracting and social support. Find a friend or relative who would like to give up smoking. This will not be difficult. Smokers often try to quit; the problem is that they are usually unsuccessful. Draw up a contract for each of you to smoke less gradually over a period of weeks (gradual programming). Use the contract format described in chapter 3. If you do not presently smoke, make your contract address your not starting to smoke and the other person's contract specific to reducing the number of cigarettes smoked per week gradually. Each of you then sign the other's contract as a witness. The support you can provide each other, and the pressure of a contract that will periodically be evaluated, can be just the motivation needed to counteract the influence of other smoking friends and relatives.

You may find exercise uncomfortable. Your muscles may ache, your clothes and body may get sweaty, and you may not enjoy the activity itself. With this attitude, you cannot be expected to maintain an exercise program even if you are motivated to begin one. After all, most people do not want to feel uncomfortable and will choose not to be so.

Use goal setting strategies to establish realistic and achievable fitness goals. If you are experiencing aches and pains, you are overtraining or exercising inappropriately. The old maxim, "no pain, no gain," has long been discarded by fitness experts. You should feel good after a workout.

You can also use selective awareness described in chapter 10. Focus on the benefits of the exercise: how it will burn up calories, make you look and feel better, help you be healthier, make the clothes you bought when you weighed less once again fit, and so forth. If you focus on the benefits rather than on the temporary discomfort caused by perspiration, you will be more likely to maintain your exercise program.

You may enjoy eating foods high in saturated fats. Many of us grew up on french fried potatoes and hot dogs or hamburgers. They taste good, are easy to prepare, and are relatively inexpensive. Unfortunately, they also put us at risk for both CHD and certain cancers.

Use reminder systems to encourage the buying and eating of healthier foods. Put notes on your refrigerator and pantry to remind you to refrain from eating certain foods when you are looking for a snack. And place a picture of a clogged artery at the top of your shopping list to remind you not to buy unhealthy foods.

You can also use covert modeling. Find a friend who eats well, who looks good, and whose behavior you would like to follow. Then observe what this friend eats. After obtaining a good picture of how this friend selects and prepares foods, model your behavior on him or her. Eat and prepare similar foods—at least those that you enjoy eating and that are also low in fat and other unhealthy food ingredients.

List roadblocks interfering with your working at preventing CHD and cancer.

Now cite behavior-change strategies that can help you overcome the roadblocks you just listed. If you need to, refer back to chapter 3 for behavior-change and motivational strategies.

1. _____

2. _____

3. _____

1. _____

2. _____

3. _____

SUMMARY

Coronary Heart Disease (CHD)

CHD is the leading cause of death in the United States. It involves a blockage of blood to the heart thereby depriving it of necessary oxygen and nutrients without which a heart attack can occur and part of the heart muscle can die. Death can even be the result.

Coronary arteries can be occluded by an accumulation of blood fats and other substances on their walls. This clogging material is known as *plaque*, and the resulting condition as *atherosclerosis*. The fatty particles that can collect on the walls of the arteries are called *lipoproteins*. Lipoproteins consist of triglycerides, a blood protein, and cholesterol.

HDLs and LDLs are produced in the liver and released into the bloodstream where they carry cholesterol that is needed by the body. Excess cholesterol carried by LDLs can accumulate on the artery walls, eventually clogging coronary arteries and causing heart disease. HDLs carry excess cholesterol back to the liver and possibly provide a protective layer of grease to help prevent a build-up of substances on the walls of the arteries. When LDL is elevated and HDL is too sparse, there is a likelihood that arteries will be clogged and CHD will be promoted.

Risk factors for CHD include diets high in fats, hypertension, obesity and overweight, stress, sedentary lifestyle, the use of tobacco, and a family history of CHD.

Physical activity is an excellent means of preventing CHD since it relates to several risk factors. It exercises the heart muscle, encourages the production of HDL, aids in the control of mild hypertension, develops cardiorespiratory endurance, reduces catecholamines produced in response to stress, helps maintain desirable weight, and discourages cigarette smoking.

Cancer

Cancer is a disease involving abnormal cell growth. These cells can spread to other parts of the body by metastasis. Cancer is the second leading cause of death in the United States. As much as 80 percent of cancer cases, however, could be prevented with a change in lifestyle.

Cancer can be caused by chemicals, environmental pollutants, radiation from the sun, or viruses. The greatest cause of cancer, however, is the use of tobacco. An estimated 75 percent of all lung cancer cases are thought to be caused by cigarette smoking, and the use of tobacco is associated with cancer of the larynx, pharynx, esophagus, pancreas, and bladder.

The number of cancer cases could be dramatically reduced if people ate diets low in fats and high in fruits and vegetables (in particular, cruciferous vegetables), refrained from smoking cigarettes, eliminated or reduced their consumption of alcohol, and decreased their exposure to the sun.

Moderate physical activity seems to protect people from developing cancer. This is particularly true for cancer of the colon, prostate, endometrium, and breast. Theories about why this relationship exists point to exercise leading to lower body fat, less production of estrogen, and increased rate of transit of food through the digestive tract.

The earlier cancer is detected, the more effective is the treatment. To identify the presence of cancer early, obtain regular medical screenings and perform regular self-examinations (such as breast and testicular self-examinations).

Other Diseases and Conditions

Exercise can also be effective in preventing or responding to other diseases. Among these are diabetes, obesity, and hypertension. Exercise uses up blood glucose and other blood fats, expends calories, and makes the heart and circulatory system operate more efficiently. As a result, exercise and diet are mainstays in the treatment and prevention of these conditions.

REFERENCES

American Heart Association. *Statement on Exercise: Benefits and Recommendations for Physical Activity Programs for All Americans.* Dallas, TX: American Heart Association, 1992.

Friedman, Meyer, and Rosenman, Ray H. *Type A Behavior and Your Heart.* Greenwich, CT: Fawcett, 1974.

Lab Activity 13.1

Is Your Blood in Tune?

INSTRUCTIONS: *The composition of your blood is very important when it comes to preventing CHD. You can easily have your physician check your blood fat levels. Sometimes this is done with a simple finger prick, but to be as accurate as possible, it should be done by having blood drawn from a vein after you have fasted for about 12 hours. Record the results of that assessment below:*

_____ Total cholesterol below 200: No further evaluation necessary, recheck in five years.

_____ Total cholesterol is more than 200: Recheck in 1 to 8 weeks.

_____ Total cholesterol is 200 to 239 (borderline high cholesterol): Evaluate risk factors to see what lifestyle changes you can make (diet, exercise, and so forth). If your physician says you are not in the high-risk category for CHD, active treatment is not necessary.

_____ Total cholesterol is above 240 (high cholesterol): Analyze and measure HDL, LDL, and triglycerides.

Once the above is completed, answer the following questions:

Yes	No	
_____	_____	**1.** Is your total cholesterol no more than 4.5 × HDL cholesterol?
_____	_____	**2.** Is your cholesterol/HDL ratio at least 5:1?
_____	_____	**3.** Is your HDL reading above 35?
_____	_____	**4.** Is your LDL cholesterol less than 160?

If the answers to these questions are "Yes," your lipid profile is good. Regardless of how your lipid profile turned out, list the important changes you can make to lower your total cholesterol and increase your HDL cholesterol over the next 12 months.

Lab Activity 13.2

Risk Factor Analysis: The Game of HEALTH

INSTRUCTIONS: *Carefully complete the following form to determine your risk of heart attack. Tabulate points, and compare your score with those below to identify your risk. Keep in mind that a high score does not mean you will develop heart disease; it is merely a guide to make you aware of your potential risk. Because no two people are alike, an exact prediction is impossible without a carefully individualized evaluation.*

	1	2	3	4	6
Heredity	No known history of heart disease	One relative with heart disease over 60 years	Two relatives with heart disease over 60 years	One relative with heart disease under 60 years	Two relatives with heart disease under 60 years
	1	**2**	**3**	**5**	**6**
Exercise	Intensive exercise, work, and recreation	Moderate exercise, work, and recreation	Sedentary work and intensive recreational exercise	Sedentary work and moderate recreational exercise	Sedentary work and light recreational exercise
	1	**2**	**3**	**4**	**6**
Age	10–20	21–30	31–40	41–50	51–65
	0	**1**	**2**	**4**	**6**
Lbs.	More than 5 lbs below standard weight	± 5 lb standard weight	6–20 lb overweight	21–35 lb overweight	36–50 lb overweight
	0	**1**	**2**	**4**	**6**
Tobacco	Nonuser	Cigar or pipe	10 cigarettes or fewer per day	20 cigarettes or more per day	30 cigarettes or more per day
	1	**2**	**3**	**4**	**6**
Habits of eating food	0% No animal or solid fats	10% Very little animal or solid fats	20% Little animal or solid fats	30% Much animal or solid fats	40% Very much animal or solid fats

◆ Your risk of heart attack:

4–9	Very remote
10–15	Below average
16–20	Average
21–25	Moderate
26–30	Dangerous
31–36	Urgent dangerous—reduce score!

Other conditions, such as stress, high blood pressure, and increased cholesterol, detract from heart health and should be evaluated by your physician.

Lab Activity 13.3

Determining Your Risk of Acquiring Cancer

INSTRUCTIONS: *Select the response that best describes you for each question and record the point value for each response selected in the space provided. Total your points for each section separately.*

Lung Cancer	**Lung**

1. Sex
   a. Male (2)
   b. Female (1)

    1. _____

2. Age
   a. 39 or less (1)
   b. 40–49 (2)
   c. 50–59 (5)
   d. 60+ (7)

    2. _____

3. Smoker (8)
   Nonsmoker (1)

    3. _____

4. Type of smoking
   a. Current cigarettes or little cigars (10)
   b. Pipe and/or cigar but not cigarettes (3)
   c. Ex-cigarette smoker (2)
   d. Nonsmoker (1)

    4. _____

5. Number of cigarettes smoked per day
   a. 0 (1)
   b. Less than 1/2 pack per day (5)
   c. 1/2–1 pack (9)
   d. 1–2 packs (15)
   e. More than 2 packs (20)

    5. _____

6. Type of cigarettes
   a. High tar/nicotine (10)[a]
   b. Medium tar/nicotine (9)
   c. Low tar/nicotine (7)
   d. Nonsmoker (1)

    6. _____

[a] High T/N = More than 20 mg tar and 1.3 mg nicotine
Medium T/N = 16–19 mg tar and 1.1–1.2 mg nicotine
Low T/N = 15 mg or less tar and 1.0 mg or less nicotine

7. Duration of smoking 7. _____
   a. Never smoked (1)
   b. Ex-smoker (3)
   c. Up to 15 years (5)
   d. 15–25 years (10)
   e. More than 25 years (20)

8. Type of industrial work 8. _____
   a. Mining (3)
   b. Asbestos (7)
   c. Uranium and radioactive products (5)

Lung Total _____

Colon/Rectal Cancer **Colon/Rectal**

1. Age 1. _____
   a. 39 or less (10)
   b. 40–59 (20)
   c. 60 and over (50)

2. Has anyone in your immediate family ever had: 2. _____
   a. Colon cancer (20)
   b. One or more polyps of the colon (10)
   c. Neither (1)

3. Have you ever had: 3. _____
   a. Colon cancer (100)
   b. One or more polyps of the colon (40)
   c. Ulcerative colitis (20)
   d. Cancer of the breast or uterus (10)
   e. None (1)

4. Bleeding from the rectum (other than obvious
   hemorrhoids or piles) 4. _____
   a. Yes (75)
   b. No (1)

Colon/Rectal Total _____

Skin Cancer **Skin**

1. Frequent work or play in the sun 1. _____
   a. Yes (10)
   b. No (1)

2. Work in mines, around coal tars, or around radioactivity 2. _____
   a. Yes (10)
   b. No (1)

3. Complexion—fair or light skin. 3. _____
   a. Yes (10)
   b. No (1)

Skin Total _____

Lab Activity 13.3 (continued)
Determining Your Risk of Acquiring Cancer

Women Only—Breast Cancer   **Breast**

   1. Age Group   1. _____
      a. 20–34 (10)
      b. 35–49 (40)
      c. 50 and over (90)

   2. Race/ethnicity   2. _____
      a. Oriental (5)
      b. African American (20)
      c. White (25)
      d. Mexican American (10)

   3. Family history   3. _____
      a. Mother, sister, aunt, or grandmother
         with breast cancer (30)
      b. None (10)

   4. Your history   4. _____
      a. Previous lumps or cysts (25)
      b. No breast disease (10)
      c. Previous breast cancer (100)

   5. Maternity   5. _____
      a. First pregnancy before 25 (10)
      b. First pregnancy after 25 (15)
      c. No pregnancies (20)

                                 Breast Total _____

Women Only—Cervical Cancer[b]   **Cervical**

   1. Age group   1. _____
      a. Less than 25 (10)
      b. 25–39 (20)
      c. 40–54 (30)
      d. 55 and over (30)

   2. Race/ethnicity   2. _____
      a. Oriental (10)
      b. Puerto Rican (20)
      c. African American (20)
      d. White (10)
      e. Mexican American (20)

   3. Number of pregnancies   3. _____
      a. 0 (10)
      b. 1 to 3 (20)
      c. 4 and over (30)

   4. Viral infections   4. _____
      a. Herpes and other viral infections or
         ulcer formations on the vagina (10)
      b. Never (1)

[b]Lower portion of uterus. These questions do not apply to women who have had total hysterectomies.

5. Age at first intercourse   5. _____
   a. Before 15 (40)
   b. 15–19 (30)
   c. 20–24 (20)
   d. 25 and over (10)
   e. Never (5)
6. Bleeding between periods or after intercourse   6. _____
   a. Yes (40)
   b. No (1)

                                                    Cervical Total _____

Women Only—Endometrial Cancer[c]   **Endometrial**
   1. Age group   1. _____
      a. 39 or less (5)
      b. 40–49 (20)
      c. 50 and over (60)
   2. Race/ethnicity   2. _____
      a. Oriental (10)
      b. African American (10)
      c. White (20)
      d. Mexican American (10)
   3. Births   3. _____
      a. None (15)
      b. 1 to 4 (7)
      c. 5 or more (5)
   4. Weight   4. _____
      a. 50 or more pounds overweight (50)
      b. 20–49 pounds overweight (15)
      c. Underweight for height (10)
      d. Normal (10)
   5. Diabetes   5. _____
      a. Yes (3)
      b. No (1)
   6. Estrogen hormone intake   6. _____
      a. Yes, regularly (15)
      b. Yes, occasionally (12)
      c. None (10)
   7. Abnormal uterine bleeding   7. _____
      a. Yes (40)
      b. No (1)
   8. Hypertension   8. _____
      a. Yes (3)
      b. No (1)

                                                    Endometrial Total _____

[c]Body of uterus. These questions do not apply to women who have had total hysterectomies.

Lab Activity 13.3 (continued)
Determining Your Risk of Acquiring Cancer

✦ Analysis of Results

Lung
1. Men have a higher risk of lung cancer than women equating them for type, amount and duration of smoking. Since more women are smoking cigarettes for a longer duration than previously, their incidence of *lung and upper respiratory tract (mouth, tongue and larynx) cancer* is increasing.
2. The occurrence of lung and *upper respiratory tract* cancer increases with age.
3. Cigarette smokers have up to twenty times or even greater risk than nonsmokers. However, the rates of ex-smokers who have not smoked for ten years approach those of nonsmokers.
4. Pipe and cigar smokers are at a higher risk for lung cancer than nonsmokers. Cigarette smokers are at a much higher risk than nonsmokers or pipe and cigar smokers. *All forms of tobacco, including chewing, markedly increase the user's risk of developing cancer of the mouth.*
5. Male smokers of less than one-half pack per day have five times higher lung cancer rates than nonsmokers. Male smokers of one to two packs per day have fifteen times higher lung cancer rates than nonsmokers. Smokers of more than two packs per day are twenty times more likely to develop lung cancer than nonsmokers.
6. Smokers of low tar/nicotine cigarettes have slightly lower lung cancer rates.
7. The frequency of lung and *upper respiratory tract* cancer increase with the duration of smoking.
8. Exposures to materials used in these industries have been demonstrated to be associated with lung cancer. Smokers who work in these industries may have greatly increased risks. Exposures to materials in other industries may also carry a higher risk.

If your lung total is:

24 or less	You have a low risk for lung cancer.
24–49	You may be a light smoker and would have a good chance of kicking the habit.
50–74	As a moderate smoker, your risks of lung and upper respiratory tract cancer are increased. If you stop smoking now, these risks will decrease.
75–over	As a heavy cigarette smoker, your chances of getting lung and upper respiratory tract cancer are greatly increased. Your best bet is to stop smoking now—for the health of it. See your doctor if you have a nagging cough, hoarseness, persistent pain or sore in the mouth or throat.

Colon/Rectal
1. Colon cancer occurs more frequently after the age of fifty.
2. Colon cancer is more common in families with a previous history of this disease.
3. Polyps and bowel diseases are associated with colon cancer.
4. Rectal bleeding may be a sign of colorectal cancer.

If your colon total is:

29 or less	You are at a low risk for colon-rectal cancer.
30–69	This is a moderate-risk category. Testing by your physician may be indicated.
70–over	This is a high-risk category. You should see your physician for the following tests: digital rectal exam, guaiac slide test, and proctosocopic exam.

Skin

1. Excessive ultraviolet causes cancer of the skin. Protect yourself with a sun screen medication.
2. These materials can cause cancer of the skin.
3. Light complexions need more protection than others.

If your skin total is:

Numerical risks for skin cancer are difficult to state. For instance, a person with dark complexion can work longer in the sun and be less likely to develop cancer than a light complected person. Furthermore, a person wearing a long-sleeve shirt and wide-brimmed hat may work in the sun and be less at risk than a person who wears a bathing suit for only a short period. The risk goes up greatly with age.

The key here is if you answer "yes" to any question, you need to protect your skin from the sun or any other toxic material. Changes in moles, warts, or skin sores are very important and need to be seen by your doctor.

Breast

If your breast total is:

Under 100	Low-risk women should practice monthly breast self-examination and have their breasts examined by a doctor as part of a cancer-related checkup.
100–199	Moderate-risk women should practice monthly breast self-examinations and have their breasts examined by a doctor as part of a cancer-related checkup. Periodic breast X-rays should be included as your doctor may advise.
200 or higher	High-risk women should practice monthly breast self-examinations and have the above examinations more often. See your doctor for the recommended (frequency of breast physical examinations or X-ray) examinations related to you.

Cervical

1. The highest occurrence is in the forty and over age group. The numbers represent the relative rates of cancer for different age groups. A forty-five-year-old woman has a risk three times higher than a twenty-year-old.
2. Puerto Ricans, Blacks, and Mexican Americans have higher rates of cervical cancer.
3. Women who have delivered more children have a higher occurrence.
4. Viral infections of the cervix and vagina are associated with cervical cancer.
5. Women with earlier intercourse and with more sexual partners are at a higher risk.
6. Irregular bleeding may be a sign of uterine cancer.

If your cervical total is:

40–69	This is a low-risk group. Ask your doctor for a Pap test. You will be advised how often you should be tested after your first test.
70–99	In this moderate-risk group, more frequent Pap tests may be required.
100 or more	You are in a high-risk group and should have a Pap test (and pelvic exam) as advised by your doctor.

Lab Activity 13.3 (continued)
Determining Your Risk of Acquiring Cancer

Endometrial

1. Endometrial cancer is seen in older age groups. The numbers by the age groups represent relative rates of endometrial cancer at different ages. A fifty-year-old woman has a risk twelve times higher than a thirty-five-year-old woman.
2. Caucasians have a higher occurrence.
3. The fewer children one has delivered the greater the risk of endometrial cancer.
4. Women who are overweight are at greater risk.
5. Cancer of the endometrium is associated with diabetes.
6. Cancer of the endometrium may be associated with prolonged continuous estrogen hormone intake. This occurs in only a small number of women. You should consult your physician before starting or stopping any estrogen medication.
7. Women who do not have cyclic regular menstrual periods are at greater risk.
8. Cancer of the endometrium is associated with high blood pressure.

If your endometrial total is:

45–59	You are at very low risk for developing endometrial cancer.
60–99	Your risks are slightly higher. Report any abnormal bleeding immediately to your doctor. Tissue sampling at menopause is recommended.
100 and over	Your risks are much greater. See your doctor for tests as appropriate.

Source: American Cancer Society, *Cancer Facts & Figures—1993.* New York: American Cancer Society, 1993, p. 12. Used by permission. © American Cancer Society, Inc.

14

Women and Physical Fitness

Chapter Objectives

By the end of this chapter, you should be able to:

1. Define and contrast terms such as essential versus storage fat and fast-twitch versus slow-twitch muscle fibers.

2. Identify gender differences in physiological performance.

3. Identify risk factors for osteoporosis.

4. Evaluate your daily intake of calcium and iron.

5. Detail the role of iron supplementation in iron-deficiency anemia versus sports anemia.

6. Evaluate the safety and benefits of exercise during pregnancy and lactation.

WHEN LIZA WAS a senior in high school 25 years ago, she had an interest in cross-country running but was discouraged from exercising by those who feared exercise would be hazardous to her health. In fact, her school had very few facilities for women and had no competitive teams for women's sports. Today Liza jogs 30 miles per week and often competes in road races. She rides in long-distance bicycle races and has begun training for her first ultramarathon at age 43. This mother of four children maintains a very active lifestyle and is in excellent physical condition. At her last class reunion, she was given the "Best Preserved" award for both men and women from her Senior class. When asked her secret, Liza responded that she began a walking program in college and simply never stopped!

In 1979 the American College of Sports Medicine (ACSM) issued a position statement regarding female participation in long-distance running. They concluded that women should not be denied the opportunity to compete in any distance for which men are allowed to compete. Women are capable of adapting to strenuous training programs and have large maximal aerobic capacities. Since that time, it has become evident that, though there are some sex differences in performance, women can improve cardiorespiratory endurance, decrease body-fat percentage, increase muscle endurance and strength, and improve performance. In fact, women of all ages can benefit from physical conditioning programs.

Such a large number of women are successfully participating in endurance exercise programs that it is evident that gender should not be a deterrent to women participating in aerobic sports. The large number of national and international female athletes who have set world records in every sport in which men commonly compete has shown that women have the ability to tolerate the physiological demands of strenuous endurance exercise.

We also know that there are many health benefits to be derived from participating in physical conditioning programs. Active women tend to be leaner, have a more positive blood lipid profile, respond more favorably to mental stress, have less high blood pressure, are less prone to cardiorespiratory and metabolic diseases, and may even be less susceptible to cancer than are sedentary women. Also, exercisers are less prone to developing crippling diseases such as osteoporosis in adult years than are nonexercisers.

In this chapter we will explore sexual differences in physiological performance and discuss the potential benefits women can derive from participating in physical conditioning programs. We will then explore special considerations for women such as osteoporosis, iron-deficiency anemia, sports anemia, menstrual disorders, pregnancy, lactation, and exercise. We want to emphasize that additional benefits, such as improved self-esteem and a sense of self-satisfaction most people derive from participation in physical conditioning programs, are certainly not sex-specific. If you have not been involved in an exercise program, get started today.

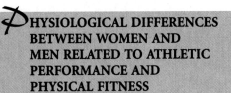

PHYSIOLOGICAL DIFFERENCES BETWEEN WOMEN AND MEN RELATED TO ATHLETIC PERFORMANCE AND PHYSICAL FITNESS

There are four major categories of sex differences in athletic performance and physical fitness that will be considered in this section. These include differences in the energy systems for both anaerobic power and maximal aerobic power, body composition, and muscular strength. On average, women weigh less and are shorter than men, but they have more fat tissue and less muscle mass. This remains true even when female athletes are matched against male athletes for any sport. Some of the differences in performance can thus be explained by the difference in physical stature.

Anaerobic Power

As mentioned earlier, the major energy systems in the body are the anaerobic and aerobic metabolism systems. Almost no research has been conducted on the anaerobic capability of female athletes. Hence, we can only discuss potential differences in performance between males and females.

The energy that is released when food is broken down in the body is not directly used by the muscles to do work. Instead, it is used to manufacture a substance called *adenosine triphosphate (ATP)*, the primary energy molecule of the body. It is either stored in small amounts in the muscles or manufactured through the process of metabolism. Only when energy is liberated from the breakdown of ATP can the cells of the body perform work.

The immediate energy system is composed of ATP and **creatine phosphate (CP)** stored in the muscles. Since much larger amounts of CP than ATP are stored in the muscle, the body can quickly make more ATP through the immediate energy system by adding the free phosphate to the **adenosine diphosphate (ADP)** molecule. This energy system is generally used for activities that are less than 30 seconds in duration and are high intensity. Research has shown

Adenosine diphosphate (ADP) A substrate present in muscle tissue that combines with phosphate to form ATP for muscle contractions.

Creatine phosphate (CP) A substrate present in muscle tissue that is broken down into its component parts (creatine and phosphate) in order to provide phosphates for the production of ATP.

Stroke volume The amount of blood pumped per beat of the heart; usually expressed in units of milliliters per beat (ml/beat).

Table 14.1 ✦ Sex Differences in VO₂ (ml O₂/kg⁻¹/min⁻¹) (fiftieth percentile)

Age	Males	Females
20–29	40.0	31.1
30–39	37.5	30.3
40–49	36.0	28.0
50–59	33.6	25.7
Over 60	30.0	22.9

Source: Data from J. H. Wilmore Pollock and S. M. Fox, *Health and Fitness Through Physical Activity.* New York: John Wiley & Sons, 1978.

that the muscular concentrations of ATP and PC are similar in women and men. Women tend to have a smaller total muscle mass due to differences in physical stature, and so their total amount of ATP and PC is less than the average male. For this reason, their total anaerobic capacity is less than that of the average male.

The lactic acid system is a second source of energy for anaerobic activities. It provides energy for high-intensity activities lasting from 30 seconds to two or three minutes in duration. Research has shown that women tend to have lower levels of lactic acid in their blood after maximal exercise than men do. This implies that the capacity of this system is lower in women than it is in men. A probable explanation for this difference is that women have a smaller total muscle mass than men.

When the capacity of both the ATP, PC, and lactic acid systems are evaluated, women have a less anaerobic capacity than do men. The effect on performance is that women have less power and less explosive capability than men do. This partially explains

Table 14.2 ✦ Sex Differences in Resting and Maximal Heart Rate (fiftieth percentile)(in beats/min⁻¹)

Age	Resting Males	Resting Females	Maximal Males	Maximal Females
20–29	64	67	192	188
30–39	63	68	188	183
40–49	64	68	181	175
50–59	63	68	171	169
Over 60	63	65	159	151

Source: Data from J. H. Wilmore Pollock and S. M. Fox, *Health and Fitness Through Physical Activity.* New York: John Wiley & Sons, 1978.

the difference in world-record performances for most weight-lifting and track and field events, such as sprint races or the shot put.

Maximal Aerobic Power

The aerobic metabolism energy system is used primarily in activities lasting longer than three minutes and is the major energy source for daily activities and endurance exercise. As with the anaerobic energy systems, the maximal aerobic power, or maximal oxygen consumption (VO₂), of females is also lower than that of males. Before puberty, there is no difference in VO₂ between girls and boys. Most researchers estimate that the VO₂ of women is 15 to 25 percent lower than that of adult males past 20 years of age. Table 14.1 shows sex differences in VO₂. As you can see, from age 20, men have consistently higher VO₂ values than do women. It is also clear that there is a consistent decline in VO₂, or maximal aerobic power, every decade past the age of 20 for both women and men. For both sexes, there is a 25 percent decline in VO₂ in the 40-plus years of life after age 20. This decrease in aerobic power is reflected in lesser endurance times among adult athletes.

There are numerous causes of the lower VO₂ in women as compared to men. Since the VO₂ is a product of oxygen delivery to the muscles times the amount of oxygen extracted from the blood by the muscles, several major systems are involved. The cardiorespiratory system is responsible for the amount of oxygen delivered to the muscles. In particular, the cardiac output determines the amount of oxygen delivered to the muscles. The maximal **stroke volume** is lower in women than in men because women have smaller hearts than men do. Also, as can be seen in Table 14.2, the maximal heart rate is also lower in women than in men regardless of age. Thus the overall output of the heart is lower in women than in men because of a lower number of beats and a smaller amount pumped by the heart with each beat.

Another factor affecting sex differences in the amount of oxygen delivered to the muscles is the total difference in blood volume and the difference in amount of hemoglobin in the blood. Women tend to have lower total blood volume than that of men. Hemoglobin is responsible for carrying oxygen in the bloodstream to the muscles. Women also have lower concentrations of hemoglobin in the blood than men do. Since the total amount of blood and its oxygen-carrying capacity are both lower in women, the maximal aerobic capacity of women is also lower than that of men.

In terms of the amount of oxygen removed from the blood to be used by the muscles, women also have less capacity because they have small muscle masses. If you compare the amount of oxygen used per unit of muscle, there is very little difference between women and men. But when the total amount of oxygen used by muscles is compared, women have less capacity. For this reason, it is important to learn different ways of expressing the VO_2 when you are examining sex differences.

The VO_2 is highest in women who participate in endurance sports. Table 14.3 shows body composition and VO_2 data for female athletes of varying ages. As can be seen on the table, women who participate in cross-country skiing have the highest measured VO_2. The next highest values occur in women engaging in activities such as the triathlon, track and field, cycling, and cross-country running. Sports with a very low aerobic capacity such as golf, have the lowest VO_2 values. It is also interesting to note that some of the highest recorded VO_2 values have been recorded in women older than 30.

Body Composition

The average adult female is 3 to 4 inches shorter, 25 to 30 lb lighter in total body weight, and has 10 to 15 lb more fat tissue than the typical adult male. No

Table 14.3 ✦ Body Composition and VO_2 Data for Female Athletes of Varying Ages

ATHLETIC GROUP OR SPORT	AGE	HEIGHT (CM)	WEIGHT (KG)	RELATIVE FAT (%)	VO_2 (ML/KG^{-1}/MIN^{-1})
Basketball	19.1	169.1	62.6	20.8	42.9
Bicycling	—	167.7	61.3	15.4	57.4
Dancing, ballet	15.0	161.1	48.4	16.4	48.9
General	21.2	162.7	51.2	20.5	41.5
Golf	33.3	168.9	61.8	24.0	34.2
Gymnastics	15.2	161.1	50.4	13.1	45.2
	19.4	163.0	57.9	23.8	36.3
Pentathlon	21.5	175.4	65.4	11.0	45.9
Racquetball	23.0	173.0	68.0	14.0	—
Skating, figure	16.5	158.8	48.6	12.5	48.9
Skiing, Alpine	19.5	165.1	58.8	20.6	52.7
Cross-country	20.2	163.4	55.9	15.7	61.5
	24.3	163.0	59.1	21.8	68.2
Swimming	19.4	168.0	63.8	26.3	37.6
Distance	—	166.3	60.9	17.1	43.2
Tennis	39.0	163.3	55.7	20.3	44.2
Track and field	19.9	161.3	52.9	19.2	57.5
	32.4	169.4	57.2	15.2	59.1
	43.8	161.5	53.8	18.3	43.4
Sprint	20.1	164.9	56.7	19.3	—
Cross-country	15.6	163.3	50.9	15.4	50.8
Discus	21.1	168.1	71.0	25.0	—
Jumpers/hurdlers	20.3	165.9	59.0	20.7	—
Shot put	21.5	167.6	78.1	28.0	—
Triathlon	—	—	—	12.6	58.7
Volleyball	19.9	172.2	64.1	21.3	43.5
Weight lifting					
Body builders	27.0	160.8	53.8	13.2	—

Source: From Jack H. Wilmore and David L. Costill, *Training for Sport and Activity: The Physiological Basis of the Conditioning Process,* 3d ed. Copyright © 1988 Wm. C. Brown Publishers Communications, Inc., Dubuque, IA. All Rights Reserved. Reprinted by permission.

Table 14.4 ✦ Sex Differences in Fat Percentage (fiftieth percentile)

AGE	MALES	FEMALES
20–29	21.6	25.0
30–39	22.4	24.8
40–49	23.4	26.1
50–59	24.1	29.3
Over 60	23.1	28.3

Source: Data from J.H. Wilmore Pollock and S. M. Fox, *Health and Fitness Through Physical Activity.* New York: John Wiley & Sons, 1978.

matter whether women and men are athletes, these differences are usually present. The average sex differences in body-fat percentage are shown in Table 14.4. In every age category, women have a higher percentage of body fat than men do. For both sexes, the body fat percentage increases as they get older.

The reason for a higher percentage of body fat in women as compared to men is based on the types of fat in the body. **Essential fat** is stored in the muscles, heart, lungs, liver, spleen, intestines, kidneys, and bone marrow. **Storage fat** includes fat tissue that protects the internal organs and the **subcutaneous fat**. The higher body-fat level of women compared to men is determined primarily by a higher percentage of sex-specific essential fat in women. Women need a minimum of 12 percent body fat to maintain their essential body-fat stores and conduct all the necessary functions for normal body metabolism, while men only need 3 percent body fat. When women reduce their body fat stores below 12 percent, menstrual disorders and hormone irregularities are likely to occur.

This higher level of body fat, coupled with a decrease in muscle mass, adversely affects physiological performance. Endurance activities are affected the most. In general, any activity that demands that body weight is supported will be most adversely affected by a high amount of body fat and a lesser amount of muscle mass. This is one reason why women tend to have poorer performances in distance running events.

Let us take another look at Table 14.3. The wide range of body-fat percentages shown illustrates the diversity among women who participate in different sports. Women who participate in some anaerobic sports have lower body-fat percentages than women who participate in aerobic sports. Thus the energy system used is not the primary criterion for estimating body-fat percentage among female athletes. Female athletes tend to manipulate their body-fat percentage in order to improve performance. The optimal percentage of body fat for the particular sport and the aesthetic value of having a low body-fat percentage are important determinants for maintaining a particular body-fat percentage for female athletes.

Muscular Strength

In general, the muscular strength in women is about 70 percent that of men. Part of the explanation for this phenomenon is that there are different types of muscle fibers that are used in different types of sports that are in two groups: **slow-twitch (ST)** and **fast-twitch (FT) fibers**.

Both women and men who participate in endurance sports have a higher percentage of ST fibers. Women and men who participate in anaerobic sports

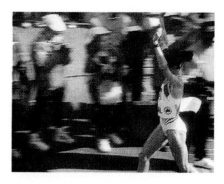

While female athletes are stronger than they ever were, their greater amounts of body fat and less muscle mass usually make it difficult for them to perform as well as men in endurance activities. (Photo Courtesy of Cable News Network.)

Essential fat The amount of fat required for normal physiological functioning.

Storage fat Fat that is stored in the adipose tissue.

Subcutaneous fat The layer of adipose tissue directly beneath the skin.

Slow-twitch (ST) fibers The type of muscle fiber used in endurance sports, which are equipped metabolically to meet the demands of aerobic activities of long duration.

Fast-twitch (FT) fibers The type of muscle fiber used in anaerobic, power sports, which are metabolically equipped to meet the demands of short-duration, high-intensity activities.

have a higher percentage of FT fibers. Actually, there is no difference between men and women in terms of who has the largest percentage of ST fibers. The sex difference appears in the *size* of the muscle fibers. Women athletes who participate in endurance sports have 66 and 71 percent of the male FT and ST fiber areas, respectively. Thus the *percentage* of fibers is similar between men and women, but the *size* of the muscle fibers is smaller among women compared to men who engage in similar training programs. This smaller total muscle mass in women causes a decrease in total muscle strength.

Have you ever wondered why women in a weight-training class do not experience the same degree of muscular **hypertrophy** as men even though they use the same training program? Both women and men will increase in strength following a weight-training program. In fact, the actual percent of increase in strength may be higher for women than it is for men after a weight-training program. Yet women seldom experience the muscular bulkiness seen in men following intense weight-training programs. The primary reason for this is that muscular hypertrophy is controlled by the male sex hormone testosterone. The level of testosterone in the blood is about ten times higher in men than it is in women. And since women have lower levels of testosterone, they will experience less muscular development, even though they will gain strength from participating in a weight-training program.

You must also remember that since women have a smaller total muscle mass than men, they will also have less muscle hypertrophy than men. Finally, since women have more subcutaneous body fat than men, much of the muscular hypertrophy they experience is masked beneath the layers of fat. As women tend to lose more body fat, they will see greater muscle definition, but there is no need to worry about becoming masculine as a result of participating in a weight-training program.

Based on the guidelines in Table 14.5, girls and young women are not prohibited from participating in any type of physical activity, simply because of their sex. Using the guidelines in the table, women

---

Hypertrophy An increase in the size of the muscle.

Trabecular bone The interior of the bone which looks like a dense lacy crystal network and makes up part of the body's calcium bank.

Table 14.5　◆　Guidelines for Female Participation in Sports

Many parents and coaches remain reluctant to allow girls and young women to participate in sports, especially strenuous sports. For this reason, the Committee on Pediatric Aspects of Physical Fitness, Recreation, and Sports established guidelines for safe participation in sports. They recommend:

1. Prepubescent children do not need to be separated according to sex before participating in sports, physical education, and recreational activities.

2. When possible, match girls for size, weight, skill, and physical maturity when they are competing, and follow customary safeguards for protection of health and safety in sports and competitive athletics.

3. Girls should not be prohibited from participating in strenuous conditioning programs in order to increase level of physical fitness, strength, agility, appearance, cardiorespiratory endurance, or mental well being. Such participation has no negative influences on menstrual cycle, future probability of getting pregnant, or childbirth.

4. Beyond puberty, girls should not compete against boys in heavy collision sports because their lower muscle mass per unit of body weight places them at increased risk of serious injury.

5. Talented female athletes should not be prohibited from participating on a team with males in an appropriate sport if the opportunity is provided for all females to participate in comparable activities.

---

can benefit from participating in endurance and anaerobic training programs just as much as men can.

SPECIAL CONSIDERATIONS FOR WOMEN: OSTEOPOROSIS

Melinda and her mom sat at the dinner table one evening talking after the evening meal. Her mom, more than 90 years old, reached across the table to pick up a spoon and suddenly screamed out in pain. When she was rushed to the hospital, it was discovered that three vertebrae in her back had shattered. Because of the nature of the breaks, the doctors were unable to completely restore the vertebrae. More than one year later, Melinda's mom was still confined to a wheelchair and had not recovered from the breaks in her spine.

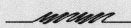

Myth and Fact Sheet

Myth	Fact
1. Women should not lift weights because they will develop large, bulky muscles.	1. Women seldom develop large bulky muscles from weight training because they have much lower levels of testosterone than that of men. In general, women also have smaller muscles and more body fat so the degree of muscle definition is more concealed in women.
2. After puberty, girls have more body fat than boys because they just do not exercise as much.	2. Estrogen secretion begins at puberty and has a major influence on body growth. Some of the changes include wider hips, larger breasts, and increased deposition of fat, particularly in the hips and thighs. Thus the greater body-fat percentage in women is partially due to changes in sex hormone production.
3. Vigorous physical activity causes iron deficiency in women.	3. There is no evidence that exercise of any intensity will cause the depletion of iron stores or iron-deficiency anemia in women who have an adequate diet. Women often confuse true iron-deficiency anemia with sports anemia. True iron-deficiency anemia can be corrected through increasing dietary iron availability. Iron supplementation, however, has no effect on sports anemia. True sports anemia reverses itself within nine weeks in an aerobic training program.
4. Contact sports such as hockey and soccer are more dangerous for women than they are for men.	4. No research has shown that women are more physiologically vulnerable to injury than their male counterparts who are involved in sports. While we know that the injury rate is often high among men who participate in contact sports, we have few data reporting the incidence of injury among women. Studies of women in sports such as basketball and field hockey show that they often have injuries similar to those suffered by men, such as sprained knees and ankles.

Melinda's mom had a crippling disease common to older women, called osteoporosis. Osteoporosis typically plagues older people. In this disease, the bones become porous and fragile and break with very little exertion as massive amounts of bone are lost. Last year, more than one million adults in the United States suffered bone breaks due to this degenerative disease.

Furthermore, at least one-third of all women aged 65 or older will suffer a fracture of the spine at some point in their lives. Such fractures are often complicated to treat because the break is usually not clean. The bone literally explodes into countless fragments that cannot be reassembled. If an artificial joint-replacement operation is not possible, the person may be confined to a wheelchair for years.

Although osteoporosis is more common in women than it is in men, this crippling disease constitutes a primary health concern for most older adults. The causes of osteoporosis are multiple and somewhat confusing as will be explained later. Though we strongly recommend that men and women meet the recommended dietary allowance (RDA) for daily calcium intake, it is not yet clear whether adequate calcium intakes can prevent osteoporosis or merely help to slow it down. There are two major types of osteoporosis that often occur.

Type I Osteoporosis

If you remove any long bone in an animal and cut it cross-sectionally, the interior of the bone would be **trabecular**. It is often used to raise the level of calcium in the blood when the daily dietary intake of calcium is insufficient. When dietary calcium intake is high, calcium is redeposited in the bone. Thus trabecular bone is very metabolically active and the amount of calcium deposited in this type of bone is partially dependent on the levels of certain hormones in the blood stream and certain vitamins and minerals in the diet.

Type I osteoporosis is typically characterized by losses of trabecular bone and is associated with low estrogen levels accompanying menopause or surgical removal of the ovaries. Type I is also identified by the kind of bone breaks that occur. The type of bone break that Melinda's mom experienced is often characteristic of Type I osteoporosis because the bones may become so fragile that even your own body weight can overburden the spine, causing the vertebrae to disintegrate and crush down. When such breaks occur, major nerves may also become pinched and cause excruciating pain in the individual. Trabecular bone loss usually begins in the third decade of life. Women experience Type I osteoporosis six times as often as men, after age 65.

Type II Osteoporosis

Cortical bone can lose its calcium deposits, but usually at a much slower rate than trabecular bone can. Cortical bone losses usually begin at age 40. In Type II osteoporosis, both cortical and trabecular bone lose their calcium deposits, but at a much slower pace. As the person ages, the vertebrae may slowly begin to compress into wedge shapes, usually painlessly, and cause the hunchback posture common in older adults. This type of osteoporosis occurs twice as often in women as in men but is seen in both sexes after age 70.

Developing Peak Bone Mass

Peak bone mass is developed up to age 24. Between the ages of 25 and 30, peak bone mass is usually maintained. However, after approximately 30 years of age, bone loss begins to occur. While this process cannot be reversed in people, the rate of bone loss can often be retarded. Hence the bones are their strongest and most dense during late teenage and early adulthood. This is important to know because you can be very successful in reducing your likelihood of developing osteoporosis right now. Once the decline in bone mineralization begins, men typically experience a lifetime bone density loss of 20 to 30 percent. Women have a more accelerated bone-mineral loss, resulting in 50 percent or more lifetime bone density losses.

As has already been described, the type of osteoporosis you may be at risk of developing depends on the type of bone affected and the rate at which that bone is lost. Other risk factors have been established, however, which may help you determine whether you may be predisposed to developing this disease.

Risk Factors

Your predisposition to developing osteoporosis depends on both environmental and hereditary factors. The single strongest predictor is age, followed by sex. Several additional risk factors include nutritional status, body weight, cigarette smoking status, racial or ethnic heritage, hormonal health, physical inactivity, and alcohol consumption. The effects of many of these risk factors are additive, but we do not know the relative contribution of each risk factor. We recommend that you eliminate as many risk factors as possible.

Age Bones lose their density as you get older because you produce less bone-building equipment and more bone-dismantling equipment. Thus it is essential that you make every effort to obtain enough calcium during young adulthood that when the bone-dismantling process begins, you will start out with optimal bone density. If you build strong bones up to the age of 24, your skeleton will remain stronger throughout the remainder of your life. In order to maximize calcium stores in the bones, the RDA has been established at 1200 milligrams (mg) per day for young adults and decreases to 800 mg per day for men and women past the age of 24. One cup of either whole or 1 percent milk contains approximately 300 mg of calcium. Thus women need to drink three or four cups of milk per day in order to meet the RDA. One cup of plain yogurt contains approximately 415 mg of calcium. Thus only three cups of yogurt are needed to meet the RDA.

Sex and Hormones Both men and women lose bone density as they get older, but women tend to lose much greater amounts than men do and are therefore more susceptible to bone breakage. After menopause, women are especially susceptible to developing osteo-

> **Cortical bone** A very dense, ivorylike bone that forms an outer shell that protects and encompasses trabecular bone; it also composes the shafts of all long bones in the body.

porosis because the ovaries decrease their estrogen output. Premenopausal women, however, who have a disease or surgery that involves the removal of their ovaries are also at very high risk because their bodies do not produce estrogen. Research has shown that young women who are long-distance runners for years are prone to athletic amenorrhea. Many of these women can only have a period following estrogen administration. If they fail to seek estrogen-replacement therapy, however, these young women become very susceptible to osteoporosis.

Obviously, men do not usually produce large amounts of the hormone estrogen. Thus, lack of estrogen cannot be used to explain the increased incidence of osteoporosis in older men. Researchers have found that men tend to suffer more fractures when their testes have been removed or when the testes begin to lose their functional capability, as often occurs as a part of the aging process. It seems feasible to assume that both female and male sex hormones contribute significantly to osteoporosis.

Racial and Ethnic Heritage African-Americans tend to have 10 percent denser bones than do white people. African-American males tend to have the greatest average peak bone mass and develop osteoporosis less frequently than any other race/sex groups. African-American females also tend to have higher average peak bone mass than their white counterparts and consequently have a lower incidence of osteoporosis. For example, hip fractures occur three times more often in white than African-American females 80 years of age or older. In the United States, other ethnic groups have lower bone density than do white people of Northern European descent, yet they do not necessarily have higher rates of osteoporosis. The implication is that while race and ethnic heritage are important predictors, lifestyle factors are also very important in determining susceptibility to osteoporosis.

Underweight and Physical Inactivity Osteoporosis occurs much more frequently in women who are underweight, even among African-American women. Very slim women are even more susceptible than very overweight women. Thus, while obesity is linked very strongly to all types of cardiorespiratory disease, osteoporosis is equally dangerous in women who are too stringent in maintaining their body weight.

For years, researchers have known that when you are confined to bed rest, your bones lose density just as the muscles atrophy. The strong relationship

Diversity Issues

Osteoporosis Risk

Researchers have learned much about the development of osteoporosis in the last 20 years. For example, people from certain ethnic backgrounds are more likely to develop this crippling disease than others. African-American men and women have denser bones than do white Americans, and they have a much lower risk of developing osteoporosis. Regardless of age, white Americans are more susceptible to developing this disease than are their African-American counterparts.

However, it is interesting to note that while other ethnic groups have less-dense bones when compared with white Americans, they do not necessarily have a higher risk of developing osteoporosis. Chinese people who live in Singapore are known to have low bone density, yet their rates of hip fractures are among the lowest in the world. Hispanic members of South and Central America have lower bone density than whites from the United States, but they also have lower rates of osteoporosis. Japanese and Chinese natives have low bone densities, but also have low rates of osteoporosis. The reason for this lack of correlation between bone density and prevalence of osteoporosis is unknown.

From these examples, it is clear that genetic makeup may predispose people to developing osteoporosis. However, the role of environmental factors cannot be ignored. ✦

between muscle strength and bone density is important because if you want to maintain strong bones, engage in weight-bearing activities. This will be discussed in more detail in a section in this chapter entitled "Prevention of Osteoporosis."

Cigarette Smoking Smokers have a higher incidence of fractures than nonsmokers. One reason for this may be that smokers tend to weigh less than nonsmokers. Also, women who smoke tend to experience menopause at an earlier age than nonsmokers do.

Alcohol Consumption Alcoholics have long been known to have less bone density than nonalcoholics.

Even men who are alcoholics tend to have more bone fractures than nonalcoholic males do. The possible link may be that alcohol causes the body to lose more fluid and so more calcium is lost in the urine. Thus calcium is leached out of the bones to maintain the blood level of calcium. Also alcoholics tend to suffer from poor general nutritional status and typically avoid foods known to be rich sources of calcium. Alcohol also tends to affect the ovaries of women, upsetting the normal hormonal balance that is necessary to maintain healthy levels of calcium in the bones.

Evidence Supporting Risk Factors As is shown in Table 14.6, researchers have well-established evidence that obesity, African ancestry, estrogen use, and high peak bone mass are related to decreased susceptibility to osteoporosis. Factors such as being of Northern European descent, older age, surgical removal of ovaries before menopause, and extensive bed rest also increase susceptibility to osteoporosis. Moderate evidence exists that heavy exercisers (with the exception of underweight amenorrheic females) have a lower incidence of osteoporosis. Simultaneously, smokers and heavy drinkers are at greater risk. More research is needed to ascertain the impact of factors such as Asian ancestry, number of live births, diabetes mellitus, and caffeine use.

Table 14.6 ✦ Risk Factors for Osteoporosis

Factors that *increase* risk include:
   Northern European ancestry
   Female sex
   Low dietary calcium intake
   Older age
   Postmenopausal status for women
   Surgical removal of ovaries before menopause
   Surgical removal of testes
   Extensive bed rest
   Increased alcohol consumption
   Cigarette smoking
   Underweight

Factors that *decrease* risk include:
   African ancestry
   High dietary calcium intake
   High peak bone mass by age 24
   Heavy chronic exercise history
   Obesity
   Estrogen use

Prevention of Osteoporosis

Exercise As was mentioned earlier in this textbook, much research has been conducted examining the impact of exercise on the development of bone density. You may have been told since you were a child that exercising is good for you because it helps you develop stronger bones. Well, that is true, and it is important that you understand why. When you engage in activities that stress the bones, they demand that the bones strengthen their structures. We know that when muscles work, they pull on the bones and signal the bones that more tissue needs to be developed. Simultaneously, the hormones that promote increases in bone mineralization also promote the making of new muscle tissue.

Most studies of athletes who participated in weight-bearing exercises have exhibited as much as a 40 percent increase in bone mineralization when compared to sedentary controls. Bone density is increased by weight-bearing activities such as jogging, walking, aerobics, stairmaster exercise, stair climbing, dancing, calisthenics, or even swimming. From this wide range of activities, it is obvious that you can increase bone density by participating in aerobic and anaerobic exercises. To reduce bone loss after reaching peak bone mass, however, aerobic activity lasting more than 30 minutes with a minimal frequency of three sessions per week should be conducted.

Calcium Nutrition There is no doubt that calcium is essential for bone and tooth formation. In fact, 99 percent of all the calcium in your body is used for these two purposes. One factor that leads to confusion in terms of setting dietary recommendations for calcium intake in relation to minimizing your risk of osteoporosis is the principle of **bioavailability**. This principle is important in your understanding of all vitamins and minerals because the amount of a mineral such as calcium obtained from your diet or even in supplements is not always absorbed. We know that the typical rate of absorption for calcium is 60 percent for infants and children, that it decreases to 50 percent during pregnancy, and drops to a startling 10 to 30 percent for adults. The rate of absorption depends on several factors. Your total dietary intake of calcium is one factor affecting bioavailability. For example, if you only eat 400 mg of calcium per day and your RDA is 800 mg, you may absorb a much higher percentage of the ingested calcium than a person who ingests 1400 mg per day. Thus low dietary intake of calcium leads to a higher absorption rate in some people. As can be seen, the principle of bioavailabili-

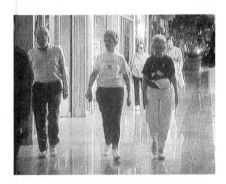

Many types of exercise help to increase bone density, thus decreasing the risk of developing osteoporosis. (Photo Courtesy of Cable News Network.)

ty can often make it difficult to determine just how much calcium is needed to prevent or retard osteoporosis.

We also cannot say that osteoporosis is a calcium-deficiency disease. The reason this statement is true is that chronically low levels of dietary calcium prior to age 24 is a strong risk factor for osteoporosis; however, high calcium intake during adulthood years is not effective in reversing bone loss when no other measures are taken. Some research has been conducted to prove that continued high intake of calcium after age 24 slows down bone loss but is still insufficient to prevent bone loss totally. A disease such as iron-deficiency anemia can be totally reversed when sufficient amounts of iron are added to the diet. Yet we have not found it to be true that increasing calcium intake will reverse osteoporosis.

Recently, researchers have found that people with high blood pressure have lower calcium intake than those with normal blood pressure. If your calcium intake is less than 300 mg per day, you have a two to three times greater risk of developing high blood pressure when compared with individuals with a daily calcium intake exceeding 1200 mg. Thus if you are at risk of developing hypertension, we recommend that you at least meet the current RDA for calcium.

Finally, we recommend that you concentrate on meeting the RDA for calcium each day. Regardless of your rate of absorption or of bone loss, meeting the RDA is your best protective measure from a dietary perspective. Unfortunately, most girls and adult women fail to meet the RDA for calcium during their bone-building years. Such girls are at a disadvantage because they will begin their adult lives with a lower bone mass and will be more prone to osteoporosis in later years. Complete Lab Activity 14.1: Osteoporosis Risk Assessment at the end of this chapter. If you are not meeting the RDA and can answer "yes" to three

or more questions in this lab activity, you are susceptible to developing osteoporosis in later years. Make the necessary changes today, and improve your quality of life later.

Suggestions for increasing the intake of calcium in your diet are given in Table 14.7 on page 310. If you have problems drinking milk or eating dairy products, you can see that several kinds of meat, fruits and vegetables, and grains are excellent sources of calcium. Strive to meet the RDA for this all-important mineral each day, and add quality to your life as you grow older.

ℐRON-DEFICIENCY ANEMIA

Have you experienced a period of several weeks when you felt chronically tired and apathetic and had a tendency to feel cold in a room where everyone else seemed to be comfortable with the temperature? **Iron-deficiency anemia** is one of the most frequently recurring nutritional problems among younger women of childbearing age. Iron deficiency occurs when the amount of iron ingested from the diet and/or the amount of iron absorbed from foods is either less than the amount of iron lost or less than the amount of iron needed to maintain all bodily functions.

Women are usually diagnosed as having **anemia** when they have a hemoglobin level of less than 12 and men when they have a level less than 14. The normal hemoglobin value for women is 14 and for men is 16.

Nutritional deficiencies, accelerated iron loss, and low bioavailability of iron affect the body's iron stores, regardless of sex. A woman's average monthly menstrual flow, however, typically results in the daily loss of 1.3 mg of iron. This is more than twice the amount of iron that men lose daily (.6 mg). For this

Bioavailability Synonymous with absorbability; refers to the individual differences in ease of absorption of nutrients.

Iron-deficiency anemia A condition that occurs when the red blood cells do not contain enough hemoglobin and consequently do not deliver enough oxygen to the tissues.

Anemia Occurs when the hemoglobin level falls below the normal reference range for individuals of the same sex and age.

Table 14.7 ✦ Suggestions for Increasing Dietary Intake of Calcium

Drink low-fat milk with meals or as a snack.

Drink orange juice that has added calcium.

Eat canned sardines or canned fish prepared with their bones.

Use milk, instead of water, when you prepare creamed soups.

Add grated cheese to salads, tacos, spaghetti, and lasagna.

Increase intake of broccoli and turnip greens.

Add powdered nonfat milk to soups, casseroles, sauces, and beverages such as cocoa.

Eat low-fat yogurt as a snack.

Encourage postmenopausal women to drink three to five cups of milk daily.

Drink buttermilk with meals or as a snack.

Make dairy products a part of your meals, especially low-fat and nonfat cheeses.

Increase intake of pork and beans and other legumes.

Eat cheese as a snack, or add a slice to your sandwiches.

Drink cocoa occasionally instead of drinking hot tea or coffee.

Encourage teenagers to drink four or more cups of milk daily.

Use low-fat or nonfat yogurt to make a low-calorie salad dressing.

Choose calcium-rich desserts, such as ice cream, custard, or pudding.

Encourage pregnant and lactating women to drink three to four cups of milk daily.

Increase intake of tofu (bean curd).

Drink fluoridated water.

Eat fortified breakfast cereals with skim milk.

Add cheese to casseroles.

reason, it is important that women in particular understand the causes of iron-deficiency anemia and are aware of dietary methods of increasing their iron intake.

Functions of Iron in the Body

Iron is used in four major ways in the body: as hemoglobin, myoglobin, ferritin, and transferrin. Approximately 75 percent of all iron in the body is a component of the proteins hemoglobin and myoglobin. Maintaining normal **hemoglobin** levels is especially important for endurance-type athletes because oxygen delivery plays a paramount role in aerobic energy production. **Myoglobin** is another iron-containing protein that helps transport oxygen directly into the muscle for the production of energy. Nearly 20 percent of iron in the body is in the form of **ferritin**. The remaining iron in the body is in the form of **transferrin**.

Causes of Iron-Deficiency Anemia

The primary cause of iron-deficiency anemia is usually inadequate iron intake, either because the total caloric intake is too low or because too much of the wrong kinds of food are consumed. Most people in the United States suffer from iron deficiency because they eat foods that are high in fats and sugar but are poor sources of iron. Also with the increase in the number of vegetarians and red-meat abstainers, many people are planning their own meals without including enough sources of absorbable iron and eventually become prone to anemia. Examples of dietary sources of iron can be found in Table 14.8.

Another major cause of iron deficiency may be poor absorption, also referred to as low bioavailability, of the iron in foods eaten. There are two types of iron in foods. **Heme iron** is the most absorbable form. Nearly 40 percent of the iron in heme sources is absorbed by the body. Typically, only 10 to 20 percent of the iron found in **nonheme iron** sources is

Table 14.8 ✦ Dietary Sources of Iron

FOOD	SERVING SIZE	IRON (MG)
Beef liver	3 oz	5.3
Beef pot roast	3 oz	3.3
Chick peas	1 cup	4.7
Chicken breast	3 oz	0.9
Chicken liver	1 each	1.7
Clams	3 oz canned	23.8
Hamburger	3 oz	2.0
Kidney beans	1 cup	3.2
Oysters	1 cup	16.6
Pinto beans	1 cup	4.5
Prune juice	1 cup	3.0
Prunes	10 med	2.1
Raisins	1 cup	3.0
Spinach	1 cup	6.4
Total (cereal)	1 cup	21.0
Tuna, canned	3 oz	2.7
Turkey, roasted	3 oz	1.7

absorbed by the body. For this reason, foods such as meats are recommended several times per week if you are diagnosed as being anemic.

There are several factors that decrease the amount of iron that is absorbed from the foods eaten. Tea and coffee contain a substance called tannic acid,

Table 14.9 ✦ Dietary sources of Vitamin C

FOOD	SERVING SIZE	VITAMIN C (MG)
Banana	1 whole	10
Broccoli spears	1 each	141
Brussel sprouts	1 cup	100
Cabbage	1 cup	25
Cantaloupe	½	113
Cranberry juice	1 cup	90
Grapefruit juice	1 cup	80
Orange	1 med	70
Orange juice	1 cup	120
Potato, baked	1 each	26
Pink grapefruit	1 each	47
Snow peas	1 cup	84
Strawberries	1 cup	84
Tomatoes	1 cup	34
Tomato juice (canned)	1 cup	45
Whole milk	1 cup	2
1% milk	1 cup	2

which decreases iron absorption. Also a high intake of wheat bran, calcium supplements, phosphates in cola drinks, and excessive fiber are known to impair iron absorption. Fortunately, there are also substances which will enhance iron absorption from foods, especially from nonheme food sources. These include ingesting any source of vitamin C at the same time that foods containing iron are ingested. Vitamin C ingested with nonheme iron sources can triple the amount of iron absorbed. Table 14.9 gives several sources of vitamin C. Remember, when you include any heme source of iron with a meal, a higher percentage of the nonheme iron is also absorbed.

It is also possible to become anemic from causes other than lack of iron in the diet. Any condition that causes increased blood losses will eventually result in anemia. The monthly menstrual cycle is thus partially responsible for the higher incidence of anemia among women. Ulcers can cause anemia when blood loss is uncontrolled. Some vitamin deficiencies can also cause anemia in an individual.

Who Is at Risk of Developing Iron-Deficiency Anemia?

Certain groups of people typically need more iron than others. Any persons experiencing a period of growth in the body usually need more iron. There-

Hemoglobin An iron-containing protein responsible for carrying oxygen throughout the bloodstream to body tissues, such as muscle, where it is used to provide energy for all forms of physical work.

Myoglobin Another iron-containing protein that helps transport oxygen directly into the muscle for the production of energy.

Ferritin A protein-rich compound that contains iron and constitutes the form in which iron is stored in the liver, the spleen, and the bone marrow.

Transferrin Another protein-rich compound that transports iron in the bloodstream.

Heme iron The form of iron found in most meats, fish, and poultry; has a high rate of absorption.

Nonheme iron The form of iron found in most plant sources of iron; has a much lower absorption rate than heme iron does.

fore, infants, children, adolescents, and pregnant women usually have increased iron needs. Because of the special role of iron in the formation of hemoglobin, some athletes also have increased iron needs. Several groups of athletes may be at risk for developing iron-deficiency anemia. These include endurance athletes, teenage athletes, athletes who do not eat red meat, female athletes, and low-body-weight athletes. If you are an athlete from one of these categories, you should examine your diet periodically to assess whether you are ingesting adequate amounts of iron. Complete Lab Activity 14.2: Assessing Your Daily Iron Intake at the end of this chapter to estimate your daily iron intake.

Were you surprised at your iron intake? It is recommended that women consume 15 mg of iron daily until menopause and that men and postmenopausal women consume 10 mg of it per day. If your intake was below these norms, you may be at risk of depleting your body's iron stores even if a blood test shows that you have a normal hemoglobin level. Include more iron-rich foods in your diet from both animal and vegetable sources.

Although some people may need to take iron supplements, the best way to ensure that you will meet your daily iron needs is to increase food sources. Table 14.8 listed several sources of dietary iron and Table 14.10 includes recommendations for boosting the amount of iron in your diet. The normal U.S. diet provides approximately 5 to 6 mg of iron for every 1000 calories ingested, so a woman who is on a very restricted caloric intake may really have problems getting enough iron from the diet alone. We recommend that women double the iron-to-calorie ratio daily by choosing iron-rich foods that are also low in calories. If you follow these guidelines, you should not have to worry about developing iron-deficiency anemia.

Stages of Iron Depletion

As has been already mentioned, it is possible to have a normal hemoglobin level but still be depleting your body's iron stores. To explain how this is possible, we need to briefly discuss the stages of iron depletion. There are three stages of iron depletion. The first stage is **depleted iron stores**. Many menstruating women, growing children, or even healthy individuals experience this initial phase of iron depletion. Researchers estimate that nearly 20 percent of all women and 3 percent of all men have no iron in their body stores.

It is estimated that millions of people suffer from iron deficiency without the benefit of a diagnosis. This second phase of iron depletion is **iron deficiency without anemia**. The hemoglobin may begin to fall to the low end of the normal range of values at this point. Since the hemoglobin level may still be considered normal, anemia is not diagnosed.

The final phase of iron depletion is referred to as **iron-deficiency anemia**. Approximately eight percent of all women and one percent of men have progressed to this final stage of anemia. A peculiar symptom of iron-deficiency anemia is **pica**. Sometimes

Table 14.10 ✦ Suggestions for Increasing Dietary Intake of Iron

Eat iron-rich foods containing vitamin C to increase absorption.

Decrease caffeinated and decaffeinated coffee intake.

Decrease hot tea and iced tea intake.

Eat beef liver.

Use cast-iron skillets when you cook whenever possible.

Purchase only fortified or iron-enriched breakfast cereals.

Increase intake of green, leafy vegetables.

Eat dry iron-enriched cereals as snacks.

Buy iron-enriched or fortified breads.

Increase intake of legumes such as kidney beans, chick peas, and lima beans.

Combine animal sources of iron with vegetable sources of iron to increase absorption.

Eat limited amounts of oysters (be careful of high dietary cholesterol intake).

Increase intake of spinach.

Eat chicken livers.

when people become anemic they develop an appetite for items such as ice, paste, and/or clay. In particular, women from low-income families are often initially diagnosed as being anemic because of the reported symptom of eating ice all the time. As soon as the hemoglobin level returns to normal, the appetite for ice or other nonnutritious items disappears. In correctly diagnosed incidences of iron-deficiency anemia, supplemental iron will be required in order to improve iron status. Large supplements of iron should only be taken under medical supervision because excesses can be toxic. If your hemoglobin level is normal, you have no history of anemia, and you ingest adequate amounts of iron in your daily caloric intake, we recommend that you avoid taking iron supplements to reduce the danger of iron toxicity.

Early diagnosis of iron-deficiency anemia is crucial because chronic anemia causes people to work less, play less, or simply do less because they just do not seem to have the energy to do much of anything. As their level of physical activity drops, many chronic problems such as obesity can arise simply because they are too tired to exercise. Also, anemic children are less productive in school and may be perceived as lazy by teachers. Teachers become reluctant to spend additional time aiding them, and the children get further behind in school. This is indeed a tragic scenario because many such problems could be avoided by simply increasing the amount of iron in the diet.

SPORTS ANEMIA

Researchers have found that female endurance athletes are especially prone to periods of iron deficiency. This type of anemia is often called *sports anemia* because of its nature. There are several proposed causes of this transient anemia that occurs in female and other endurance athletes, particularly during the early phases of a training program. One suspected factor is **hemodilution**. When a person begins a very heavy aerobic training program, there is an increase in the plasma volume and an increase in the total amount of hemoglobin produced. There is a greater proportional increase in the plasma volume, however, than in the hemoglobin; and it appears that the hemoglobin level is lower. In simpler terms, the blood is less concentrated and the athlete has less hemoglobin for every 100 milliliters (ml) of blood. Thus, with less oxygen being delivered to the tissues with every heart beat, the athlete appears anemic. This condition is usually transient and usually lasts

from approximately two to eight weeks during the initial training period.

Another possible cause of sports anemia is a diet inadequate in iron, especially heme sources of iron. Exercisers who consume large quantities of junk food may meet the caloric requirements to maintain their body weight, in spite of strenuous training schedules. The iron-to-calorie ratio, however, may in fact be very low. In one report, 42 percent of the female distance runners studied were modified vegetarians. They ingested less than 200 g of meat a week. This excessively low intake of such a rich source of heme iron partially explains the inability of many female athletes to meet the suggested intake of iron. We recommend that coaches regularly include the assessment of iron status as a part of the medical screening for all athletes.

Recent research has shown that exercisers lose significant amounts of iron through sweating. As the level of fitness increases, however, a smaller amount of iron is lost. In spite of this positive training adaptation, exercisers still lose significant amounts of iron through their sweat. Since this is unavoidable, we recommend that endurance exercisers increase dietary iron during heavy periods of training.

Finally, sports anemia may be caused by the rupture of red blood cells. Red blood cells are sometimes destroyed when the soles of the feet, or similar body tissues, make very high impact contact with a hard surface.

Depleted iron stores The initial state of iron depletion whereby you become vulnerable to low iron stores but you do not experience any adverse physiological effects.

Iron deficiency without anemia The second phase of iron depletion where some adverse physiological effects occur such as chronic fatigue, decreased physical work capacity, and diminished productivity due to a reduced hemoglobin level.

Iron-deficiency anemia The final phase of iron depletion, which occurs when all forms of iron in the body are low.

Pica A craving for nonfood substances which occurs as a symptom of iron-deficiency anemia.

Hemodilution An increase in the plasma volume (fluid portion of blood) that exceeds the increase in the total amount of hemoglobin produced, creating symptoms of anemia.

Any combination of these factors will likely result in the transient anemia which plagues some endurance athletes. Since women often have lower normal values of hemoglobin than men, very strenuous exercise is of some concern. It is important to realize that true sports anemia cannot be reversed with iron supplementation. Sports anemia appears to be a temporary response to exercise, thus no treatment is required.

MENSTRUATION AND EXERCISE

Exercise and Menstrual Disorders

Many female athletes engaging in intense chronic aerobic exercise have reported abnormal menstrual cycles. While much research has been conducted to find the causes of this phenomenon, we still are unable to define clearly who will have abnormal menstrual cycles and why. Most women and nonendurance athletes have **eumenorrhea**. However, with chronic endurance exercise, an increased percentage of female athletes report **oligomenorrhea**. Some researchers estimate that 5 to 40 percent of female athletes, depending on the sport, are oligomenorrheic. This value is compared to 10 to 12 percent in the general female population. One research project reported that 45 percent of female track and cross-country runners who ran more than 80 miles per week experienced irregular menstrual cycles. A smaller percentage report amenorrhea. Only 2 to 3 percent of women in the general population are amenorrheic. Yet in activities such as distance running, as many as 34 percent of women are reported to be amenorrheic. The incidence of amenorrhea decreases to 23 percent of joggers, and is only 4 percent among a nonrunning control group. Runners were defined as running more than 30 miles per week at very hard intensity. Joggers ran from 5 to 30 miles per week, but all at low-to-moderate intensity.

As shown in numerous studies, the decrease in menstrual function is often directly related to the intensity and duration of exercise. For women engaging in very intense training programs such as ballet dancing, figure skating, distance running, gymnastics, and cycling, irregular menstruation may be the norm rather than the exception. Some female athletes have reported the absence of menstruation for months or even years while engaging in high-intensity endurance exercise.

Possible Causes of Menstrual Disorders among Female Athletes

What is it about chronic participation in aerobic exercise that leads to abnormal menstrual function? Actually, neither the cause nor the long-term consequences of oligomenorrhea or secondary amenorrhea are known. Researchers, however, have discovered several possible reasons for this phenomenon. Numerous studies link the intensity of exercise with abnormal menstrual function. Athletes that perform at higher levels of intensity appear to be more susceptible to oligomenorrhea.

Athletes who lose large amounts of weight through the reduction of body-fat stores are more prone to amenorrhea. Researchers report that a loss of 33 percent body fat or even a 10 to 15 percent reduction in body weight will induce amenorrhea. As was shown earlier in the chapter, female athletes in nearly all endurance sports have much lower body-fat percentages than the general nonathletic population. For example, body-fat levels of less than 12 percent have been reported for world-class marathon runners.

The storage and metabolism of the female sex hormone estrogen is related to the amount of body fat stored. Hence as body-fat stores decrease, so does estrogen production. With low levels of estrogen available, the follicular phase of the menstrual cycle is affected and menstruation may be abnormal or may cease totally. Menstrual irregularities may thus be caused by changes in the levels of circulating sex hormones, as the level of body fat decreases.

It is difficult to separate the effects of exercise from those of the emotional stresses associated with intense physical training. We know that athletes who train hardest, tend to perform at a higher level. This higher level of performance and competition generally leads to more stress. When the athlete is exposed to more psychological stress, hormone production is also affected.

You can easily see that explaining the causes of amenorrhea can be complicated. High levels of training lead to low body-fat stores. High levels of training also lead to increased psychological stress. Low fat stores cause reductions in hormone production. High levels of psychological stress also cause changes in levels of circulating hormones. These factors combined have all been associated with menstrual irregularities. It is impossible to determine the relative contribution of each factor, however, when you are assessing menstrual irregularities among female athletes.

Performance and Competition during Menstruation

Surveys show that many female athletes are concerned about the potential effects of the menstrual cycle on performance during competition. Results of several studies show that there is considerable individual variation in these effects. Some women are totally unaffected by their menstrual cycle, but others have problems during the premenstrual phase and the initial-flow phase. **Dysmenorrhea** was more often reported by those women.

Some women have even reported improvement in performance in the short period immediately postflow. The number of women who report difficulties with performance is approximately equal to those who report no effect of menstruation on their level of performance. Hence individual variations must always be considered. In general, most young athletes are unaffected by menstruation. Endurance athletes tend to report more adverse effects of the menstrual cycle on their levels of performance. Track and field athletes, especially sprinters, appear to be least affected by menstruation during performance.

Physiologically, no research projects report significant cardiorespiratory or metabolic changes either at rest or during maximal exercise in any phase of the menstrual cycle. A limited number of studies report minor changes at rest during certain phases of the cycle. None, however, reported any physiological fluctuations during exercise.

Some physicians advise women not to swim while menstruating. Yet there is no physiological basis supporting this advice. Researchers have shown that there is no bacterial contamination of the water in the pool when women swim while menstruating. We also know that there have been no signs of bacterial infections in the reproductive organs. When women use tampons while swimming, all indications are that they are not susceptible to contracting bacterial infections, and no one is susceptible to contracting infections as a result of their menses.

In conclusion, based on current data, we have no reason to suggest that women avoid physical activity of any type during any phase of the menstrual cycle. If a woman feels any physical discomfort, she should not feel compelled to exercise. She should experience no physiological fluctuations during performance as a result of menstruation.

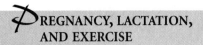

PREGNANCY, LACTATION, AND EXERCISE

Exercise during Pregnancy

In recent years, more physicians are advising physically active women to remain active during pregnancy. Because of this, the American College of Obstetrics and Gynecology (ACOG) established guidelines of exercise during pregnancy and postpartum (see Table 14.11 on page 316).

There is still some debate about whether participation in athletics has an adverse effect on childbirth. A recent extensive review by Lokey and associates (1991) of all major research papers concerning pregnant women summarized several findings with respect to the safety of exercise during pregnancy, effects of exercise on delivery, and guidelines for participation in exercise. Most of the studies support the finding that athletes had fewer complications of pregnancy than did nonathletes. Also, exercisers who remained active during pregnancy weighed less, gained less weight during pregnancy, and delivered smaller babies than nonexercising women. The duration of labor was shorter and exercising women appeared to tolerate labor pain better than nonexercising women did. Athletes had fewer cesarean sections and less tissue ruptures during delivery than nonathletes. Although all women decreased their amount of total work as the pregnancy progressed, many remained active up to the day of delivery.

While most studies report no adverse effects on pregnancy, especially for women who were already physically active, it is still recommended that pregnant women seek the advice of their personal physicians before engaging in endurance exercise programs. It is also strongly recommended that women avoid heavy-lifting exercises and avoid the use of any restrictive belts, such as would be used to lift weights, during pregnancy. The use of such items could restrict uterine blood flow and adversely affect the fetus.

Finally, most studies reported that women tend to exercise at least 3 times per week during pregnancy at an average heart rate of 144 beats per minute. The total amount of exercise done by pregnant athletes exceeded the minimal limits established as safe

---

Eumenorrhea Regularly occurring menstrual cycles.

Oligomenorrhea Reduced, scanty, or irregular menstruation.

Dysmenorrhea Painful menstrual cycles.

Table 14.11 ✦ ACOG Exercise Guidelines

Pregnancy and Postpartum

1. Regular exercise (at least three times per week) is preferable to intermittent activity. Competitive activities should be discouraged.

2. Vigorous exercises should not be performed in hot, humid weather or during a period of illness within the fetus.

3. Ballistic movements (jerky, bouncy motions) should be avoided. Exercise should be done on a wooden floor or a tightly carpeted surface to reduce shock and provide a sure footing.

4. Deep flexion or extension of joints should be avoided because of connective tissue laxity. During pregnancy, connective tissue tends to loosen. This leads to increased risk of injury. Activities that require jumping, jarring motions, or rapid changes in direction should be avoided because of joint instability.

5. Vigorous exercise should be preceded by a five-minute period of muscle warmup. This can be accomplished by slow walking or stationary cycling with low resistance.

6. Vigorous exercise should be followed by a period of gradually declining activity that includes gentle stationary stretching. Because connective-tissue laxity increases the risk of joint injury, stretches should not be taken to the point of maximum resistance.

7. Heart rate should be measured at times of peak activity. Target heart rates (THRs) and limits established in consultation with the physician should not be exceeded.

8. Care should be taken to rise gradually from the floor to avoid orthostatic hypotension. In practical terms, the blood pressure can drop quickly when you move from a horizontal (lying down) to a vertical (standing up) position. Some form of activity involving the legs should be continued for a brief period after standing in order to maintain the blood pressure.

9. Liquids should be taken liberally before and after exercise to prevent dehydration. If necessary, activity should be interrupted to replenish fluids.

10. Women who have had sedentary lifestyles should begin with physical activity of very low intensity and advance activity levels very gradually.

11. Activity should be stopped and your physician consulted if any unusual symptoms appear.

Pregnancy Only

1. Maternal heart rate should not exceed 140 beats per minute.

2. Strenuous activities should not exceed 15 minutes in duration.

3. No exercise should be performed in the supine position after the fourth month of gestation is completed.

4. Exercises that employ the Valsalva maneuver should be avoided. This technique includes any activity that involves breathholding while lifting or moving a heavy object, and you should refrain from this kind of activity in order to avoid big increases in blood pressure.

5. Caloric intake should be adequate to meet not only the extra energy needs of pregnancy but also those of the exercise performed.

6. Maternal core temperature should not exceed 100.4 degrees Fahrenheit.

by the ACOG. None of the female athletes involved, however, experienced complications during pregnancy, and the birthweights of their babies were similar to those of nonathletes. To decide on a safe exercise prescription, tailor your exercise program to your current level of fitness, and always seek the advice of your physician. The onset of any complications may necessitate the discontinuance of exercise during pregnancy.

Benefits of Exercise on Weight Reduction after Pregnancy

Have you ever heard a woman complain of developing "thunder thighs" that she seemed to be unable to get rid of after having a baby? It is true that women tend to store more body fat in the hips and thighs while they are pregnant. When they do not become physically active and do not breastfeed their babies, it is very difficult for many of them to lose all the weight they gained during the pregnancy. Researchers have found that women who maintain an exercise program during and after pregnancy are much more likely to reduce the thunder thighs than those who are not active. What role does physical activity play in this puzzle?

When we eat fat, it is broken down and packaged in the liver in the form of a triglyceride. Triglycerides are then combined with lipoproteins (fat carriers) because triglycerides cannot dissolve directly in the blood. Lipoproteins then carry the triglycerides through the blood stream to the fat cells all over the body. At the entrance to the fat cell, there is an enzyme called lipoprotein lipase (LPL) whose job is to break apart the lipoprotein and the triglyceride. Triglyceride, or fat, is then transported to the fat cell where it is stored, and the lipoprotein continues traveling through the bloodstream.

The enzyme LPL plays a major role in increased fat stores during pregnancy. When the body-fat stores get low, the activity of this enzyme increases so that more fat is stored in the fat cells. In addition, during the early stages of pregnancy, LPL activity in the thighs increases so that more fat is stored in these areas. This is a protective mechanism for the mother because more fat will be needed in these areas to provide the energy to make milk when the mother begins breastfeeding. Milk production actually requires a great deal of energy. So this extra body fat is constantly being broken down to provide energy as long as the mother continues breastfeeding. Thus when women breastfeed, they break down more of the fat

Fitness Heroes

Delisa Walton-Floyd was a track athlete at the University of Tennessee in Knoxville in 1983. She was ranked among the top three U.S. women in the 800-meter event for five years and had broken her own personal record several times.

Because this was the final training and competitive season before the 1984 Olympics, Delisa maintained her athletic discipline even when she became pregnant. As her pregnancy progressed, she never ran less than three miles per day. During the last six weeks of her pregnancy, Delisa developed symptoms of toxemia and gained a great deal of weight. This would have discouraged many athletes, but not Delisa. She was so determined to continue training that she walked the three miles every day, with her mother by her side to make sure she was okay.

When Ebonie was born, everyone commended Delisa on her diligence in pursuing her physical conditioning program, but there were secret fears that she would not make the 1984 Olympic team. Within six weeks, however, Delisa was back on the track every day. As the weeks passed, she lost all the weight she had gained during pregnancy. Because of her discipline and determination, Delisa made it to the final rounds of the Olympic trials and placed fourth for the U.S. team in the 800-meter race. In little more than six months after the birth of her child, she had restored her fitness to an even higher level than before and became an Olympian. ✦

that is stored in the hips and thighs and lose weight quicker.

Also, endurance exercise will trigger the breakdown of fat in the hips and thighs for women who have delivered babies. As you get involved in an exercise program, more fat is released from those fat stores to provide the energy for long-duration activity. But just dieting alone in order to lose thunder thighs is totally ineffective because cutting down on your calories without exercising will not trigger the stubborn fat cells to burn the fat stored within them. Remember to encourage women who are considering getting pregnant or who have recently had a baby to get involved in a physical activity program in order to maintain their body-fat percentage!

Behavioral Change and Motivational Strategies

There are many things that might interfere with your ability and motivation to exercise, and you may find it difficult to eat enough calcium-rich and iron-rich food. Here are some barriers (roadblocks) and strategies for overcoming them.

Roadblock	Behavioral Change Strategy
You are a 20-year-old female on a cross-country team. You have been a long-distance runner since you were 13 years old. You are proud of the fact that you maintain strict dietary habits that include the avoidance of most dairy products. You also have only 10 percent body fat. During the past year you have had two stress fractures. You no longer enjoy exercise because of the fractures.	During the seven years of intensive endurance training you have placed a lot of stress on your body. There are three potential explanations for your stress fractures during the past year. First, the intensive training schedule for seven years has probably weakened your bones because of the constant impact on your lower extremities. You may have overworked your bones and not given your body enough time to rest. Secondly, since you do not eat many dairy products and your body weight is so low, you probably have very little calcium stored in your bones. You could actually be at risk of developing osteoporosis even at such a young age because of the depleted calcium stores in your body. Finally, since your percent body fat is so low, you are probably producing a low amount of estrogen. This makes your bones even more brittle. We recommend that you decrease your training schedule and include more time for rest. You may even consider taking several weeks off during the noncompetitive season. You also need to increase your calcium intake. Review Table 14.7 for tips on how to increase the amount of calcium in your diet.
You are a 21-year-old woman in a moderate-intensity training program. You take a step aerobics class three times a week. For years, you have had very heavy menstrual cycles. You have become a vegetarian during the past year in an effort to better your health status. You eat 1200 calories a day in order to return to the body weight you had at the age of 17. Six months after beginning your aerobics class, you find that you are constantly fatigued.	Your major concern is replenishing your body's iron stores because of the increased amount of iron you lose each month during your period. Since you are a vegetarian, your major sources of iron come from nonheme foods, which have a low absorption rate. Hence even though you may be eating enough iron, you are probably only absorbing a very small percentage. Complete Lab Activity 14.2: Assessing Your Daily Iron Intake. Double your iron-to-calorie ratio by eating iron-rich foods that are also low in calories. By doing this, you will help avoid the depletion of your body's iron stores while staying within your daily caloric intake. You may also need to take a multivitamin supplement that includes iron. Seek the advice of your personal physician, and get a total medical checkup that includes a blood profile before going any further.

Roadblock	Behavioral Change Strategy
You are an 18-year-old white female who avoided physical education in high school. You have always been considered underweight so you did not think you needed to exercise. You have lactose intolerance (which means you cannot drink milk and cannot eat some dairy products). When you completed Lab Activity 14.1: Osteoporosis Risk Assessment, you found that you are only getting 400 mg of calcium per day. Your grandmother has a disease called *osteoporosis* that you really did not know much about until you took this class. Now you are wondering if it is too late to begin an exercise program to decrease your risk of developing osteoporosis in later years.	You have four major risk factors for developing osteoporosis, including being a white female, having a sedentary lifestyle, a family history of osteoporosis, and a calcium deficiency. The good news is that you still have six years to increase your bone density and strengthen your bones. So you need to immediately begin an endurance physical-conditioning program that involves moderate exercise a minimum of three times per week. You may also consider beginning a strength-training program because weight lifting also increases bone density. You also need to examine Table 14.7 to find ways to increase the amount of calcium in your diet. Your physician may recommend that you take a calcium supplement.

Recently two products called Lactaid and DairyEase have been developed to allow people with lactose intolerance to drink milk. Since milk is such an excellent source of calcium and is in a form which has a high absorption rate, we suggest you try these products to allow you to ingest dairy products. You cannot do much to change your family history, but if you start an exercise program and maintain it, and increase your calcium intake to build the strongest bones possible during these next six years, you will greatly reduce your likelihood of getting osteoporosis.

Roadblock	Behavioral Change Strategy
List roadblocks that may keep you from exercising that may be affected by your nutritional status.	Cite behavioral-change strategies that can help you overcome the roadblocks you just listed.
1. _____	1. _____
2. _____	2. _____
3. _____	3. _____

SUMMARY

Physiological Differences between Women and Men Related to Athletic Performance and Physical Fitness

On the average, women weigh less and are shorter, but they have more fat tissue and less muscle mass than men do. This remains true even when female athletes are matched against male athletes for any given sport. There are many differences in the energy systems and physical stature of women and men.

The two anaerobic energy systems are called ATP and PC, which comprise the immediate energy and the lactic acid or anaerobic glycolysis systems. No sex differences exist with the immediate energy system in terms of the muscle concentrations of ATP and PC. Since women tend to have a smaller total muscle mass than men do, their anaerobic capacity is less.

Women also have lower levels of lactic acid than men do at the end of maximal exercise. This is primarily because they have a smaller muscle mass.

Thus, there are no significant biological differences between males and females with respect to anaerobic performance.

After puberty, men tend to have an average of 20 percent higher VO$_2$. This is primarily because women have smaller hearts and less blood volume so that they are not able to deliver as much oxygen to the tissues. Also, women have a smaller muscle mass so they are able to draw less oxygen from the blood to be used aerobically.

After puberty women have a higher percentage of essential body fat than men do because of increased estrogen production. This increased fat is stored in the hips and thighs and most internal organs of the body. Women also have high subcutaneous body-fat stores. An optimal body-fat percentage can be determined based on individual differences and level of performance.

In general, the muscular strength of women is about two-thirds that of men. Although there is no genetic difference in the percentage of muscle fibers between the sexes, there is a difference in the size of the muscle fibers. Men tend to have larger muscle fibers than women do, and this leads to greater strength.

Guidelines for Female Participation in Sports

The Committee on Pediatric Aspects of Physical Fitness, Recreation, and Sports established guidelines for safe participation in sports. They recommend that girls and boys can be allowed to play together until puberty because of similarities in physique and cardiorespiratory endurance. After puberty, whenever possible, match girls according to size, weight, and skill when they are competing. Girls should not be prohibited from participating in strenuous sports. After puberty, girls should not compete against boys in heavy collision sports. Finally, girls can be allowed to participate on the same team as boys when heavy collision is not possible during the activity. These guidelines support the safety of allowing females of all ages to participate in physical activity programs.

Special Considerations for Women

Women are more susceptible than men to certain conditions, including osteoporosis, iron-deficiency anemia, sports anemia, and menstrual disorders. All such conditions can have a debilitating effect on exercise capacity. Also, pregnancy and lactation cause physiological changes which may affect exercise tolerance. Simultaneously, exercise is beneficial for regaining fitness and restoring physique after pregnancy.

Osteoporosis is commonly known as adult bone loss. Many postmenopausal women are plagued with this disease. Peak bone mass is developed up to age 24 years. After age 30, bone loss begins to occur, regardless of how dense the bones are. Risk factors such as being female, old age, being amenorrheic, being of Northern European ancestry, being underweight, smoking cigarettes, drinking alcohol, and sedentary living make individuals more prone to developing osteoporosis.

It is important to maintain the RDA for calcium, especially in the bone-building years. Women should ingest 1200 mg per day up to age 24 and men and women past age 24 should ingest 800 mg per day. Weight-bearing activities have been shown to increase bone density. Hence, maintenance of a lifetime physical activity program is crucial to retarding and preventing this disease.

In iron-deficiency anemia, the red blood cells do not contain enough hemoglobin. Most of the iron in the body is a component of the protein hemoglobin. Hemoglobin is used to carry oxygen throughout the bloodstream to the body tissues where it provides energy for all forms of physical work.

The major cause of iron-deficiency anemia is usually inadequate iron intake. Increased blood loss also leads to such deficiency, as does poor absorption of the iron in foods. Heme iron is found in most meats, fish, and poultry and has the highest rate of absorption. Nonheme iron is in most plant sources and has a much lower absorption rate.

Infants, children, adolescents, and pregnant women usually have increased iron needs. Premenopausal women need to consume 15 mg of iron daily. Men and postmenopausal women need to consume 10 mg per day.

Iron-deficiency anemia occurs in three stages. The first stage is depleted iron stores. During this stage, there are no adverse physiological effects. The second stage is iron deficiency without anemia. At this point the hemoglobin level may be reduced to the low end of normal. In the final phase, iron-deficiency anemia, hemoglobin levels drop and chronic fatigue is induced. Some women experience symptoms called *pica*. They have the tendency to eat ice, clay, and/or paste as a result of the iron deficiency.

This transient anemia is not treatable by iron supplementation and often occurs during the early phases of a strenuous endurance-training program.

True sports anemia is reversible by the end of the ninth week of training. Athletes who experience decreased iron absorption and increased iron loss through the menstrual cycle are more susceptible to both iron-deficiency and sports anemias.

Amenorrhea is a common occurrence among many female endurance athletes. It occurs in approximately one-third of female distance runners. The exact cause of amenorrhea is unknown, but is suspected to be related to the intensity of exercise. As weekly training mileage increases, so does the prevalence of amenorrhea. At higher levels of competition, more psychological stress occurs, which affects hormone production. As the level of hormones such as estrogen is reduced, menstrual disorders are more likely to occur. Menstruation itself has not been shown to adversely affect physical training or competition. In many cases, oligomenorrhea and amenorrhea are reversed as training intensity decreases.

A greater number of physicians are advising women to remain physically active during pregnancy. Women may have shorter labor and tolerate the pain better. Athletes may have fewer complications of pregnancy than nonathletes. Exercisers may weigh less and be less likely to need cesarean sections than nonexercisers. A woman should seek the advice of her personal physician before initiating an exercise program.

During the early stages of pregnancy, the fat cells in the body are stimulated to increase the amount of fat stored, especially in the hips and thighs. If women fail to breastfeed their babies and do not exercise, many of them end up with thunder thighs which cannot be reduced through dieting alone.

REFERENCE

Lokey, E.A., Z.U. Tran, C.L. Wells, B.C. Myers, A.C. Tran. "Effects of Physical Exercise on Pregnancy Outcomes: A Meta-Analytic Review." *Medicine and Science in Sports and Exercise,* Vol. 23, No. 11, pp. 1234–1239, 1991.

Lab Activity 14.1

Osteoporosis Risk Assessment

✦ **Step One**   Write in the number of servings of the following foods you consume daily (1 cup = 8 oz). Multiply the number of servings (column 1) by the given number of mg of calcium per serving (column 2). Now total the numbers in the last column. This number is your daily calcium intake from dairy products.

FOOD	SERVING SIZE	(1) NUMBER OF SERVINGS	(2) CALCIUM (MG) PER SERVING	(1) × (2) DAILY CALCIUM INTAKE
Milk	1 cup	_____	× 300 =	_____
Yogurt	1 cup	_____	× 300 =	_____
Cheese	1 slice	_____	× 200 =	_____
Cottage cheese	½ cup	_____	× 70 =	_____
Ice cream	1 cup	_____	× 180 =	_____

Daily calcium intake from dairy products: _____

✦ **Step Two**   Write in the number of servings of the following foods you consume weekly (column 1). Multiply that number by the given number of mg of calcium (column 2) and add these amounts to get a total. This number is your weekly calcium intake from nondairy products.

FOOD	SERVING SIZE	(1) NUMBER OF SERVINGS	(2) CALCIUM (MG) PER SERVING	(1) × (2) WEEKLY CALCIUM INTAKE
Broccoli	1/2 cup	_____	× 65 =	_____
Baked beans	1/2 cup	_____	× 65 =	_____
Pizza	1 slice	_____	× 100 =	_____
Soup (made with milk)	1 cup	_____	× 170 =	_____
Sardines	3 oz	_____	× 375 =	_____
Canned salmon	4 oz	_____	× 300 =	_____
Shrimp	3 oz	_____	× 100 =	_____

Weekly calcium intake from nondairy foods (except soup base): _____

Now divide your weekly calcium intake from nondairy foods by 7: $\dfrac{\rule{2cm}{0.4pt}}{7}$ = _____

✦ **Step Three**   Add your daily calcium intake from section 1 and your weekly calcium intake divided by 7 from section 2. The total of these two figures is your average daily calcium intake.

Daily calcium intake from dairy foods   = _____

+ Weekly calcium intake from other foods divided by 7   = _____

Average daily calcium intake   = _____

✦ **Step Four**   Compare your average daily calcium intake to:

Women and men aged 11 to 24 years = 1200 mg/day
Women and men aged 25 years and older = 800 mg/day

Some researchers recommend that premenopausal women ingest 1000 mg of calcium per day and that postmenopausal women ingest 1500 mg of calcium per day. Seek the advice of your personal physician before taking amounts in excess of the 1989 RDA.

✦ **Step Five**   Answer the following questions. If you answer "yes" to three or more questions, you are at risk for developing osteoporosis.

1. Has anyone in your family suffered a hip or vertebral (back) fracture?

Yes _____   No _____   Relationship: _____

2. Is your ethnic background Northern European?

Yes _____   No _____

3. Do you exercise less than 3 times a week for 30 minutes each time?

Yes _____   No _____

4. Do you regularly take antacids? (Aluminum increases calcium excretion. Anyone who takes an aluminum-containing antacid regularly should switch to one with no aluminum.)

Yes _____   No _____   Brand name: _____

5. Do you consume carbonated beverages? Yes _____   No _____

Number per day: _____   Type: _____

A calcium-to-phosphorus ratio of 1:1 is needed to avoid calcium depletion. Some research has shown that because of significant changes in the American diet, most people's calcium-to-phosphorus ratio is now close to 1:2. This excessive consumption of phosphorus is thought to leach more calcium out of the bones, resulting in increased bone loss.

One significant source of phosphorus is most carbonated beverages. Excessive consumption of these beverages must be considered when assessing dietary risk of osteoporosis. Check labels for phosphorus content, and substitute skim or whole milk when possible.

6. Do you not take any calcium supplements?

Yes _____ (I do *not* take calcium supplements.)

No _____ (I *do* take calcium supplements.)

Number per day: _____   Type: _____

Source: A. Larson and S. Shannon, "Decreasing the Incidence of Osteoporosis-Related Injuries through Diet and Exercise," *Geritopics,* 8 (1985):2, 5–9. Reprinted from *Geritopics* with the permission of the American Physical Therapy Association.

Lab Activity 14.2

Assessing Your Daily Iron Intake

✦ **Step One** For each item on this list of several sources of heme and nonheme iron, write in the number of servings you consume daily. Multiply the number of servings (column 1) by the given number of mg of iron per serving (column 2). Now total the numbers in the last column. This number is your daily iron intake from heme and nonheme food sources.

FOOD	SERVING SIZE	(1) NUMBER OF SERVINGS	(2) IRON (MG) PER SERVING	(1) × (2) DAILY IRON INTAKE
Good Sources of Iron				
Beef liver	3 oz	_____	5.3	_____
Chicken liver	1 each	_____	1.7	_____
Clams	3 oz canned	_____	23.8	_____
Oysters	1 cup	_____	16.6	_____
Corned beef	3 oz	_____	1.8	_____
Pork loin	3 oz	_____	1.0	_____
Prune juice	1 cup	_____	3.0	_____
Prunes	10 med	_____	2.1	_____
Raisins	1 cup	_____	3.0	_____
Lima beans	1 cup	_____	4.5	_____
Kidney beans	1 cup	_____	3.2	_____
Pinto beans	1 cup	_____	4.5	_____
Black-eyed peas	1 cup	_____	4.3	_____
Chick peas	1 cup	_____	4.7	_____
Soybeans	1 cup	_____	8.8	_____
Sunflower seeds	1/4 cup	_____	2.4	_____
Almonds	1 cup	_____	5.0	_____
Cashews	1 cup	_____	6.0	_____
Total cereal	1 cup	_____	21.0	_____
Most cereal	2/3 cup	_____	9.0	_____
Raisin bran	1/2 cup	_____	4.5	_____
Cheerios	1 cup	_____	3.6	_____

Food	Serving Size	(1) Number of Servings	(2) Iron (mg) Per Serving	(1) × (2) Daily Iron Intake
Fair Sources of Iron				
Tuna, canned	3 oz	_____	2.7	_____
Salmon	3 oz	_____	0.9	_____
Shrimp	6 med	_____	2.6	_____
Sardines	3 oz	_____	2.5	_____
Veal	3 oz	_____	1.0	_____
Chicken, breast	3 oz	_____	0.9	_____
Turkey, roasted	3 oz	_____	1.7	_____
Rabbit	3 oz	_____	2.0	_____
Liverwurst	1 oz	_____	1.5	_____
Beef pot roast	3 oz	_____	3.3	_____
Hamburger	3 oz	_____	2.0	_____
Ham	3 oz	_____	1.2	_____
Hot dog	1 each	_____	0.7	_____
Fish stick	1 oz	_____	0.1	_____
Walnuts	1 cup	_____	3.0	_____
Pecans	1 cup	_____	2.3	_____
Peanuts	1 cup	_____	2.6	_____
Peanut butter	1 tbsp	_____	0.3	_____
Apricots, dried	¼ cup	_____	1.2	_____
Bananas	1 each	_____	1.1	_____
Strawberries	1 cup	_____	0.6	_____
Watermelon	1 slice	_____	0.8	_____
Canned peaches	1 cup	_____	0.7	_____
Nectarines	1 each	_____	0.2	_____
Potato	1 med	_____	2.8	_____
Green beans	1 cup	_____	1.1	_____
Green peas	1 cup	_____	2.6	_____
White rice	½ cup	_____	0.9	_____
Whole wheat bread	1 slice	_____	1.0	_____
Egg noodles	1 cup	_____	2.5	_____
Corn flakes	1¼ cup	_____	1.8	_____

Food	Serving Size	(1) Number of Servings	(2) Iron (mg) Per Serving	(1) × (2) Daily Iron Intake
Oatmeal, cooked	1 cup	_____	1.6	_____
Bagel	1 each	_____	1.8	_____
Collard greens	1 cup	_____	0.2	_____
Spinach	1 cup	_____	6.4	_____
Mustard greens	1 cup	_____	1.7	_____
Turnip greens	1 cup	_____	1.7	_____
Broccoli	1 cup	_____	1.3	_____
Corn	1 ear	_____	0.5	_____
Eggs	1 each	_____	0.7	_____
Flour, enriched	1 cup	_____	3.2	_____
Flour, unenriched	1 cup	_____	0.9	_____

Others:

_____	_____	_____	_____	_____
_____	_____	_____	_____	_____
_____	_____	_____	_____	_____
_____	_____	_____	_____	_____
_____	_____	_____	_____	_____
_____	_____	_____	_____	_____

* The number of mg of iron per serving is calculated by using the average values from several nutrition textbooks.

This is your daily intake from iron (heme and nonheme) sources _____ mg/day

◆ **Step Two**   Review your food sources of iron and make a list of heme compared to non-heme sources in the space provided.

Heme Iron

Source	Amount (mg)
_____	_____
_____	_____
_____	_____
_____	_____
_____	_____
_____	_____
Total (mg)	_____

Nonheme Iron

Source	Amount (mg)
_____	_____
_____	_____
_____	_____
_____	_____
_____	_____
_____	_____
Total (mg)	_____

1. From which source are you obtaining most of your dietary iron?

   Heme _____   Nonheme _____

2. What is the significance of differentiating between heme and nonheme sources of iron in your diet?

   _____

   _____

   _____

   _____

✦ **Step Three**   Compare your average daily iron intake with:

Premenopausal women   = 15 mg/day
Postmenopausal women   = 10 mg/day

Men aged 11 to 18 years = 12 mg/day
Men aged 18 and older   = 10 mg/day

✦ **Step Four**   Answer the following questions. If you answer "yes" to three or more questions, you may need to take an iron supplement. Please seek the advice of your personal physician before doing so.

	Yes	No
1. Does most of your daily iron come from nonheme sources?	_____	_____
2. Does anyone in your family have a history of iron-deficiency anemia?	_____	_____
Relationship: _____		
3. Do you exercise more than 3 times a week for 45 minutes or longer?	_____	_____
4. Do you drink more than two glasses of iced tea each day?	_____	_____
5. Do you drink more than two carbonated sodas each day?	_____	_____
6. Do you take calcium supplements?	_____	_____
7. Do you have heavy menstrual cycles?	_____	_____

15

Designing a Program Unique for You: A Lifetime of Fitness

Chapter Objectives

By the end of this chapter, you should be able to:

1. Identify your fitness goals.

2. Select physical activities to meet your fitness goals.

3. Design an exercise program that is appropriate for you now and that can be continued and/or adapted for many years to come.

4. List criteria for evaluating an exercise club and selecting exercise equipment to purchase.

5. Describe how you can keep fit as you age.

WHEN MANDY WAS an infant she crawled around her playpen and on the carpet endlessly. A full day of that type of exercise tired her out and she had no problem sleeping through the night. When she started school, Mandy participated in physical education and soon learned sports skills she used to become physically fit and healthy. She became enamored with soccer, in particular, and joined a recreational soccer league that played on the weekends. By the time she enrolled in college, Mandy was interested in weight training and aerobic dance classes. She used the college's exercise room to lift weights and signed up for an aerobic dance class to meet the physical education course requirement before graduation. Mandy is now in her sixties and no longer interested in aerobic dance, is not in condition to play soccer, and cannot lift the amount of weight she could when younger. Yet, Mandy still exercises regularly. She walks daily and joins her contemporaries in the pool for aqua aerobics four days a week. She found that the local Y has a weight room with a staff person qualified to advise her on the type of weight training best for someone of her age and in her condition, so she even weight trains three days a week. In a very real sense, Mandy is still enrolled in physical education, only this time with a different type of instructor.

Today there are some excellent physical education instructors who understand the nature of physical fitness and how it relates to health and wellness. There has been this kind of instructor for many years. Unfortunately, there are many inadequate physical education instructors who force individuals to run long distances even though they are not in shape to do so or who only teach how to play softball, basketball, or football. These inadequate instructors teach individuals to hate running as it tires them out for the rest of the day and creates aches and pains where they do not even know they have body parts. The team sports, on the other hand, may be great fun, but once the class is over, it is nearly impossible to get 22 people together to play football, 18 people to play softball, or even 10 people to play basketball. Of course, there are co-ed softball leagues, and pick-up basketball games at the local YMCA or community center, and some people still meet on the weekends to play touch football. And yet, most of us would prefer physical activities that require less organization. That may be why we join health clubs and weight train. Or why we take up jogging and swimming. Or why we play tennis or golf. These lifetime sports activities can be done alone or at most require only one other person. And our bodies can withstand the activity even into our later years.

Today, more and more physical education courses of study include instruction on tennis, golf, weight training, and badminton, while not neglecting more aerobically intensive physical activities such as basketball, soccer, football, and jogging. What is more, they sometimes even add a health and wellness perspective to the courses.

In this concluding chapter of this book, we provide you with the information you need to continue your fitness program for the rest of your life. We do this by helping you determine your fitness goals and by then showing you how to achieve them. We even help you evaluate fitness and health clubs and identify what you should look for when purchasing exercise equipment.

IDENTIFYING YOUR FITNESS GOALS

Why do you want to engage in physical activity? Some people just want to be healthy. Others want to look good, to have energy, to develop strength, or to compete for the sake of competing. It stands to reason that if you do not know why you participate in physical fitness activities, you cannot select activities that will help you meet your goals. Determine your fitness goals by completing Lab Activity 15.1: Why I Want to Be Physically Fit at the end of this chapter.

HEALTH PROMOTION AND DISEASE PREVENTION

One of your fitness goals is probably to maintain good health. We have already discussed the fact that this requires more than just exercise. For example, you know that in order to remain healthy, you need to eat nutritionally, to use stress-management techniques to prevent illness and disease, and to refrain from using chemical substances that can harm you (such as tobacco and illicit drugs). When you do all this, you can prevent, or at least postpone, the onset of cardiovascular diseases (such as coronary heart disease and stroke) as well as precursors of these diseases (such as high blood pressure). You can also decrease your risk of contracting cancer or other life-threatening diseases. But beyond merely preventing illness and disease, you can also enhance your well being by engaging in a variety of lifestyle behaviors. Although we will now focus on exercise behaviors, do not neglect to consider other lifestyle behaviors when designing a total fitness program for yourself. We will return to this at the conclusion of this chapter.

FITNESS ACTIVITIES TO HELP YOU ACHIEVE YOUR GOALS

There is a seemingly endless array of physical activities in which you can participate. Now that you have completed Lab Activity 15.1: Why I Want to Be Physically Fit and have a better idea of why you want to exercise, it will be easier for you to choose one of these activities. We will describe several of the more popular and effective exercise options in this section. If we missed your favorite activity, we apologize but be comforted by knowing a trip to the library will probably disclose all you ever wanted to know about it.

Walking

Walking is an excellent way to keep fit without putting undue stress on your connective tissue and bones. Studies have shown that adults who walk for exercise 2½ to 4 hours a week tend to have less than half the prevalence of elevated serum cholesterol as those who do not walk or exercise regularly. Walking can develop cardiorespiratory endurance (especially if the speed of the walking is brisk) and is effective as a calorie burner. What is more, walking is an activity in which all ages can participate. Finally, walking can have psychological benefits as well: it can help to reduce anxiety and depression.

The President's Council on Physical Fitness and Sports offers some tips to help you develop an efficient walking style:

- Hold your head erect, and keep your back straight and abdomen flat. Your toes should point straight ahead and your arms should swing loosely at your sides.
- Land on the heel of your foot and roll forward to drive off the ball of your foot. Walking only on the balls of your feet or flatfooted may cause fatigue and soreness.
- Take long, easy strides, but do not strain for distance. When walking up or down hills or at a very rapid pace lean forward slightly.
- Breathe deeply (with your mouth open, if that is more comfortable).

To help you to begin a walking program, follow the regimen in Table 15.1.

Table 15.1 ♦ A Walking Program

Week One

Walk briskly for 5 minutes. (Do not walk so briskly that you become breathless.)

Walk slowly for 3 minutes.

Walk briskly for 5 minutes.

Repeat for a total of about 30 minutes of walking.

Week Two

Same as week one. If you can pick up the pace a little without becoming breathless, do so.

Week Three

Same as week one but increase brisk walking to 8 minutes at a time. Increase time for a total of about 40 minutes of walking.

Week Four

Same as week three. If you can pick up the pace a little without becoming breathless, do so.

After four weeks, increase brisk walking for as long as it is comfortable.

Jogging and Running

If walking is too slow for you, try **jogging** or **running**. With either you can get a comparable workout in a shorter period of time. Unfortunately, jogging puts stress on your body, subjecting you to a greater chance of injury than walking does. Foot, ankle, knee, and back problems can develop. Yet with the proper precautions (good shoes and not doing more than you are in condition to do) jogging injuries can be minimized.

Having the right running shoes is important if you choose to jog. There are many shoes from which to choose. We will discuss how to purchase shoes in which to run or jog later in this chapter. Personnel in stores selling running shoes can help you select a shoe right for you, but *you* need to be the final judge. If the shoe feels comfortable and provides enough support, that is probably the right shoe for you.

The President's Council on Physical Fitness and Sports points out that running for fitness is different than running for speed and power. When you run for fitness, you should maintain a comfortable, economical running style:

- Run in an upright position, avoiding excessive forward lean. Keep your back as straight as you comfortably can and keep your head up. Do not look down at your feet.
- Carry your arms slightly away from your body, with your elbows bent so your forearms are roughly parallel to the ground. Occasionally shake and relax your arms to prevent tightness in your shoulders.
- Land on the heel of your foot and rock forward to drive off the ball of your foot. If this proves difficult, try a more flat-footed style. Running only on the balls of your feet will tire you quickly and make your legs sore.
- Keep your stride relatively short. Do not force your pace by reaching for extra distance.
- Breathe deeply with your mouth open.

One concern about either walking or running is safety. Recognizing the need to advise runners how to

Jogging Running at a 9-minute-per-mile pace or slower.

Running Running faster than 9 minutes per mile.

exercise to limit vulnerability, the Road Runners Club of America offers these tips in their booklet entitled *Women Running: Run Smart. Run Safe:*

Stay Alert

- Do not wear headphones. If you wear them you will not hear an approaching car or an approaching attacker.
- Run against traffic so that you can observe approaching vehicles.
- Practice identifying characteristics of strangers and memorizing license tags.
- Tune into your environment, not out of it.

Avoid Isolation

- Run in familiar areas.
- Run with a partner or dog.
- Write down or leave word about the direction of your run. Tell friends and family of your favorite running routes.
- Befriend neighbors and local businesses.

Use Your Intuition

- Trust your intuition about an area or a person, avoiding any place or person you are unsure of.
- Use discretion in acknowledging verbal harassment by strangers. Look directly at others and be observant, but keep your distance and keep moving.
- Call police immediately if something happens to you or someone else or if you notice anyone out of the ordinary.

Be Prepared

- Carry identification or write your name, phone number, and blood type on the inside of your running shoe.
- Do not wear jewelry.
- Carry a noisemaker.
- Be prepared to scream and break the silence.
- Wear reflective material.
- Know the location of telephones.
- Vary your route.

Jogging or running costs relatively little (good running shoes are the only major expense), can be done almost anywhere (indoors or out of doors), and is an excellent aerobic exercise.

Rope Jumping

When one of the authors was 13, he fell head over heels in love with 12-year-old blonde-haired, adorable, vivacious Jill, heart-poundingly, palm-perspiringly, any-spare-time-spent-with-her love. The problem was that Steven was also in love with Jill. In the competition to win Jill's heart, Steven and he learned how to jump rope that summer. While their friends played basketball and softball, they jumped rope with Jill. They were frantic not to be seen by their friends in this sissy activity. If their other friends had seen them, they would have died.

Well, no longer crippled by that thought, we learned that the gender you were born with need not stop you from participating in any enjoyable activity, and that rope jumping is an excellent way of developing cardiorespiratory endurance, strength, agility, coordination, and a sense of wellness. Here are some pointers for rope jumping:

1. Determine the best length for your rope by standing on the center of the rope. The handles should reach from armpit to armpit.
2. When you are jumping, keep your arms close to your body with your elbows almost touching your sides. Have your forearms out at right angles, and turn the rope by making small circles with your hands and wrists. Keep your feet, ankles, and knees together.
3. Relax. Do not tense up. Enjoy yourself.
4. Keep your body erect, with your head and eyes up.
5. Start slowly.
6. Land on the balls of your feet, bending your knees slightly.
7. Maintain a steady rhythm.
8. Jump just one or two inches from the floor.
9. Try jumping to music and maintaining the rhythm of the music.
10. When you get good, improvise. Create new stunts. Have fun.

See Table 15.2 for recommended rope-jumping stunts. Why not get a jump rope and try them out?

Table 15.2 ✦ Basic Single Short Rope Skills

1. **Basic Jump**
   1. Jump on both feet.
   2. Land on balls of feet.
   3. Jump once for each revolution of rope.

   Tips: Keep feet, ankles and knees together.
   Cue: JUMP - JUMP - JUMP

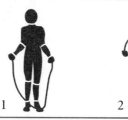

2. **Side Swing**
   1. Swing rope to left side.
   2. Repeat to the right side.
   3. Swing rope alternately from side to side.

   Tips: Hold one rope handle in each hand.
        Keep hands together, keep feet together.
   Cue: LEFT - RIGHT - LEFT - RIGHT

 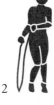 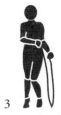

3. **Double Side Swing and Jump**
   1. Swing rope to left side.
   2. Swing rope to right side.
   3. Jump over rope.

   Tips: Keep hands together on side swings,
        keep feet together.
   Cue: LEFT - RIGHT - JUMP

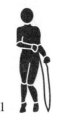 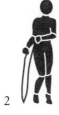 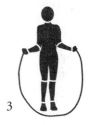

4. **Single Side Swing and Jump**
   1. Swing rope to left side.
   2. Jump over rope.
   3. Swing rope to right side.
   4. Jump over rope.

   Tips: Hold one rope handle in each hand.
        Keep hands together on side swings,
        keep feet together.
   Cue: LEFT - JUMP - RIGHT - JUMP

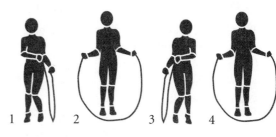

5. **One-Handed Side Swing (Twirl)**
   1. Hold both handles in left hand.
   2. Twirl rope on left side.
   3. Repeat to right side.

   Tips: Keep rope parallel to side of body.
        Practice on both sides.
   Cue: SWING - SWING

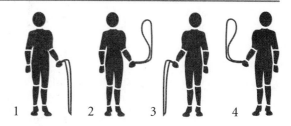

6. **Skier**
   1. Jump left.
   2. Jump right.

   Tips: Feet move laterally 4-6" to each side,
        keep feet together.
   Cue: LEFT - RIGHT

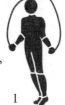 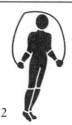

Source: Reproduced with permission. *Jump Rope for Heart Curriculum Guide,* 1991. Copyright American Heart Association.

Table 15.2 ✦ Basic Single Short Rope Skills *(continued)*

7. Bell
1. Jump forward.
2. Jump backward.

Tips: Feet move 4-6" forward and backward as a bell clapper, keep feet together.
Cue: FORWARD - BACK

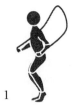 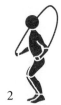

8. Side Straddle
1. Jump to straddle position.
2. Return to basic jump.

Tips: Spread feet shoulder width apart as rope passes under.
Cue: APART - TOGETHER

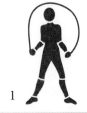 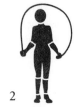

9. Scissors (Forward Straddle)
1. Jump to stride position with left foot forward.
2. Jump and reverse position of feet.

Tips: Feet should be 8-12" apart.
Cue: LEFT - RIGHT

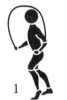 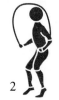

10. Straddle Cross
1. Jump to straddle position.
2. Jump to crossed legs.

Tips: Feet shoulder width apart. Alternate leg in front with each cross.
Cue: APART - CROSS

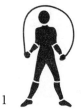 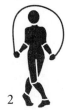

11. Wounded Duck
1. Jump, toes and knees together, heels spread.
2. Jump, heels together, toes and knees spread.

Tips: Alternate toes together and heels together.
Cue: TOES - HEELS

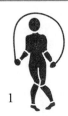 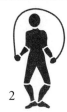

12. Criss Cross
1. Cross arms until elbows touch and jump.
2. Open rope and perform basic jump.

Tips: Handles in extended position. Keep hands down low on the cross.
Cue: CROSS - OPEN

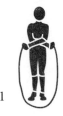 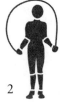

13. Full Turn (one complete circle with rope in front)
1. Turn body to left with left side swing.
2. Facing rope, continue to turn body left a full turn, lifting the rope up.
3. Jump rope forward.

Tips: Follow rope, keep rope in front of body. May also turn to right.
Cue: SWING - TURN - LIFT - JUMP

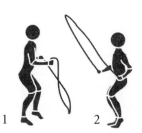 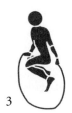

Table 15.2 ✦ Basic Single Short Rope Skills *(continued)*

14. Heel to Heel
1. Jump and touch left heel to floor in front.
2. Jump and touch right heel to floor in front.

Tips: Heel touches are forward.
Cue: HEEL - HEEL - HEEL

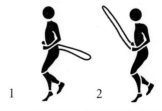

15. Toe to Toe
1. Hop on left foot, touch right toe to floor in back.
2. Hop on right foot, touch left toe to floor in back.

Tips: Keep body over weighted foot.
Cue: TOE - TOE - TOE

 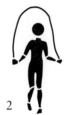  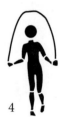

16. Heel-Toe
1. Hop on left foot, touch right heel forward.
2. Hop on left foot again, touch right toe backward.
3. Repeat on opposite side.

Tips: Heel-toe as in a polka.
Cue: HEEL - TOE - HEEL - TOE

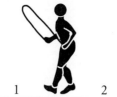

17. Kick Swing
1. Hop on left foot, swing right leg forward.
2. Hop on right foot, swing left leg forward.

Tips: Repeat directions sideward and backward.
Cue: KICK - KICK - KICK

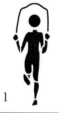 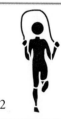

18. Toe Touch
1. Hop on left foot, touch right toe to right.
2. Hop on right foot, touch left toe to left.

Tips: Keep feet close to floor.
Cue: RIGHT - LEFT

 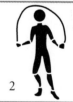

19. Double Toe Touch
1. Hop on right foot, touch left toe to left about 6".
2. Hop on right foot again, touch left toe to left about 12".
3. Repeat with right toe 6" and 12".

Tips: Keep feet close to floor. Bring foot in to avoid rope between toe touches.
Cue: LEFT - LEFT - RIGHT - RIGHT

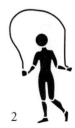

20. Forward 180 (half turn to backward jumping position)
1. Side swing left, half turn body to left.
2. Jump over backward turning rope.

Tips: Turn body to follow rope. May be performed to left or right.
Cue: JUMP - TURN - JUMP BACKWARDS

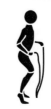 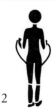

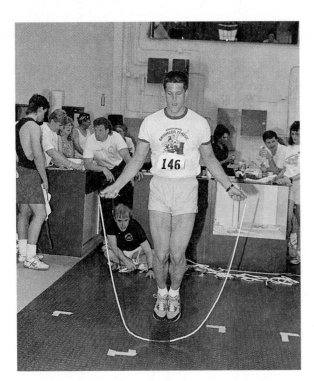

Rope skipping is an excellent cardiovascular exercise, and can be done just about anywhere at any time. (Photo courtesy of the Aspen Hill Club.)

Swimming

Swimming is both popular and a very good physical fitness activity. What's more, it enhances physical fitness while diminishing the chances of injury. That is because it limits the amount of weight your body must bear. When you are submerged up to the neck in water, you experience an apparent loss of 90 percent of your weight. If you weigh 130 pounds, when you are in water up to your neck, your feet and legs have to support a weight of only 13 pounds. Therefore, you are less apt to injure your legs and feet.

Many people who use swimming for conditioning do lap swimming, that is, they swim back and forth. When you are lap swimming, you should periodically check your heart rate to determine if you are at your target. But lap swimming is not appropriate for everyone. Backyard pools usually are not large enough. Most residential pools are no longer than 36 feet (ft) by 17 ft, with approximately 600 square ft of water surface, starting at 3 to 8.5 ft in depth. In a swimming pool of this size, a workout must be adjusted considerably from that usually practiced in the typical school, college, or athletic club pool. Otherwise swimming in the backyard pool becomes largely diving in, gliding across, and climbing out. For the typical person, it means only inactive bathing. But

swimming pools, regardless of size have a high potential as exercise facilities. This potential can be realized as individuals learn how to exercise in limited water areas.

The President's Council on Physical Fitness and Sports recommends an exercise program for limited water areas in its booklet *Aqua Dynamics.* The program involves standing water drills (for example, alternate toe touching, side straddle hopping, toe bounding, and jogging in place), poolside standing drills (such as stretching the arms out, pressing the back flat against the wall, and raising the knees to the chest), gutter-holding drills (such as knees to chest, hop twisting, front and back flutter kicking, and side flutter kicking), bobbing, and treading water. If you have your own pool and feel it is too small for lap swimming, you might write to the President's Council on Physical Fitness and Sports, Washington, DC 20201, for the *Aqua Dynamics* booklet. Another good source is Jane Katz's article, "The W.E.T. Workout," which was published in the June 1986 issue of *Shape* magazine, or you can contact your nearest health club, YMCA, or JCC to see if they have water aerobics classes.

Tennis

As with all fitness activities, duration and intensity will determine how much your tennis game contributes to your physical fitness and wellness. A doubles match generally results in less of a workout than does a singles match. In fact, a doubles match will use up to 330 calories (cal) per hour, whereas a singles match will use up to 390 cal per hour.

The contribution of tennis to wellness, however, is another matter. As we have stated so often in this book, even if your physical health is improved, if the other components of your health suffer, you have not improved your health. Playing tennis may improve the efficiency of your heart, but if your attitude and behavior on the court loses you friends, results in your not enjoying yourself, or frustrates you, you would be better off not playing at all. In spite of exercising, you are making yourself *less well.* Two solutions make the most sense to us: Either approach tennis with a different attitude, or select a less competitive exercise to engage in regularly.

When stroking the ball, if you roll over the shot too much (too much topspin), you can contribute to tennis elbow. Using too much wrist in the shot will lead you to roll over; instead you should stroke through the ball with your wrist locked. If tennis elbow does develop, you can switch to a lighter racket

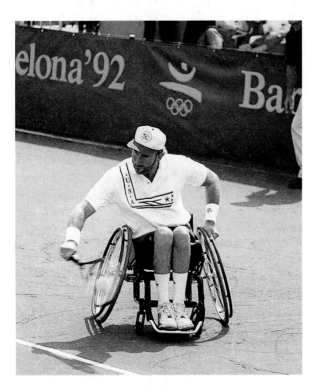

Tennis can contribute to overall fitness, muscular strength, and flexibility. (Photo Courtesy of Wendy Parks/National Foundation of Wheelchair Tennis.)

Fitness Heroes

In 1993, at the age of 85, Johnny Kelley ran his sixty-first Boston Marathon. He is a Boston hero. He has run the marathon almost every year since 1928 and he won the marathon in both 1935 and 1945. As he runs the course every year, Bostonians and others recognize him and cheer enthusiastically.

In 1993, Johnny Kelley was honored with a 7-foot statue, depicting him in two stages of his remarkable life. The statue stands tall in downtown Boston—a constant reminder that no matter how old you are, you are never too old to exercise. ✦

to aggravate the elbow less. Applying ice after playing will also help.

A warmup that includes stretching is a must. Tennis involves dynamic, quick movements with a great deal of stretching to reach the ball. Therefore, if you are not flexible enough, you may be prone to muscle and connective-tissue injury, such as muscle pulls or sprained ligaments.

Racketball, Handball, and Squash

The indoor racket sports can be excellent ways to develop and maintain fitness. That is because they contribute to cardiorespiratory endurance, muscular strength and endurance of the legs, flexibility, agility, balance and coordination, and weight control. They are also usually fun. Yet there is danger involved in these sports. Every year, over 3000 eye injuries result from them. That need not be the case if players wear appropriate eye protectors. Eye protectors should offer a complete shield (do not use the kind with narrow bands with opening between them) and be made of polycarbonate.

Another risk involved in these sports can be found in the environment in which they are played.

To exercise in a hot room can be hazardous unless you take certain precautions. You should drink plenty of water before starting to play and intermittently take breaks to replenish the water you lose through perspiration. You should not play longer than you are in condition to play; to overdo it in a hot room can be risky. Know when to stop.

Last, you must be in good physical condition before engaging in these sports. Since they are highly competitive, they are usually played in a hot environment, and they involve dynamic (stop and go) and stretching movements. If you are not in good physical condition, you may injure yourself. If you *are* in good condition, these sports are excellent activities to help you remain fit.

Aerobic Dance

One of the best fitness activities is dance, especially if you're serious about your training. Look at the bodies of dancers. They are remarkably muscular, incredibly supple, and ready to meet the demands strenuous exercise places on their hearts and circulatory and respiratory systems. Dance is one good way to develop and maintain physical fitness.

The traditional dance programs were tap, ballet, and modern dance. In recent years a different form of dance has swept the country and become a significant part of the fitness movement. It combines calisthenics and a variety of dance movements, all done to music, and is called aerobic dance. The term, coined by Jacki Sorenson in 1979, involves choreographed routines that include walking, jumping, hopping, bouncing, kicking, and various arm movements designed to develop cardiorespiratory endurance, flexibility, and muscular strength and endurance. Dancing to music is an enjoyable activity for many people who would not otherwise seek to exercise. And since aerobic dance is often done in groups, the social contact makes it even more enjoyable.

To maximize the fitness benefits of aerobic dance, you should maintain the dancing for approximately 35 to 45 minutes and work out three or four times a week. In addition, you should check periodically to see if you are maintaining your target heart rate (THR). Since many communities offer aerobic dance classes (some may be called Dancercize or Jazzercise) through YM/YWCAs, Jewish community centers, colleges, local schools, and even on morning television programs, maintaining a regular dance regimen should not be difficult. The only equipment you will need is a good pair of aerobic dance shoes with good shock absorbency, stability, and outer sole flexibility and clothes to work out in. One caution: Do not dance on a concrete floor, since the constant pounding could result in shin splints. A wooden floor is ideal.

Low-Impact Aerobics

Several factors associated with aerobic dance has led some experts to question the manner in which it is usually conducted. A study by the American Aerobics Association found 80 percent of its teachers and students were getting injured during workouts, and another questionnaire administered to aerobic instructors found 55 percent reported significant injuries. Among the causes of these injuries are bad floors (too hard), bad shoes (too little shock absorbency and stability), and bad routines offered by poorly trained instructors. With the popularity of aerobics, it is not surprising what is done in its name. Even a *pet aerobics* routine has been developed for the pudgy dog or cat. It is therefore no surprise that many aerobics instructors are poorly trained and teach routines that are inappropriate and injury producing, using surfaces that cause high-impact injuries.

To respond to these concerns, several things have happened. One is the certification of aerobics instructors. Organizations, such as the American College of Sports Medicine (ACSM), the Aerobics and Fitness Association of America, National Dance-Exercise Instructor's Training Association, Ken Cooper's Aerobics Way, and the Aerobic Center, have all instituted certification programs for aerobics instructors. Unfortunately, the requirements for certification by

these organizations vary greatly. Some form of certification, however, is probably better than none.

Another attempt at limiting the injuries from aerobics is the development of *low-impact* aerobic routines. Low-impact aerobics features one foot on the ground at all times and the use of light weights. The idea is to cut down on the stress to the body caused by jumping and bouncing while at the same time deriving the muscle toning and cardiorespiratory benefits of high-impact aerobics. These routines have become more and more popular as the risk of injury from high-impact aerobics has become better known. Something called *chair aerobics* has even been developed. It involves routines done while the participant is seated in a chair. Low-impact aerobics are not totally risk-free. Injuries to the upper body caused by the circling and swinging movements with weights are not infrequent. Many of these injuries can be treated at home, however, and are not serious. With any form of physical activity, there is always the chance of injury. The benefits to the cardiorespiratory system and the rest of the body—benefits that we have described in this book—are often worth the slight chance of injury.

A recent aerobic dance development is *step aerobics,* which involves stepping up and down on a small platform (step) to the rhythm of music and the directions of an instructor. The workout can vary from mild to extremely intense depending on the speed, the movements, and the duration of the exercise. Double step aerobic routines have been developed that involve the use of two platforms. Step aerobic classes are usually offered at the same places aerobic dance classes are conducted. If you are interested in double step aerobics, you can read an article about it in the May 1993 issue of *American Health* magazine (page 92).

Bicycling

To begin a bicycle exercise program, you obviously need a bicycle. A good 10-speed bike will cost approximately $300. You can get an adequate 10-speed or a mountain bike (a sturdier bike) for less, however, if you shop around or buy one secondhand. You will also need a helmet to protect your head from injury should you fall. Gloves with padded palms can also make your ride more comfortable. In addition, think about adding pant clips and/or clothes designed specifically for biking.

Of course, you can exercise with any bike—it need not have 10 speeds or be a mountain bike—if you choose. A good bike, however, will allow you to

Figure 15.1 ✦ Seat Adjustment When Riding
a Stationary Bike

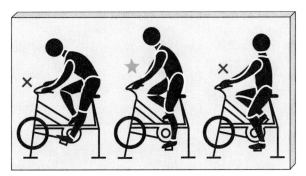

Correct seat height is depicted in the middle drawing. The seat on the left is too high, and the one on the right is too low. Maintain a slight bend in the lower leg when vertical.

take trips that add to the enjoyment of biking in addition to enhancing overall health and wellness.

When you are biking, follow this advice:

- Keep your elbows slightly bent.
- Lower your upper body for a streamlined position.
- Do not grip the handlebars too tightly.
- Wear bright clothing so motorists can easily see you.
- Obey all traffic laws.
- Always lean into the turn.
- Learn and use hand signals that indicate which way you are turning.
- Leave the radio at home so you can focus on the road and hear cars and other potential hazards.

Figure 15.2 ✦ Handlebar Adjustment When
Riding a Stationary Bike

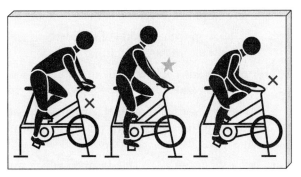

Correct handlebar adjustment is depicted in the middle drawing.

- Keep your bike in good working order, well oiled with grease and dirt removed from around the chain and gears.

Some people bike for terrific exercise and yet go nowhere. They use a stationary bike. Many health clubs have computerized stationary bikes that can be set for various kinds of riding (for example, hilly or high speed) and for various distances. Still other people remove a wheel from their bicycle, raise the frame, and bike indoors during the winter months. There is equipment you can buy called a wind trainer that does this for you.

When you ride a stationary bike, you need to pay attention to adjusting the seat and handlebars so that they are just right. To work your leg muscles properly, your knee should be slightly bent when the pedal is in the fully down position (see Figure 15.1). Too great a bend or too little a one will result in inefficient use of the leg muscles. The handlebars should be adjusted so you are relaxed and leaning slightly forward (see Figure 15.2).

Select the Right Activity

Even though you find an exercise that is enjoyable and helps you meet your fitness goals, that does not mean you will stay with it. It just means you are *more likely* to maintain your exercise program. It also does not necessarily mean you will even begin the program. One way to exercise even when you are not in the mood or when you doubt its benefits is to employ self-talk. This is when you identify your negative thoughts and convert them to positive ones. Lab Activity 15.2: Developing a New Mind Set about Exercise at the end of this chapter shows you how to use self-talk.

Furthermore, some sports will better match your personality than others. To identify which sports those are, complete Lab Activity 15.3, Which Sports Match Your Personality at the end of this chapter.

BEING A FITNESS CONSUMER

To remain fit your whole life, you need to know how to be an effective fitness consumer. You need to know how to select a health/fitness club, and to buy the right equipment.

Selecting an Exercise Club

Joining a health/fitness club is an excellent strategy for beginning and/or maintaining your exercise pro-

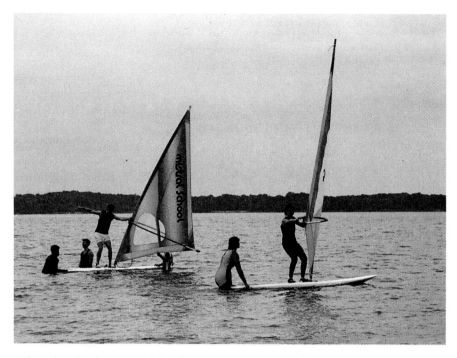

When choosing fitness activities, do not limit yourself by choosing only typical ones. (Photo Courtesy of the Aspen Hill Club.)

gram. The club will encourage your participation in several ways. First, once you shell out the membership fee, you will want to get your money's worth. Second, after working out a few times, you will probably meet other people at the club whom you would like to get to know better. That social contact is reinforcing, and the subtle peer pressure to be there—"Hey, Betty, where were you last Wednesday?"—may be just enough to get you to the club when you do not feel like working out.

Since a health/fitness club can be expensive, inconvenient to get to, or both, you should select the one you join carefully. It should meet your needs, be safe, and be supportive of your exercise goals. Table 15.3 provides you with a way to evaluate a club and decide whether it is right for you.

Purchasing Exercise Equipment

There are some fitness activities that require little, if any, equipment. Just a pair of running shoes, shorts, a

> **Pronate** Rolling the foot inward when it is pushing off.
>
> **Supinate** Rocking the foot to the outside when it is pushing off.

top, and socks is usually enough for jogging. On the other hand, you cannot play tennis without a tennis racket nor bike without a bicycle. In this section, we make brief comments to help you make sensible decisions when you purchase exercise equipment.

Athletic Shoes The major criteria to use when selecting athletic shoes are comfort and support. Here are a few suggestions that will help you purchase the right shoe (and the left one, too, for that matter):

- Recognize whether you **pronate** or **supinate.** Buy a shoe made specifically for either pronators or supinators.

- Shop for shoes late in the day. Your feet tend to swell at that time. No sense buying a shoe that fits snugly in the morning when you usually, or even occasionally, exercise in the afternoon.

- Try shoes on with the kind of socks you usually wear when you are exercising.

- Buy shoes with uppers made of leather or nylon that breathe.

- Look for brands of shoes that come in different widths if you have an exceptionally narrow or wide foot.

- Get a shoe with a last (the form on which the shoe is made) made for your size foot. That means most women ought to buy shoes made

Table 15.3 ✦ Is This the Club for Me?

To decide whether a particular fitness facility is the one you want to join, check as many of the following as apply.

A. The Staff

_____ Do professional staff members have the appropriate educational background and/or certification from a nationally recognized professional organization?

_____ Are all staff members certified in cardiopulmonary resuscitation (CPR)?

_____ Does the specialty staff have the appropriate credentials?

_____ Are adequate staff available in the exercise and activity areas?

_____ Are staff members friendly and helpful?

_____ Are all staff in uniform and wearing some type of identification?

_____ Does the staff provide each new member of the facility with an orientation and instruction to using the areas and equipment in the facility?

_____ Does the staff provide an avenue for ongoing communication between members and themselves?

B. Facility and Equipment

_____ Does the facility have the necessary types and quantity of equipment to enable you to achieve your personal program goals?

_____ Does the facility have the necessary activity areas to enable you to achieve your personal program goals?

_____ Does the facility have sufficient equipment so that enough is available at the time of day you'll be using it?

_____ Are all activity areas regularly cleaned and maintained?

_____ Is all equipment regularly cleaned and maintained?

_____ Are all unsafe conditions and equipment malfunctions remedied promptly?

_____ Is the equipment arranged within an activity area in such a way that maximizes its safety and effectiveness?

_____ Are the surrounding outdoor areas that lead to the facility well illuminated?

_____ Does the facility have adequate parking?

_____ Are childcare facilities available if you need them?

C. Programming

_____ Does the facility offer structured exercise activity programs?

_____ Are the structured exercise programs based on sound principles of exercise prescription and exercise physiology?

_____ Does the facility offer personalized exercise programs tailored specifically to your needs and interests?

_____ Does the facility offer structured exercise programs which address the specific fitness component(s) in which you are interested?

_____ If you have a special medical condition does the facility offer programs which address those needs?

_____ Does the facility offer exercise and recreational programs at convenient times?

_____ Does the facility offer either unstructured or structured recreational programming in an activity in which you are interested?

Table 15.3 ✦ Is This the Club for Me? *(continued)*

_____ Does the facility offer programs for specific age groups, such as children and the elderly?

_____ Does the facility offer instruction in an activity you would like to learn?

_____ Does the facility offer specifically focused health promotion programs?

_____ Does the facility provide the option of evaluating your fitness level before you begin an exercise program?

D. Safety Issues

_____ Does the facility refer at-risk individuals to appropriate medical personnel for clearance?

_____ Does the facility have users complete a risk/benefit disclosure form when they initially join the facility?

_____ Does the facility offer ongoing monitoring of all facility users?

_____ Does the facility have a written emergency plan which is available for review?

_____ Does the facility have a first aid kit that is properly stocked and available at all times?

_____ Are all areas in the facility free from physical hazards?

_____ Are all activity areas in the facility free from environmental hazards?

_____ Is the equipment maintained, suitable for use and well cared for?

_____ Is the staff CPR certified and is at least one first aid certified individual on duty at all times?

E. General Business Practices

_____ Does the facility management provide a grace period in which users can cancel their memberships and receive a full refund on their payments?

_____ Does the facility provide a trial membership or guest pass that allows the prospective user to utilize the facility prior to joining?

_____ Does the facility provide written literature on its facilities, services, programs, and pricing which you can take with you after visiting the club?

_____ Does the facility allow you time to make the decision to purchase a membership?

_____ Does the facility management provide a written set of rules and policies which governs the club's dealings with users?

_____ Does the facility management survey its members periodically to determine their interests and needs?

_____ Does the facility provide a feedback system by which members can express their concerns or needs as they apply to the club?

_____ Does the facility have a system of communication that informs its users of any changes in services, policies, etc. on a periodic basis?

_____ Is the facility a member of a nationally recognized trade organization related to their business?

After completing this checklist, only you can decide if the club is right for you. No club is perfect. Can you live with the club's deficits? Are its benefits worth putting up with its shortcomings?

Source: Reprinted with permission of American College of Sports Medicine, *ACM's Health/Fitness Facilities Consumer Selection Guide.* Indianapolis, IN: American College of Sports Medicine, 1992.

for women, and men shoes made for men because women's and men's lasts differ.

- Shop at a store with experienced salespeople. Discuss your particular concerns with them. For example, if you want a shoe with shock absorption, one that is extra wide, or one that will hold up, the salesperson should be able to recommend a shoe that has the characteristics you are looking for. If you want a shoe for tennis or basketball or some other sport, an experienced salesperson should be able to help with that also.

- When trying the shoes on, perform some of the moves you will when exercising in them. Jump or twist or bend or stretch. Make sure the shoe is comfortable during these movements.

- Once you decide which shoe you want to buy, check the price at different stores or from several athletic shoe distributors. You can do this by telephone quite easily. Also, check the back of sports magazines for distributors who discount the price of shoes.

Orthotics Some people have problems with their feet that need correcting when they are exercising. They may have leg imbalances (one leg longer than the other) or they may pronate or supinate. Orthotic devices can be placed in athletic shoes to correct these problems and allow people to exercise in comfort. They also diminish the risk of injury. Orthotics come in rigid or soft forms. The rigid orthotic, made of plastic, is usually recommended, but a podiatrist or orthopedic physician may have reason to advise a soft one. Ready-made inserts are available in drugstores and sporting goods shops and may be all that is needed in some cases. Since each foot is different from every other foot, however, if you have a problem, it is wise to consult an expert.

Bicycles There are many different kinds of bikes: city bikes, all-terrain mountain bikes, touring bikes, racing bikes, and so forth. An experienced salesperson can guide you to the right type of bike depending on the use you wish to make of it. When you buy a bike (usually somewhere between $300 and $1200) factor in the cost of a helmet, a water bottle, a repair kit for flat tires, shorts, shoes, and gloves. That means approximately another $300. Purchase the bike at a store that offers good service and is staffed by professionals who *really* know bikes. When you think you are interested in a particular bike, test ride it. Also, test ride others for comparison. Try all the gears. Do

they shift easily? Do the brakes work well? How does it corner? Purchasing the right bike is important to the enjoyment you will experience biking, and consequently, to whether you will maintain your exercise program.

Home Exercise Equipment Some people prefer to exercise alone. If you can afford to purchase home-exercise equipment, you might consider buying a stationary bike (maybe one with a built-in computer), a recumbent bicycle (a stationary bike that is low to the floor so your legs are straight out instead of hanging down), a climber (imitating stair climbing), a rower, a cross-country ski machine, a treadmill, and/or

---

Diversity Issues

Health Club Discrimination

When selecting a health and fitness facility, it is important to be aware of any discriminatory policies of the club. Some clubs discriminate by ethnicity, gender, race, and sexual preference.

One national chain recently admitted to discriminatory practices against African-Americans. When they asked about joining, African-Americans were given a hurried tour of the facility, they were not told of the membership discounts available to them, and were told that there was a long waiting list for membership. These factors made it appear as though the facility were overpriced and unavailable, and discouraged African-Americans from joining.

When thinking about joining a health and fitness club, observe the membership for diversity in ethnicity, gender, race, and age. This diversity will make the club a more interesting place in which to exercise. Sameness, while sometimes comforting, may not be as interesting or educational as diversity.

Also observe the staff. Does it include people of different races, genders, cultural backgrounds, and ages?

More and more people are realizing that they can do something about discrimination. After all, clubs need members. If people like you refuse to join because of discriminatory practices, these clubs will soon be out of business unless they change their ways. Becoming aware of these problems can help you become part of the solution! ◆

weights. Since this equipment can be quite expensive, you should be careful to buy exercise equipment that will help you meet your fitness goals safely.

The following should be considered when you are deciding what equipment to purchase.

- **What are your fitness goals?** If you are trying to develop cardiorespiratory endurance, you would be better advised to buy a treadmill or stationary bike than weights.
- **Who is going to use the equipment?** If more than one person will exercise with this equipment, it needs to be easily adjustable.
- **How much space do you have?** You might have room for a stationary bike but not if you are going to add a rower. In this case, you will need to decide which piece of equipment you most want.
- **How much can you spend?** In a perfect world, money would not be of concern, but this is not a perfect world so you will need to decide the best way to spend your limited resources.

Try out the equipment before buying it. Is the seat comfortable? Is the climbing motion smooth? Is the machine sturdy? Is it fun to do? Do you get the type of workout you want?

KEEPING FIT AS YOU AGE

The Andean village of Vilcabamba in Ecuador and the community of Abkhagia in Georgia share an unusual reputation. They are places where people supposedly live longer and remain more vigorous in old age than is the case in most places. What factors contribute to the unusual longevity of people in these communities, where men and women who are well beyond 100 years of age are common? In the United States, the average life expectancy is in the 70s (depending on such factors as gender, ethnicity, education, and socioeconomic status), and there are only slightly more than 3 centenarians per 100,000 persons.

Clearly, genetic factors play a major role. This is true in the communities just cited. Many of the elderly had parents who also lived to be quite old. And yet when researchers studied these communities intensely, they found other factors related to longevity. Elders are held in high esteem. They receive encouragement to work and be productive community members. Their efforts are appreciated and valued. These 100-year-old individuals eat low-calorie diets, about 1800 calories a day compared to the 3300-calorie diet of the average American. These communities are located in remote and mountainous regions and tend to be agricultural. That means that daily living requires significant climbing and descending steep slopes and vigorous physical activity.

Exercise for the Elderly

We are generally less physically active than the centenarians just described. Therefore, we need to plan regular exercise. If we do, we will not only live longer, we will also live better. We will be less ill, less dependent on other people, more pain-free, and more psychologically healthy.

Planning exercise for elderly people requires some special considerations:

- Skeletal structures are more prone to fracture (especially in older women).

Table 15.4 ♦ Good Physical Activities for the Elderly

ACTIVITY	HOW OFTEN	DURATION
Walking	3 times per week	3/4 hour
Swimming	3 times per week	1/2 hour
Dancing	2 times per week	Sets of 20 minutes with intervals of rest
Stretching/Calisthenics	Every day	10–15 minutes
Golf	2 or 3 times per week	As long as necessary to complete 9 or 18 holes
Horseshoe pitching	According to desire	1/2 hour
Shuffleboard	According to desire	1 hour
Bocce	According to desire	1 hour
Croquet	According to desire	1 hour

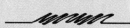

Myth and Fact Sheet

Myth	Fact
1. Jogging is a better physical fitness activity than is walking.	1. Walking is as good an activity to develop physical fitness as any other. You just have to walk for a longer time to get comparable benefits.
2. Jogging leads to all sorts of injuries.	2. You can limit injuries from jogging if you take certain precautions. Wear the appropriate athletic shoes and do not overdo your workout.
3. Rope jumping is for wimps.	3. You can get a great workout while having fun if you know several rope-jumping stunts.
4. Most health/fitness clubs are the same as all others.	4. Health/fitness clubs differ in a number of significant ways. Some clubs do not have enough equipment or enough variety of equipment. Others do not have adequately trained staff, do not offer a safe environment in which to exercise, or cost too much.
5. Elderly people do not need to exercise.	5. Everyone can benefit from regular exercise. Not only can exercise help elderly people maintain their physical fitness, it can also enhance their social, mental, emotional, and spiritual health, thereby helping to maintain their overall wellness.

- Connective tissue is more dense, and ligaments and tendons less elastic. Range of motion may be significantly limited.
- Muscle mass is somewhat diminished, and reaction and reflex times slower.

For these reasons, Careful assessment should be made before prescribing exercise for an elderly individual. Wrenching and twisting movements should be avoided. So should sudden starting and stopping or changing direction. Slow, rhythmic stretching activities are best. And frequent rests should be built into the program.

Walking is an excellent activity for older people, especially in groups where they can socialize. Supervised swimming or exercises in the water are other good activities since they decrease weight bearing and tend to be fun. Also, do not forget dancing, which can enhance fitness goals when it is done rigorously. See Table 15.4 for one possible program for elders.

Benefits of Exercise for Elders

Exercising will increase longevity and provide older people with a more fulfilling life. It can also enhance wellness when exercising with other people (social health), when exercising out of doors and appreciating the surroundings (spiritual health), when exercising with family members and learning to control emotions that interfere with performing the activity (emotional health), and when reading and learning about the particular exercise and its benefits (mental health). In addition, exercise can postpone the inevitable changes associated with aging. Table 15.5 shows which physical activities relate to which of these aging changes.

Table 15.5 ✦ Aging Effects and Physical Activities That May Postpone or Reduce Them

Effects	Physical activities
1. Reduced cardiac output	Aerobic activities, jogging, swimming, cycling
2. Lowered pulmonary ventilation	Exercises that stretch rib cage joints, aerobic activities of moderate-to-high intensity
3. Elevated blood pressure	Aerobic activities, jogging, swimming, cycling
4. Decrease in muscular strength	Weight training (resistance training)
5. Decrease in muscular endurance	Aerobic dance, calisthenics
6. Decrease in flexibility	Stretching, bending
7. Increase in percentage of stored body fat	Jogging, running, swimming, cycling
8. Loss of skin elasticity	Weight training (to maintain muscle tone and fill skin out)

Behavioral Change and Motivational Strategies

There are many things that might interfere with your ability to maintain a lifetime of physical fitness, health, and wellness. Here are some barriers (roadblocks) and strategies for overcoming them.

Roadblock	Behavioral Change Strategy
There will be occasions when you will decide not to work out. Either you will be too busy, too tired, or too interested in doing something else. It is interesting to note that the most effective behavioral-change programs allow for periodic deviation from the goal. That is understandable when you consider a dieter who diets for two months but has an ice cream sundae one weekend. Those who recognize that a deviation is just that, that it need not mean the diet is ruined, are more likely to continue dieting. Those who believe once they go off their diet they have failed are likely to cease dieting after eating the sundae. It is similar with exercise. It is okay to not exercise when you are supposed to, as long as this does not happen frequently. If it happens often, you need to make an adjustment in your exercise program.	Make a list of the benefits and disadvantages of the exercise(s) that make up your routine. List as many benefits and disadvantages as you can, big ones and little ones. Now go over the list and decide: 1. Are the benefits worth the potential disadvantages? 2. Are there other physical activities that can give me similar benefits with fewer disadvantages? Or less important or significant disadvantages? 3. Are there ways I can decrease the barriers to my engaging in a fitness program? For example, can I exercise closer to home (using chaining to my advantage)? Or exercise with a friend (social support)? 4. What changes do you need to make to maintain an exercise regimen?
You have participated in competitive athletics all your life and have maintained a high level of fitness by doing so. Now you are getting older and the competition is potentially harmful. You are getting bumped around too much and getting injured. In addition, winning is not as important to you as it was when you were younger. Now maintaining fitness, health, and wellness are your exercise goals.	You need to find noncompetitive physical activities that can help you achieve your new fitness goals. Ask friends who are noncompetitive what they do for exercise. Use their help (social support). You can also use covert techniques. Imagine yourself participating in noncompetitive activities and reward yourself by thinking of a relaxing image or pleasant thought (covert rehearsal). If that is too much unlike you, imagine someone you know who is not competitive engaging in a noncompetitive physical activity and then substitute yourself for that person (covert modeling).
You dislike exercising but you know it is good for you. You need to find ways to continue your fitness program. You are afraid you will give it up before too long.	You can use self-monitoring by keeping a record of the times you engage in exercise activities. Then boast to friends in a nice way about sticking with your program. You can also make a contract with yourself that if you exercise at least three times a week for at least 20 or 30 minutes each time, you will reward yourself. Think up really rewarding rewards. Rewards that are realistic and feasible as well as worth striving for will be most effective. You may also want to question your choice of exercise activity. Exercise should be fun or else you are likely to discontinue it before too long. What other activities can you substitute for what you have been doing that would be more fun but still help you achieve your fitness goals?

Roadblock	Behavioral Change Strategy
List roadblocks interfering with your maintaining a lifetime of physical fitness, health, and wellness. 1. _____ 2. _____ 3. _____	Cite behavioral-change strategies that can help you overcome the roadblocks you just listed. If you need to, refer back to chapter 3 for behavioral-change and motivational strategies. 1. _____ 2. _____ 3. _____

CONCLUSION: SOME LAST WORDS ON WELLNESS

- To be well, pay attention to your body. If you do, you will know when it is doing fine, and when it needs special care.

- Pay attention to your mind. When you choose an activity to include in your fitness routine, chose one that is enjoyable, one you look forward to doing. Not only will this improve the chances of your continuing the activity, it will also increase your wellness by making you feel good.

- Pay attention to your spirit too. Gain spiritual health from your fitness selections. Feel closer to nature or to a supreme being. Feel connected to your past and your future. To do so is to move toward high-level wellness.

- Be aware of the effects of your fitness choices on your mental and social health. Do your choices add to your knowledge? To your learning? Do they improve your relationships or help you establish new ones?

- Remember that improving one component of your health to the neglect of the others is not being well. Wellness is coordinating and integrating your physical fitness activities with the mental, social, emotional, and spiritual parts of your life.

We can think of no better image to leave you with than that of the Special Olympics—athletic competition for the mentally and physically challenged. These athletes try their best, train long and hard, and feel good about participating and competing. What better example of wellness is there? The learning (mental health) that must precede the competition, the good feelings developed between athletes and their coaches and competitors (social health), the satisfaction derived from trying one's best (emotional health), and the sense of oneness and closeness developed in competition (spiritual health), not to mention the physical fitness level needed to participate in the first place (physical health), provide evidence of the wellness of these competitors. They may not be totally healthy, but they certainly are *well*.

We wish for all of you the same degree of wellness, and we hope this book helps you achieve it.

SUMMARY

Identifying Your Fitness Goals

There are many reasons people engage in physical activity. Some do so for their health, others to look good, or to have energy, and still others to develop strength or because they enjoy the competition. In order to select activities to meet your fitness goals, you need to identify why you want to become fit.

Fitness Activities to Help You Achieve Your Goals

There are many physical activities that can contribute to the development of physical fitness; among these activities are walking, jogging, running, rope jumping, swimming, tennis, racketball, handball, squash, aerobic dance, low-impact aerobics, and bicycling. Some of these help develop cardiorespiratory endurance; others, muscular strength or muscular endurance; and still others, other components of physical fitness. In choosing an activity in which to engage regularly, make sure it matches your personality. You may be sociable, spontaneous, disciplined, aggressive, competitive, able to concentrate well, a risk-taker, or a combination of two or more of these traits. Since people's personalities differ, their choices of exercise will differ.

Being a Fitness Consumer

When you are deciding whether a health/fitness club is right for you, determine if the facility and the equipment are such that they can be used to achieve your fitness goals. The staff should be well trained and the equipment abundant enough so you will not have to wait too long to use it. Safety procedures should be in place so your chances of being injured are minimized. And the club should be easily accessible to you (with adequate parking, not too far from where you live or work, and with a membership fee within your budget).

Purchasing athletic equipment should be done thoughtfully so you do not waste your money. When buying athletic shoes, choose shoes that are comfortable and consistent with any foot problems you may have (for example, if you pronate or supinate). If orthotics are needed because of a foot abnormality, a podiatrist should be consulted, although, in some cases, ready-made shoe inserts are all that is needed. There are many different kinds of home exercise equipment you can purchase. These include stationary bikes, climbers, rowers, cross-country ski machines, treadmills, and weights. In deciding what home exercise equipment to purchase, you should determine your fitness goals, who is going to use the equipment, the space you have available to house the equipment, and how much you have to spend.

Keeping Fit as You Age

Exercise can help you live longer and live better. It also staves off some of the effects of aging. For example, it can help with reduced cardiac output, lowered pulmonary ventilation, elevated blood pressure, a decrease in muscular strength and endurance, a decrease in flexibility, an increase in body fat, and a loss of skin elasticity. Furthermore, exercise is an excellent way for elders to enhance their overall wellness.

REFERENCES

Katz, Jane. "The W.E.T. Workout." *Shape* (June 1986): 82–88.

President's Council on Physical Fitness and Sports, *Aqua Dynamics.*

Road Runners Club of America, *Women Running: Run Smart. Run Safe.* Used with permission.

Winters, Catherine. "For Step Aerobic Addicts, a Challenging New Workout: Doing the Two-Step." *American Health* (May 1993): 92.

Lab Activity 15.1

Why I Want to Be Physically Fit

INSTRUCTIONS: *There are many reasons why people engage in physical activity in an effort to become physically fit. If you know why you exercise, you will be able to choose activities that help you achieve your goals. To determine the reason(s) why you exercise, rank order the statements below.*

✦ **I Exercise Because**

_____ I want to lose or maintain my weight.

_____ I want to look good.

_____ I want to have a healthy heart and lungs.

_____ I want to be strong.

_____ I want to make new friends or socialize with my present friends.

_____ I want to channel my aggression positively.

_____ I like competition.

_____ I like to be out in natural surroundings.

_____ I want to develop enough energy not to be tired during the day.

_____ I want to be flexible.

_____ I want to have fun.

✦ **Interpretation of Results**

Consult Table 4.2 on page 66 to match the reasons you exercise with the benefits of the various physical activities. For example, if you exercise to lose weight, consider activities such as aerobic dance, basketball, or bicycling. If you exercise to make friends, play softball or volleyball.

If you exercise to look good, weight train. Matching your fitness goals with activities that can help you achieve those goals is the best way of assuring you will maintain your exercise program. Conversely, if you exercise regularly but do not achieve your goals because you have chosen the wrong physical activities, you will probably not continue with your program.

Mix and match activities so you achieve more than one of your goals. That way you will further increase the probability that you will become a lifetime participant in physical fitness activities.

Lab Activity 15.2

Developing a New Mind Set about Exercise

INSTRUCTIONS: *When people try to develop a new habit, they are often plagued by thoughts of failure. During the early stages of your new exercise program, you can become your own worst enemy. Examine the list of excuses. Do any of these look familiar to you? Take a minute to prepare your own list of self-defeating thoughts about exercise. Prepare a list of positive thoughts, too.*

Learn to use these lists wisely. When self-defeating thoughts enter your mind, counteract them immediately with positive ones. Write your list of positive thoughts on a card, and carry it in your wallet or purse so you can refer to it when you are about to avoid a scheduled exercise session. List both long-term benefits (such as more energy, weight loss, and prevention of disease) and more immediate benefits (such as using up calories and feeling good).

Negative Thought about Exercise

1. I'm too busy to exercise today. I'm working too hard anyway and need a break.

2. I'm too tired to exercise today, and if I do work out, I won't have enough energy to do other things I must do.

3. I missed my workout today. I might as well forget all this fitness stuff. I do not have the self-control to keep at it.

4. None of my friends are fit or trim and they don't worry about it. I am not going to worry either.

5. I am already over the hill. I should just let myself go and enjoy life more.

Positive Thoughts about Exercise

1. I can find time to exercise today. I just have to think about my routine and plan carefully.

2. I may feel tired today, but I will do a light exercise routine instead of the heavy one I usually do. If I keep working out on a regular basis, I will build my stamina so I will not feel so tired during the day.

3. Just because I missed one exercise session does not mean that I should give up. I'm not going to let this small setback ruin everything I've accomplished.

4. What my friends do about exercising has nothing to do with my exercise habits. I'll make additional friends who do exercise.

5. I can get in shape and stay there. All I have to do is stick to my schedule. Knowing I can control my behavior is something I can enjoy every day.

Negative Thought about Exercise

1. _____

2. _____

3. _____

4. _____

Positive Thoughts about Exercise

1. _____

2. _____

3. _____

4. _____

Source: Jerrold S. Greenberg and George B. Dintiman, *Exploring Health: Expanding the Boundaries of Wellness.* Englewood Cliffs, NJ: Prentice Hall, 1992, p. 225.

Lab Activity 15.3

Which Sports Match Your Personality?

INSTRUCTIONS: *Fitness experts tell us that if you match your personality with your choice of exercise, the chances are you will stay with your program. Here is a way to do that. Read the description of each psychosocial personality variable, and then rate yourself on the scorecard that follows.*

Sociability: Do you prefer doing things on your own or with other people? Do you make friends easily? Do you enjoy parties?

Spontaneity: Do you make spur-of-the-moment decisions, or do you plan in great detail? Can you change direction easily, or do you get locked in once you make up your mind?

Discipline: Do you have trouble sticking with things you find unpleasant or trying, or do you persist regardless of the obstacles? Do you need a lot of support, or do you just push on alone?

Aggressiveness: Do you try to control situations by being forceful? Do you like pitting yourself against obstacles, or do you shy away when you must assert yourself physically or emotionally?

Competitiveness: Are you bothered by situations that produce winners and losers? Does your adrenaline flow when you're challenged, or do you back off?

Mental Focus: Do you find it easy to concentrate, or do you have a short attention span? Can you be single-minded? How good are you at clearing your mind of distractions?

Risk-Taking: Are you generally adventurous, physically and emotionally, or do you prefer to stick to what you know?

Scorecard				
Fill in the appropriate circles and connect them with a line.				
Very High ◄――――► Very Low				
Sociability	O O O O O			
Spontaneity	O O O O O			
Discipline	O O O O O			
Aggressiveness	O O O O O			
Competitiveness	O O O O O			
Mental Focus	O O O O O			
Risk-taking	O O O O O			

Walking

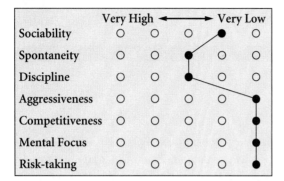

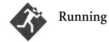 **Running**

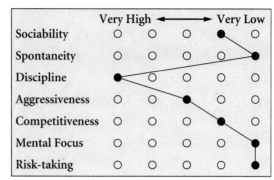

 Cycling

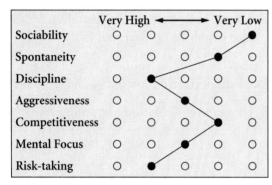

 Weight Training

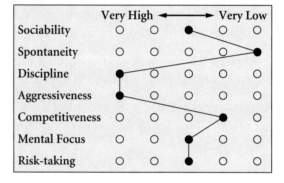

✦ Understanding Your Score

To see how well your profile matches your sport or exercise activity, look at the four sample profiles in this lab activity. If you have the typical personality of a runner, walker, cyclist, or bodybuilder, your profile should look similar to one of these profiles. If your athletic preference lies elsewhere, turn to the "Your Personality/Your Sport" chart to see where your activities rank on each characteristic. Then compare these rankings with how you scored yourself.

Compared to running, for example, walking is more spontaneous and less aggressive. (It is also safer, in terms of physical stress.) Racquet sports are high in sociability, spontaneity, competitiveness, and focus but low in discipline. Swimming is fairly high in discipline and low in sociability, spontaneity, and aggressiveness.

If you've been having trouble sticking to a fitness program, these charts may help explain why. If you're still looking for a sport, use your findings as a guide.

Source: James Gavin, "Your Brand of Sweat," *Psychology Today,* March 1989, pp. 50–57. Reprinted with permission from *Psychology Today* magazine, copyright © 1989 (Sussex Publishers, Inc.).

Your Personality/Your Sport

Higher ←——— ———→ Lower

SOCIABILITY
Running · Weight Training · Tennis · Golf · Tennis · Martial Arts · Downhill Skiing · Aerobics · Dance · Weight Training · Cross-country Skiing | Walking · Running · Cycling · Yoga · Swimming

SPONTANEITY
Weight Training · Cycling · Tennis · Martial Arts · Dance · Aerobics · Walking · Cross-country Skiing | Swimming · Yoga · Running · Golf

DISCIPLINE
Tennis · Swimming · Yoga · Aerobics · Walking · Dance · Cross-country Skiing · Weight Training | Golf · Downhill Skiing

AGGRESSIVENESS
Tennis · Martial Arts · Weight Training · Tennis · Downhill Skiing · Golf · Cycling · Running · Cross-country Skiing | Aerobics · Dance · Swimming · Walking · Yoga

COMPETITIVENESS
Tennis · Golf · Downhill Skiing · Martial Arts · Dance · Running · Weight Training · Cycling · Cross-country Skiing | Swimming · Aerobics · Walking · Yoga

MENTAL FOCUS
Tennis · Golf · Downhill Skiing · Yoga · Weight Training · Cycling · Aerobics · Cross-country Skiing · Swimming | Swimming · Aerobics · Walking

RISK-TAKING
Dance · Golf · Tennis · Martial Arts · Downhill Skiing · Golf · Cycling · Weight Training · Dance · Cross-country Skiing | Running · Walking · Aerobics · Swimming · Yoga · Running · Walking

355

Caloric Expenditure per Minute for Various Activities

BODY WEIGHT

	90	99	108	117	125	134	143	152	161	170	178	187	196	205	213	222	231	240	249	257	266	275
Archery	3.1	3.4	3.7	4.0	4.5	4.6	4.9	5.2	5.5	5.8	6.1	6.4	6.7	7.0	7.3	7.6	7.9	8.2	8.5	8.5	9.1	9.4
Badminton (recreation)	3.4	3.8	4.1	4.4	4.8	5.1	5.4	5.6	6.1	6.4	6.8	7.1	7.4	7.8	8.1	8.3	8.8	9.1	9.4	9.8	10.1	10.4
Badminton (competition)	5.9	6.4	7.0	7.6	8.1	8.7	9.3	9.9	10.4	11.0	11.6	12.1	12.7	13.3	13.9	14.4	15.0	15.6	16.1	16.7	17.3	17.9
Baseball (player)	2.8	3.1	3.4	3.6	3.9	4.2	4.5	4.7	5.0	5.3	5.5	5.8	6.1	6.4	6.6	6.9	7.2	7.5	7.7	8.0	8.3	8.6
Baseball (pitcher)	3.5	3.9	4.3	4.6	5.0	5.3	5.7	6.0	6.4	6.7	7.1	7.4	7.8	8.1	8.5	8.8	9.2	9.5	9.9	10.2	10.6	10.9
Basketball (half-court)	2.5	3.3	3.5	3.8	4.1	4.4	4.7	4.9	5.3	5.6	5.9	6.2	6.4	6.7	7.0	7.3	7.5	7.6	8.2	8.5	8.8	9.0
Basketball (moderate)	4.2	4.6	5.0	5.5	5.9	6.3	6.7	7.1	7.5	7.9	8.3	8.8	9.2	9.6	10.0	10.4	10.8	11.2	11.6	12.1	12.5	12.9
Basketball (competition)	5.9	6.5	7.1	7.7	8.2	8.8	9.4	10.0	10.6	11.1	11.7	12.3	12.9	13.5	14.0	14.6	15.0	15.2	16.3	16.9	17.5	18.1
Bicycling (level) 5.5 mph	3.0	3.3	3.6	3.9	4.2	4.5	4.8	5.1	5.4	5.6	5.9	6.2	6.5	6.8	7.1	7.4	7.7	8.0	8.3	8.6	8.9	9.2
Bicycling (level) 13 mph	6.4	7.1	7.7	8.3	8.9	9.6	10.2	10.8	11.4	12.1	12.7	13.4	14.0	14.6	15.2	15.9	16.5	17.1	17.8	18.4	19.0	19.6
Bowling (nonstop)	4.0	4.4	4.8	5.2	5.6	5.9	6.3	6.7	7.1	7.5	7.9	8.3	8.7	9.1	9.5	9.8	10.2	10.6	11.0	11.4	11.8	12.2
Boxing (sparring)	3.0	3.3	3.6	3.9	4.2	4.5	4.8	5.1	5.4	5.6	5.9	6.2	6.5	6.8	7.1	7.4	7.7	8.0	8.3	8.6	8.9	9.2
Calisthenics	3.0	3.3	3.6	3.9	4.2	4.5	4.8	5.1	5.4	5.6	5.9	6.2	6.5	6.8	7.1	7.4	7.7	8.0	8.3	8.6	8.9	9.2
Canoeing, 2.5 mph	1.8	1.9	2.0	2.2	2.3	2.5	2.7	3.0	3.2	3.4	3.6	3.7	3.9	4.1	4.7	4.4	4.6	4.8	5.0	5.1	5.3	5.5
Canoeing, 4.0 mph	4.2	4.6	5.0	5.5	5.9	6.3	6.7	7.1	7.5	7.9	8.3	8.7	9.2	9.4	10.0	10.5	10.8	11.2	11.6	12.0	12.4	12.9
Dance, modern (moderate)	2.5	2.8	3.0	3.2	3.5	3.7	4.0	4.2	4.5	4.7	5.0	5.2	5.4	5.7	5.9	6.2	6.4	6.7	6.9	7.2	7.4	7.6
Dance, modern (vigorous)	3.4	3.7	4.1	4.4	4.7	5.1	5.4	5.7	6.1	6.4	6.7	7.1	7.4	7.7	8.1	8.4	8.7	9.1	9.4	9.7	10.1	10.4
Dance, fox-trot	2.7	2.9	3.2	3.4	3.7	4.0	4.2	4.5	4.7	5.0	5.3	5.5	5.8	6.0	6.3	6.6	6.8	7.1	7.3	7.6	7.9	8.1
Dance, rumba	4.2	4.6	5.0	5.4	5.8	6.2	6.6	7.0	7.4	7.8	8.2	8.6	9.0	9.4	9.8	10.2	10.6	11.0	11.5	11.9	12.3	12.6
Dance, square	4.1	4.5	4.9	5.3	5.7	6.1	6.5	6.9	7.3	7.8	8.1	8.5	8.9	9.3	9.7	10.1	10.5	10.9	11.3	11.7	12.1	12.4
Dance, waltz	3.1	3.4	3.7	4.0	4.3	4.6	4.9	5.2	5.5	5.8	6.1	6.4	6.7	7.0	7.3	7.6	7.9	8.2	8.5	8.8	9.1	9.4
Fencing (moderate)	3.0	3.3	3.6	3.9	4.2	4.5	4.8	5.1	5.4	5.6	6.0	6.2	6.5	6.8	7.1	7.4	7.7	8.0	8.3	8.6	8.9	9.2
Fencing (vigorous)	6.2	6.8	7.4	8.0	8.6	9.2	9.8	8.7	11.0	11.6	12.2	12.8	13.4	14.0	14.6	15.2	15.8	16.4	17.0	17.6	18.2	18.8
Football (moderate)	3.0	3.3	3.6	4.0	4.2	4.5	4.8	5.1	5.4	5.7	6.0	6.2	6.5	6.8	7.1	7.4	7.7	8.0	8.3	8.6	8.9	9.2
Football (vigorous)	5.0	5.5	6.0	6.4	6.9	7.4	7.9	8.4	8.9	9.4	9.8	10.3	10.8	11.3	11.8	12.3	12.8	13.2	13.7	14.2	14.7	15.2
Golf, twosome	3.3	3.6	3.9	4.2	4.5	4.8	5.2	5.5	5.8	6.1	6.4	6.7	7.1	7.4	7.7	8.0	8.3	8.6	9.0	9.3	9.6	10.0
Golf, foursome	2.4	2.7	2.9	3.2	3.4	3.6	3.9	4.1	4.3	4.6	4.8	5.1	5.3	5.5	5.8	6.0	6.2	6.5	6.7	7.0	7.2	7.4
Handball	5.9	6.4	7.0	7.6	8.1	8.7	9.3	9.9	10.4	11.0	11.6	12.1	12.7	13.3	13.9	14.4	15.0	15.6	16.1	16.7	17.3	17.9
Hiking, 40-lb pack, 3.0 mph	4.1	4.5	4.9	5.3	5.7	6.1	6.5	6.9	7.3	7.7	8.1	8.5	8.9	9.3	9.7	10.1	10.5	10.9	11.3	11.7	12.1	12.5
Horseback riding (walk)	2.0	2.3	2.4	2.6	2.8	3.0	3.1	3.3	3.5	3.7	3.9	4.1	4.3	4.5	4.7	4.9	5.1	5.3	5.5	5.7	5.8	6.0
Horseback riding (trot)	4.1	4.4	4.8	5.2	5.6	6.0	6.4	6.8	7.2	7.6	8.0	8.4	8.8	9.2	9.6	10.0	10.4	10.8	11.2	11.6	12.0	12.4
Horseshoe pitching	2.1	2.3	2.5	2.7	3.0	3.3	3.4	3.6	3.8	4.0	4.2	4.4	4.6	4.8	5.0	5.2	5.4	5.6	5.8	6.0	6.3	6.5
Judo, Karate	7.7	8.5	9.2	10.0	10.7	11.5	12.2	13.0	13.7	14.5	15.2	16.0	16.7	17.5	18.2	19.0	19.7	20.5	21.2	22.0	22.7	23.5

BODY WEIGHT

Activity	90	99	108	117	125	134	143	152	161	170	178	187	196	205	213	222	231	240	249	257	266	275
Mountain climbing	6.0	6.5	7.2	7.8	8.4	9.0	9.6	10.1	10.7	11.3	11.9	12.5	13.1	13.7	14.3	14.8	15.4	16.0	16.6	17.2	17.8	18.4
Paddleball, racquetball	5.9	6.4	7.0	7.6	8.1	8.7	9.3	9.9	10.4	11.0	11.6	12.1	12.7	13.3	13.9	14.4	15.0	15.6	16.1	16.7	17.3	17.9
Pool, billiards	1.1	1.2	1.3	1.4	1.5	1.6	1.7	1.8	1.9	2.0	2.1	2.2	2.4	2.5	2.6	2.7	2.8	2.9	3.0	3.1	3.2	3.3
Push ups	4.3	4.7	5.1	5.6	6.0	6.4	6.8	7.2	7.7	8.1	8.5	8.9	9.4	9.8	10.2	10.6	11.0	11.5	11.9	12.3	12.7	13.2
Racquetball	6.0	6.6	7.2	7.8	8.3	8.9	9.5	10.1	10.7	11.3	11.9	12.5	13.1	13.7	14.2	14.8	15.4	16.0	16.6	17.2	17.8	18.4
Rowing (recreation)	3.0	3.3	3.6	3.9	4.2	4.5	4.8	5.1	5.4	5.6	6.0	6.2	6.5	6.8	7.1	7.5	7.7	8.0	8.3	8.6	8.9	9.2
Rowing (machine)	8.2	9.0	9.8	10.6	11.4	12.2	13.0	13.8	14.6	15.4	16.2	17.0	17.8	18.6	19.4	20.2	21.0	21.8	22.6	23.4	24.2	25.0
Running, 11-min mile, 5.5 mph	6.4	7.1	7.7	8.3	9.0	9.6	10.2	10.8	11.5	12.1	12.7	13.4	14.0	14.6	15.2	15.9	16.5	17.1	17.8	18.4	19.0	19.6
Running, 8.5-min mile, 7 mph	8.4	9.2	10.0	10.8	11.7	12.5	13.3	14.1	14.9	15.7	16.6	17.4	18.2	19.0	19.8	20.7	21.5	22.3	23.1	23.9	24.8	25.6
Running, 7-min mile, 9 mph	9.3	10.2	11.1	12.0	12.9	13.9	14.8	15.7	16.6	17.5	18.4	19.3	20.2	21.1	22.1	23.0	23.9	24.8	25.7	26.6	27.5	28.4
Running, 5-min mile, 12 mph	11.8	13.0	14.1	15.3	16.4	17.6	18.7	19.9	21.0	22.2	23.3	24.5	25.6	26.8	27.9	29.1	30.2	31.4	32.5	33.7	34.9	36.0
Sailing	1.8	2.0	2.1	2.3	2.4	2.7	2.8	3.0	3.2	3.4	3.6	3.8	3.9	4.1	4.3	4.4	4.6	4.8	5.0	5.1	5.3	5.5
Sit ups	4.3	4.7	5.1	5.6	6.0	6.4	6.8	7.2	7.7	8.1	8.5	8.9	9.4	9.8	10.2	10.6	11.0	11.5	11.9	12.3	12.7	13.2
Sprinting	13.8	15.2	16.6	17.9	19.2	20.5	21.9	23.3	24.7	26.1	27.3	28.7	30.0	31.4	32.7	34.0	35.4	36.8	38.1	39.4	40.3	42.2
Skating (moderate)	3.4	3.8	4.1	4.4	4.8	5.1	5.4	5.8	6.1	6.4	6.8	7.1	7.4	7.8	8.1	8.3	8.8	9.1	9.4	9.8	10.1	10.4
Skating (vigorous)	6.2	6.8	7.4	8.0	8.6	9.2	9.8	10.4	11.0	11.6	12.2	12.8	13.4	14.0	14.6	15.2	15.8	16.4	17.0	17.6	18.2	18.8
Skiing (downhill)	5.8	6.4	6.9	7.5	8.1	8.6	9.2	9.8	10.3	10.9	11.4	12.0	12.6	13.1	13.7	14.3	14.8	15.4	16.0	16.5	17.1	17.7
Skiing (level, 5 mph)	7.0	7.7	8.4	9.1	9.8	10.5	11.1	11.8	12.5	13.2	13.9	14.6	15.2	15.9	16.6	17.3	18.0	18.7	19.4	20.0	20.7	21.4
Skiing (racing downhill)	9.9	10.9	11.9	12.9	13.7	14.7	15.7	16.7	17.7	18.7	19.6	20.6	21.6	22.6	23.4	24.4	25.4	26.4	27.4	28.3	29.3	30.2
Snowshoeing (2.3 mph)	3.7	4.1	4.5	4.8	5.2	5.5	5.9	6.3	6.7	7.0	7.4	7.8	8.1	8.5	8.8	9.2	9.6	9.9	10.3	10.6	11.0	11.4
Snowshoeing (2.5 mph)	5.4	5.9	6.5	7.0	7.5	8.0	8.6	9.1	9.7	10.2	10.7	11.2	11.8	12.3	12.8	13.3	13.9	14.4	14.9	15.4	16.0	16.5
Soccer	5.4	5.9	6.4	6.9	7.5	8.0	8.5	9.0	9.6	10.1	10.6	11.1	11.6	12.2	12.7	13.2	13.7	14.3	14.8	15.3	15.8	16.3
Squash	6.2	6.8	7.5	8.1	8.7	9.3	9.9	10.5	11.1	11.7	12.3	12.9	13.5	14.2	14.8	15.4	16.0	16.6	17.2	17.8	18.4	19.0
Stationary running, 140 counts/min	14.6	16.1	17.5	18.9	20.4	21.8	23.2	24.6	26.1	27.5	28.9	30.4	31.8	33.2	34.6	36.1	37.5	38.9	40.4	41.8	43.2	44.6
Swimming, pleasure 25 yds/min	3.6	4.0	4.3	4.7	5.0	5.4	5.7	6.1	6.4	6.8	7.1	7.5	7.8	8.2	8.5	8.9	9.2	9.6	10.0	10.3	10.6	11.0
Swimming, back, 20 yd/min	2.3	2.6	2.8	3.0	3.2	3.5	3.7	3.9	4.1	4.2	4.6	4.8	5.0	5.3	5.5	5.7	6.0	6.2	6.4	6.6	6.9	7.1
Swimming, back, 30 yd/min	3.2	3.5	3.8	4.1	4.4	4.7	5.1	5.4	5.7	6.0	6.3	6.6	6.9	7.2	7.4	7.9	8.2	8.5	8.8	9.1	9.4	9.7
Swimming, back, 40 yd/min	5.0	5.5	5.8	6.5	7.0	7.5	7.9	8.5	8.9	9.4	9.9	10.4	10.9	11.4	11.9	12.3	12.8	13.3	13.8	14.3	14.8	15.3
Swimming, breast, 20 yd/min	2.9	3.2	3.4	3.8	4.0	4.3	4.6	4.9	5.1	5.4	5.7	6.0	6.3	6.5	6.8	7.1	7.4	7.7	7.9	8.2	8.5	8.8
Swimming, breast, 30 yd/min	4.3	4.8	5.2	5.7	6.0	6.4	6.9	7.3	7.7	8.1	8.6	9.0	9.4	9.9	10.3	10.8	11.1	11.5	11.9	12.4	13.0	13.3
Swimming, breast, 40 yd/min	5.8	6.3	6.9	7.5	8.0	8.6	9.2	9.7	10.3	10.8	11.4	12.0	12.5	13.1	13.7	14.2	14.8	15.4	15.9	16.5	17.0	17.6

BODY WEIGHT

	90	99	108	117	125	134	143	152	161	170	178	187	196	205	213	222	231	240	249	257	266	275
Swimming, butterfly, 50 yds/min	7.0	7.7	8.4	9.1	9.8	10.5	11.1	11.9	12.5	13.2	13.9	14.6	15.2	15.9	16.6	17.3	18.0	18.7	19.4	20.0	20.7	21.4
Swimmng, crawl, 20 yd/min	2.9	3.2	3.4	3.8	4.0	4.3	4.6	4.9	5.1	5.4	5.7	5.8	6.3	6.5	6.8	7.1	7.3	7.7	7.9	8.2	8.5	8.8
Swimming, crawl, 45 yd/min	5.2	5.8	6.3	6.8	7.3	7.8	8.3	8.8	9.3	9.8	10.4	10.9	11.4	11.9	12.4	12.9	13.4	13.9	14.4	15.0	15.5	16.0
Swimming, crawl, 50 yd/min	6.4	7.0	7.6	8.3	8.9	9.5	10.1	10.7	11.4	12.0	12.6	13.2	13.9	14.5	15.1	15.7	16.3	17.0	17.4	17.9	18.8	19.5
Table tennis	2.3	2.6	2.8	3.0	3.2	3.5	3.7	3.9	4.1	4.2	4.6	4.8	5.0	5.3	5.5	5.7	6.0	6.2	6.4	6.6	6.9	7.1
Tennis (recreation)	4.2	4.6	5.0	5.4	5.8	6.2	6.6	7.0	7.4	7.8	8.2	8.6	9.0	9.4	9.8	10.2	10.6	11.0	11.5	11.9	12.3	12.6
Tennis (competition)	5.9	6.4	7.0	7.6	8.1	8.7	9.3	9.9	10.4	11.0	11.6	12.1	12.7	13.3	13.9	14.4	15.0	15.6	16.1	16.7	17.3	17.9
Timed calisthenics	8.8	9.6	10.5	11.4	12.2	13.1	13.9	14.8	15.6	16.5	17.4	18.2	19.1	19.9	20.8	21.5	22.5	23.9	24.2	25.1	25.9	26.8
Volleyball (moderate)	3.4	3.8	4.0	4.4	4.8	5.1	5.4	5.8	6.1	6.4	6.8	7.1	7.4	7.8	8.1	8.3	8.8	9.1	9.4	9.8	10.1	10.4
Volleyball (vigorous)	5.9	6.4	7.0	7.6	8.1	8.7	9.3	9.9	10.4	11.0	11.6	12.1	12.7	13.3	13.9	14.4	15.0	15.6	16.1	16.7	17.3	17.9
Walking (2.0 mph)	2.1	2.3	2.5	2.7	2.9	3.1	3.3	3.5	3.7	4.0	4.2	4.4	4.6	4.8	5.0	5.2	5.4	5.6	5.8	6.0	6.2	6.4
Walking (4.5 mph)	4.0	4.4	4.7	5.1	5.5	5.9	6.3	6.7	7.1	7.5	7.8	8.2	8.6	9.0	9.4	9.8	10.1	10.6	10.9	11.3	11.7	12.0
Walking 110–120 steps/min	3.1	3.4	3.7	4.0	4.3	4.7	5.0	5.3	5.6	5.9	6.2	6.5	6.8	7.1	7.4	7.7	8.0	8.3	8.6	8.9	9.2	9.5
Waterskiing	4.7	5.1	5.6	6.1	6.5	7.0	7.4	7.9	8.3	8.8	9.3	9.7	10.2	10.6	11.1	11.5	12.0	12.5	12.9	13.4	13.8	14.3
Weight training	4.7	5.1	5.7	6.2	6.7	7.0	7.5	7.9	8.4	8.9	9.4	9.9	10.3	10.8	11.1	11.7	12.2	12.6	13.1	13.5	14.0	14.4
Wrestling	7.7	8.5	9.2	10.0	10.7	11.5	12.2	13.0	13.7	14.5	15.2	16.0	16.7	17.5	18.2	19.0	19.7	20.5	21.2	22.0	22.7	23.5

From Consolazio, Johnson and Pecora, *Physiological Measurements of Metabolic Functions in Man*, McGraw-Hill.

Nutritional Information for Selected Foods

Food item	Serving size	Grams	Calories	Protein (g)	Carbohydrate (g)	Fat (g)	Cholesterol (mg)	Sodium (mg)
Beverages								
Alcoholic								
Beer								
Regular	12 fl oz	360	150	1	13	0	0	18
Light	12 fl oz	355	95	1	5	0	0	11
Gin, rum, vodka, whiskey								
80-proof	1½ fl oz	42	95	0	Tr	0	0	Tr
86-proof	1½ fl oz	42	105	0	Tr	0	0	Tr
90-proof	1½ fl oz	42	110	0	Tr	0	0	Tr
Wines								
Dessert	3½ fl oz	103	140	Tr	8	0	0	9
Table								
Red	3½ fl oz	102	75	Tr	3	0	0	5
White	3½ fl oz	102	80	Tr	3	0	0	5
Carbonated								
Club soda	12 fl oz	355	0	0	0	0	0	78
Cola type								
Regular	12 fl oz	369	160	0	41	0	0	18
Diet, artificially sweetened	12 fl oz	355	Tr	0	Tr	0	0	32[a]
Ginger ale	12 fl oz	366	125	0	32	0	0	29
Grape	12 fl oz	372	180	0	46	0	0	48
Lemon-lime	12 fl oz	372	155	0	39	0	0	33
Orange	12 fl oz	372	180	0	46	0	0	52
Pepper type	12 fl oz	369	160	0	41	0	0	37
Root beer	12 fl oz	370	165	0	42	0	0	48
Fruit drinks, noncarbonated								
Canned								
Fruit punch drink	6 fl oz	190	85	Tr	22	0	0	15
Grape drink	6 fl oz	187	100	Tr	26	0	0	11
Pineapple-grapefruit juice drink	6 fl oz	187	90	Tr	23	Tr	0	24
Frozen lemonade concentrate, diluted with 4⅓ parts water by volume	6 fl oz	185	80	Tr	21	Tr	0	1

Tr = trace amount.

[a]Blend of aspartame and saccharin; if only saccharin is used, sodium is 75 mg; if only aspartame is used, sodium is 23 mg.

Information summarized from *Nutritive Value of Foods,* Superintendent of Documents, US Government Printing Office, Washington, DC, Revised 1981.

FOOD ITEM	SERVING SIZE	GRAMS	CALORIES	PROTEIN (G)	CARBOHYDRATE (G)	FAT (G)	CHOLESTEROL (MG)	SODIUM (MG)
Dairy products								
Butter. See **Fats and Oils**								
Cheese								
Cheddar								
Cut pieces	1 oz	28	115	7	Tr	9	30	176
	1 in	17	70	4	Tr	6	18	105
Shredded	1 cup	113	455	28	1	37	119	701
Creamed (cottage cheese, 4% fat):								
Large curd	1 cup	225	235	28	6	10	34	911
Small curd	1 cup	210	215	26	6	9	31	850
With fruit	1 cup	226	280	22	30	8	25	915
Lowfat (2%)	1 cup	226	205	31	8	4	19	918
Cream	1 oz	28	100	2	1	10	31	84
Feta	1 oz	28	75	4	1	6	25	316
Mozzarella, made with								
Whole milk	1 oz	28	80	6	1	6	22	106
Part skim milk (low moisture)	1 oz	28	80	8	1	5	15	150
Muenster	1 oz	28	105	7	Tr	9	27	178
Parmesan, grated	1 oz	28	130	12	1	9	22	528
Provolone	1 oz	28	100	7	1	8	20	248
Swiss	1 oz	28	105	8	1	8	26	74
Pasteurized process cheese								
American	1 oz	28	105	6	Tr	9	27	406
Swiss	1 oz	28	95	7	1	7	24	388
Pasteurized process cheese food, American	1 oz	28	95	6	2	7	18	337
Pasteurized process cheese spread, American	1 oz	28	80	5	2	6	16	381
Cream, sweet								
Half-and-half (cream and milk)	1 cup	242	315	7	10	28	89	98
	1 tbsp	15	20	Tr	1	2	6	6
Light, coffee or table	1 cup	240	470	6	9	46	159	95
	1 tbsp	15	30	Tr	1	3	10	6
Cream, sour	1 cup	230	495	7	10	48	102	123
	1 tbsp	12	25	Tr	1	3	5	6
Ice cream. See **Milk desserts, frozen**								
Milk								
Whole (3.3% fat)	1 cup	244	150	8	11	8	33	370
Low-fat (2% fat)	1 cup	244	120	8	12	5	18	377
Low-fat (1% fat)	1 cup	244	100	8	12	3	10	381
Nonfat (skim)	1 cup	245	85	8	12	Tr	4	406

FOOD ITEM	SERVING SIZE	GRAMS	CALORIES	PROTEIN (G)	CARBOHYDRATE (G)	FAT (G)	CHOLESTEROL (MG)	SODIUM (MG)
Dairy products *(continued)*								
Chocolate milk (commercial)								
Regular	1 cup	250	210	8	26	8	31	149
Low-fat (2% fat)	1 cup	250	180	8	26	5	17	151
Low-fat (1% fat)	1 cup	250	160	8	26	3	7	152
Milk beverages								
Cocoa and chocolate-flavored beverages								
Prepared (8-oz whole milk plus ¾-oz powder)	1 serving	265	225	9	30	9	33	176
Eggnog (commercial)	1 cup	254	340	10	34	19	149	138
Malted milk, chocolate	¾ oz	21	85		18	1	1	49
Prepared (8 oz whole milk plus ¾-oz powder)	1 serving	265	235	9	29	9	34	168
Shakes, thick								
Chocolate	10-oz container	283	335	9	60	8	30	314
Vanilla	10-oz container	283	315	11	50	9	33	270
Milk desserts, frozen								
Ice cream, vanilla								
Regular (about 11% fat)	1 cup	133	270	5	32	14	59	116
Yogurt								
Made with low-fat milk								
Fruit-flavored[b]	8-oz container	227	230	10	43	2	10	133
Plain	8-oz container	227	145	12	16	4	14	159
Made with nonfat milk	8-oz container	227	125	13	17	Tr	4	174
Made with whole milk	8-oz container	227	140	8	11	7	29	105
Eggs								
Eggs, large (24 oz per dozen):								
Cooked								
Fried in margarine	1 egg	46	90	6	1	7	211	162
Hard-cooked, shell removed	1 egg	50	75	6	1	5	213	62
Poached	1 egg	50	75	6	1	5	212	140
Scrambled (milk added) in margarine	1 egg	61	100	7	1	7	215	171

[b]Carbohydrate content varies widely because of amount of sugar added and amount of added flavoring. Consult the label if more precise values for carbohydrate and calories are needed.

FOOD ITEM	SERVING SIZE	GRAMS	CALORIES	PROTEIN (G)	CARBOHYDRATE (G)	FAT (G)	CHOLESTEROL (MG)	SODIUM (MG)
Fats and oils								
Butter (4 sticks per lb)								
Stick	½ cup	113	810	1	Tr	92	247	933[c]
Tablespoon (⅛ stick)	1 tbsp	14	100	Tr	Tr	11	31	116[c]
Pat (1-in square, ⅓ in high; 90 per lb)	1 pat	5	35	Tr	Tr	4	11	41[c]
Margarine								
Regular (about 80% fat)								
Stick	½ cup	113	810	1	1	91	0	1066[d]
Tablespoon (⅛ stick)	1 tbsp	14	100	Tr	Tr	11	0	132
Pat (1-in square, ⅓ in high; 90 per lb)	1 pat	5	35	Tr	Tr	4	0	47[d]
Oils, salad or cooking								
Corn	1 tbsp	14	125	0	0	14	0	0
Olive	1 tbsp	14	125	0	0	14	0	0
Peanut	1 tbsp	14	125	0	0	14	0	0
Safflower	1 tbsp	14	125	0	0	14	0	0
Sunflower	1 tbsp	14	125	0	0	14	0	0
Salad dressings								
Blue cheese	1 tbsp	15	75	1	1	8	3	164
French								
Regular	1 tbsp	16	85	Tr	1	9	0	188
Low-calorie	1 tbsp	16	25	Tr	2	2	0	306
Italian								
Regular	1 tbsp	15	80	Tr	1	9	0	162
Low-calorie	1 tbsp	15	5	Tr	2	Tr	0	136
Mayonnaise								
Regular	1 tbsp	14	100	Tr	Tr	11	8	80
Thousand island								
Regular	1 tbsp	16	60	Tr	2	6	4	112
Low-calorie	1 tbsp	15	25	Tr	2	2	2	150
Fish and shellfish								
Crab meat, canned	1 cup	135	135	23	1	3	135	1350
Fish sticks, frozen, reheated (stick, 4 by 1 by ½ in)	1 stick	28	70	6	4	3	26	53
Flounder or sole, baked, with lemon juice and butter	3 oz	85	120	16	Tr	6	68	145
Ocean perch, breaded, fried[e]	1 fillet	85	185	16	7	11	66	138
Salmon								
Baked (red)	3 oz	85	140	21	0	5	60	55
Smoked	3 oz	85	150	18	0	8	51	1700
Scallops, breaded, frozen, reheated	6 scallops	90	195	15	10	10	70	298

[c]For salted butter; unsalted butter contains 12 mg sodium per stick, 2 mg per tbsp, or 12 mg per pat.

[d]For salted margarine.

[e]Dipped in egg, milk, and bread crumbs; fried in vegetable shortening.

FOOD ITEM	SERVING SIZE	GRAMS	CALORIES	PROTEIN (G)	CARBOHYDRATE (G)	FAT (G)	CHOLESTEROL (MG)	SODIUM (MG)
Fish and shellfish *(continued)*								
Shrimp, French fried (7 medium)[f]	3 oz	85	200	16	11	10	168	384
Trout, broiled, with butter and lemon juice	3 oz	85	175	21	Tr	9	71	122
Tuna, canned, drained solids								
Oil pack, chunk light	3 oz	85	165	24	0	7	55	303
Water pack, solid white	3 oz	85	135	30	0	1	48	468
Tuna salad[g]	1 cup	205	375	33	19	19	80	877
Fruits and fruit juices								
Apples								
Raw								
Unpeeled, without cores, 3¼-in diam (about 2 per lb with cores)	1 apple	212	125	Tr	32	1	0	Tr
Peeled, sliced	1 cup	110	65	Tr	16	Tr	0	Tr
Apple juice, bottled or canned	1 cup	248	115	Tr	29	Tr	0	7
Apricots								
Raw, without pits (about 12 per lb with pits)	3 apricots	106	50	1	12	Tr	0	1
Bananas, raw, without peel								
Whole (about 2½ per lb with peel)	1 banana	114	105	1	27	1	0	1
Sliced	1 cup	150	140	2	35	1	0	2
Blueberries, raw	1 cup	145	80	1	20	1	0	9
Cherries, sweet, raw, without pits and stems	10 cherries	68	50	1	11	1	0	Tr
Grapefruit, raw, without peel, membrane, and seeds (3¾-in diam. 1 lb 1 oz, whole, with refuse)	½ grapefruit	120	40	1	10	Tr	0	Tr
Grapes, European type (adherent skin) raw, Thompson seedless	10 grapes	50	35	Tr	9	Tr	0	1

[f]Dipped in egg, milk, and bread crumbs; fried in vegetable shortening.

[g]Made with drained, chunk light tuna, celery, onion, pickle relish, and mayonnaise-type salad dressing.

Food item	Serving size	Grams	Calories	Protein (g)	Carbohydrate (g)	Fat (g)	Cholesterol (mg)	Sodium (mg)
Fruits and fruit juices *(continued)*								
Melons, raw, without rind and cavity contents								
Cantaloupe, orange-fleshed (5-in diam, 2⅓ lb, whole, with rind and cavity contents)	½ melon	267	95	2	22	1	0	24
Honeydew (6½-in diam, 5¼ lb, whole, with rind and cavity contents)	⅟₁₀ melon	129	45	1	12	Tr	0	13
Nectarines, raw, without pits (about 3 per lb with pits)	1 nectarine	136	65	1	16	1	0	Tr
Oranges, raw, whole, without peel and seeds (2⅝-in diam, about 2½ per lb, with peel and seeds)	1 orange	131	60	1	15	Tr	0	Tr
Orange juice								
Raw, all varieties	1 cup	248	110	2	26	Tr	0	2
Canned, unsweetened	1 cup	249	105	1	25	Tr	0	5
Peaches, raw								
Whole, 2½-in diam, peeled, pitted (about 4 per lb with peels and pits)	1 peach	87	35	1	10	Tr	0	Tr
Sliced	1 cup	170	75	1	19	Tr	0	Tr
Pears, raw, with skin, cored, Bartlett, 2½-in diam (about 2½ per lb with cores and stems)	1 pear	166	100	1	25	1	0	Tr
Pineapple, raw, diced	1 cup	155	75	1	19	1	0	2
Pineapple juice, unsweetened, canned	1 cup	250	140	1	34	Tr	0	3
Plums, without pits, raw, 2⅛-in diam (about 6½ per lb with pits)	1 plum	66	35	1	9	Tr	0	Tr
Raisins, seedless, cup, not pressed down	1 cup	145	435	5	115	1	0	17
Raspberries, raw	1 cup	123	60	1	14	1	0	Tr
Strawberries, raw, capped, whole	1 cup	149	45	1	10	1	0	1

Food item	Serving Size	Grams	Calories	Protein (g)	Carbohydrate (g)	Fat (g)	Cholesterol (mg)	Sodium (mg)
Fruits and fruit juices (*continued*)								
Watermelon, raw, without rind and seeds, piece (4 by 8-in wedge with rind and seeds; 1/16 of 32 2/3-lb melon, 10 by 16 in)	1 piece	482	155	3	35	2	0	10
Grain products								
Bagels, plain or water, enriched, 3 1/2-in diam[h]	1 bagel	68	200	7	38	2	0	245
Breads								
French or vienna bread, enriched[i]								
Slice								
French, 5 by 2 1/2 by 1 in	1 slice	35	100	3	18	1	0	203
Vienna 4 3/4 by 4 by 1/2 in	1 slice	25	70	2	13	1	0	145
Italian bread, enriched								
Slice, 4 1/2 by 3 1/4 by 3/4 in	1 slice	30	85	3	17	Tr	0	176
Mixed grain bread, enriched[i]								
Slice (18 per loaf)	1 slice	25	65	2	12	1	0	106
Pita bread, enriched, white, 6 1/2-in diam	1 pita	60	165	6	33	1	0	339
Pumpernickel (2/3 rye flour, 1/3 enriched wheat flour)[j]								
Slice, 5 by 4 by 3/8 in	1 slice	32	80	3	16	1	0	177
Rye bread, light (2/3 enriched wheat flour, 1/3 rye flour)[j]								
Slice, 4 3/4 by 3 3/4 by 7/16 in	1 slice	25	65	2	12	1	0	175
Wheat bread, enriched[j]								
Slice (16 per loaf)	1 slice	25	65	2	12	1	0	138
Whole-wheat bread[j]								
Slice (18 per loaf)	1 slice	28	70	3	13	1	0	180
Breakfast cereals								
All-Bran (about 1/3 cup)	1 oz	28	70	4	21	1	0	320
Cap'n Crunch (about 3/4 cup)	1 oz	28	120	1	23	3	0	213

[h]Egg bagels have 44 mg cholesterol and 22 IU or 7 RE vitamin A per bagel.

[i]Made with vegetable shortening.

[j]Made with vegetable shortening.

FOOD ITEM	SERVING SIZE	GRAMS	CALORIES	PROTEIN (G)	CARBOHYDRATE (G)	FAT (G)	CHOLESTEROL (MG)	SODIUM (MG)
Grain products (*continued*)								
Cheerios (about 1¼ cup)	1 oz	28	110	4	20	2	0	307
Corn Flakes (about 1¼ cup)								
Kellogg's	1 oz	28	110	2	24	Tr	0	351
Toasties	1 oz	28	110	2	24	Tr	0	297
40% Bran Flakes								
Kellogg's (about ¾ cup)	1 oz	28	90	4	22	1	0	264
Post (about ⅔ cup)	1 oz	28	90	3	22	Tr	0	260
Froot Loops (about 1 cup)	1 oz	28	110	2	25	1	0	145
Lucky Charms (about 1 cup)	1 oz	28	110	3	23	1	0	201
100% Natural Cereal (about ¼ cup)	1 oz	28	135	3	18	6	Tr	12
Product 19 (about ¾ cup)	1 oz	28	110	3	24	Tr	0	325
Raisin Bran								
Kellogg's (about ¾ cup)	1 oz	28	90	3	21	1	0	207
Post (about ½ cup)	1 oz	28	85	3	21	1	0	185
Special K (about 1⅓ cup)	1 oz	28	110	6	21	Tr	Tr	265
Sugar Frosted Flakes, Kellogg's (about ¾ cup)	1 oz	28	110	1	26	Tr	0	230
Wheaties (about 1 cup)	1 oz	28	100	3	23	Tr	0	354
Cakes prepared from cake mixes with enriched flour[k]								
Angelfood, piece, 1/12 of cake	1 piece	53	125	3	29	Tr	0	269
Devil's food with chocolate frosting								
Piece, 1/16 of cake	1 piece	69	235	3	40	8	37	181
Cupcake, 2½-in diam	1 cupcake	35	120	2	20	4	19	92
Cakes prepared from home recipes using enriched flour								
Carrot, with cream cheese frosting[l]								
Piece, 1/16 of cake	1 piece	96	385	4	48	21	74	279
Pound								
Slice, 1/17 of loaf	1 slice	30	120	2	15	5	32	96
Cheesecake								
Piece, 1/12 of cake	1 piece	92	280	5	26	18	170	204

[k]Excepting angel food cake, cakes were made from mixes containing vegetable shortening and frostings were made with margarine.

[l]Made with vegetable oil.

FOOD ITEM	SERVING SIZE	GRAMS	CALORIES	PROTEIN (G)	CARBOHYDRATE (G)	FAT (G)	CHOLESTEROL (MG)	SODIUM (MG)
Grain products *(continued)*								
Cookies made with enriched flour								
Brownies with nuts, commercial, with frosting, 1½ by 1¾ by ⅞ in	1 brownie	25	100	1	16	4	14	59
Chocolate chip, commercial, 2¼-in diam, ⅜ in thick	4 cookies	42	180	2	28	9	5	140
Oatmeal with raisins, 2⅝-in diam, ¼ in thick	4 cookies	52	245	3	36	10	2	148
Peanut butter cookie, from home recipe 2⅝-in diam[m]	4 cookies	48	245	4	28	14	22	142
Corn chips	1-oz package	28	155	2	16	9	0	233
Crackers[n]								
Graham, plain, 2½-in square	2 crackers	14	60	1	11	1	0	86
Melba toast, plain	1 piece	5	20	1	4	Tr	0	44
Saltines[o]	4 crackers	12	50	1	9	1	4	165
Wheat, thin	4 crackers	8	35	1	5	1	0	69
Croissants, made with enriched flour, 4½ by 4 by 1¾ in	1 croissant	57	235	5	27	12	13	452
Doughnuts, made with enriched flour								
Cake type, plain, 3¼-in diam, 1 in high	1 doughnut	50	210	3	24	12	20	192
Yeast-leavened, glazed, 3¾-in diam, 1¼ in high	1 doughnut	60	235	4	26	13	21	222
English muffins, plain, enriched	1 muffin	57	140	5	27	1	0	378
French toast, from home recipe	1 slice	65	155	6	17	7	112	257

[m]Made with vegetable shortening.

[n]Crackers made with enriched flour except for rye wafers and whole-wheat wafers.

[o]Made with lard.

FOOD ITEM	SERVING SIZE	GRAMS	CALORIES	PROTEIN (G)	CARBOHYDRATE (G)	FAT (G)	CHOLESTEROL (MG)	SODIUM (MG)
Grain products *(continued)*								
Macaroni, enriched, cooked (cut lengths, elbows, shells), firm stage (hot)	1 cup	130	190	7	39	1	0	1
Muffins made with enriched flour, 2½-in diam, 1½ in high, from home recipe								
Blueberry[m]	1 muffin	45	135	3	20	5	19	198
Bran	1 muffin	45	125	3	19	6	24	189
Corn	1 muffin	45	145	3	21	5	23	169
Noodles (egg noodles), enriched, cooked	1 cup	160	200	7	37	2	50	3
Noodles, chow mein, canned	1 cup	45	220	6	26	11	5	450
Pancakes, 4-in diam								
Buckwheat, from mix (with buckwheat and enriched flours), egg and milk added	1 pancake	27	55	2	6	2	20	125
Plain								
From home recipe using enriched flour	1 pancake	27	60	2	9	2	16	115
From mix (with enriched flour), egg, milk, and oil added	1 pancake	27	60	2	8	2	16	160
Pies, pie crust made with enriched flour, vegetable shortening, 9-in diam								
Apple, piece, ⅙ of pie	1 piece	158	405	3	60	18	0	476
Blueberry, piece, ⅙ of pie	1 piece	158	380	4	55	17	0	423
Cherry, piece, ⅙ of pie	1 piece	158	410	4	61	18	0	480
Lemon meringue, piece, ⅙ of pie	1 piece	140	355	5	53	14	143	395
Pecan, piece, ⅙ of pie	1 piece	138	575	7	71	32	95	305

[m]Made with vegetable shortening.

Food item	Serving size	Grams	Calories	Protein (g)	Carbohydrate (g)	Fat (g)	Cholesterol (mg)	Sodium (mg)
Grain products *(continued)*								
Popcorn, popped								
Airpopped, unsalted	1 cup	8	30	1	6	Tr	0	Tr
Popped in vegetable oil, salted	1 cup	11	55	1	6	3	0	86
Sugar syrup coated	1 cup	35	135	2	30	1	0	Tr
Pretzels, made with enriched flour								
Stick, 2¼ in long	10 pretzels	3	10	Tr	2	Tr	0	48
Twisted, dutch, 2¾ by 2⅝-in	1 pretzel	16	65	2	13	1	0	258
Rice								
Brown, cooked, served hot	1 cup	195	230	5	50	1	0	0
White, enriched								
Cooked, served hot	1 cup	205	225	4	50	Tr	0	0
Instant, ready-to-serve, hot	1 cup	165	180	4	40	0	0	0
Rolls, enriched								
Commercial								
Dinner, 2½-in diam, 2 in high	1 roll	28	85	2	14	2	Tr	155
Frankfurter and hamburger (8 per 11½-oz pkg.)	1 roll	40	115	3	20	2	Tr	241
Hard, 3¾-in diam, 2 in high	1 roll	50	155	5	30	2	Tr	313
Hoagie or submarine, 11½ by 3 by 2½ in	1 roll	135	400	11	72	8	Tr	683
Spaghetti, enriched, cooked								
Firm stage, "al dente," served hot	1 cup	130	190	7	39	1	0	1
Tender stage, served hot	1 cup	140	155	5	32	1	0	1
Tortillas, corn	1 tortilla	30	65	2	13	1	0	1
Waffles, made with enriched flour, 7-in diam								
From home recipe	1 waffle	75	245	7	26	13	102	445
From mix, egg and milk added	1 waffle	75	205	7	27	8	59	515
Legumes, nuts, and seeds								
Almonds, shelled								
Whole	1 oz	28	165	6	6	15	0	3
Beans, dry								
Black	1 cup	171	225	15	41	1	0	1
Lima	1 cup	190	260	16	49	1	0	4
Pea (navy)	1 cup	190	225	15	40	1	0	13
Pinto	1 cup	180	265	15	49	1	0	3

FOOD ITEM	SERVING SIZE	GRAMS	CALORIES	PROTEIN (G)	CARBOHYDRATE (G)	FAT (G)	CHOLESTEROL (MG)	SODIUM (MG)
Legumes, nuts, and seeds *(continued)*								
Black-eyed peas, dry, cooked (with residual cooking liquid)	1 cup	250	190	13	35	1	0	20
Brazil nuts, shelled	1 oz	28	185	4	4	19	0	1
Cashew nuts, salted								
Dry roasted	1 oz	28	165	4	9	13	0	181[p]
Roasted in oil	1 oz	28	165	5	8	14	0	177[q]
Lentils, dry, cooked	1 cup	200	215	16	38	1	0	26
Mixed nuts, with peanuts, salted								
Dry roasted	1 oz	28	170	5	7	15	0	190[r]
Roasted in oil	1 oz	28	175	5	6	16	0	185[r]
Peanuts, roasted in oil, salted	1 oz	28	165	8	5	14	0	122[s]
Peanut butter	1 tbsp	16	95	5	3	8	0	75
Peas, split, dry, cooked	1 cup	200	230	16	42	1	0	26
Pistachio nuts, dried, shelled	1 oz	28	165	6	7	14	0	2
Refried beans, canned	1 cup	290	295	18	5 1	3	0	1228
Sesame seeds, dry, hulled	1 tbsp	8	45	2	1	4	0	3
Sunflower seeds, dry, hulled	1 oz	28	160	6	5	14	0	1
Meat and meat products								
Beef, cooked[t]								
Cuts braised, simmered, or pot roasted								
Relatively fat, such as chuck blade								
Lean and fat, piece, 2½ by 2½ by ¾ in	3 oz	85	325	22	0	26	87	53
Relatively lean, such as bottom round								
Lean and fat, piece, 4⅛ by 2¼ by ½ in	3 oz	85	220	25	0	13	81	43
Ground beef, broiled, patty, 3 by ⅝ in								
Lean	3 oz	85	230	21	0	16	74	65
Regular	3 oz	85	245	20	0	18	76	70

[p]Cashews without salt contain 21 mg sodium per cup or 4 mg per oz.

[q]Cashews without salt contain 22 mg sodium per cup or 5 mg per oz.

[r]Mixed nuts without salt contain 3 mg sodium per oz.

[s]Peanuts without salt contain 22 mg sodium per cup or 4 mg per oz.

[t]Outer layer of fat was removed to within approximately ½ inch of lean. Deposits of fat within the cut were not removed.

Food item	Serving size	Grams	Calories	Protein (g)	Carbohydrate (g)	Fat (g)	Cholesterol (mg)	Sodium (mg)
Meat and meat products *(continued)*								
Roast, oven cooked, no liquid added								
Relatively fat, such as rib								
Lean and fat, 2 pieces, 4⅛ by 2¼ in	3 oz	85	315	19	0	26	72	54
Relatively lean, such as eye of round								
Lean and fat, 2 pieces, 2½ by 2½ by ⅜ in	3 oz	85	205	23	0	12	62	50
Steak								
Sirloin, broiled								
Lean and fat, piece, 2½ by 2½ by ¾ in	3 oz	85	240	23	0	15	77	53
Lamb, cooked								
Chops (3 per lb with bone)								
Arm, braised Lean and fat	2.2 oz	63	220	20	0	15	77	46
Loin, broiled Lean and fat	2.8 oz	80	235	20	0	16	78	62
Leg, roasted Lean and fat, 2 pieces, 4⅛ by 2¼ by ¼ in	3 oz	85	205	22	0	13	78	57
Rib, roasted Lean and fat, 3 pieces, 2½ by 2½ by ¼ in	3 oz	85	315	18	0	26	77	60
Pork, cured, cooked								
Bacon								
Regular	3 medium slices	19	110	6	Tr	9	16	303
Canadian-style	2 slices	46	85	11	1	4	27	711
Ham, light cured, roasted Lean and fat, 2 pieces, 4⅛ by 2¼ by ¼ in	3 oz	85	205	18	0	14	53	1009
Luncheon meat								
Canned, spiced or unspiced, slice, 3 by 2 by ½ in	2 slices	42	140	5	1	13	26	541
Chopped ham (8 slices per 6-oz pkg)	2 slices	42	95	7	0	7	21	576

Food item	Serving size	Grams	Calories	Protein (g)	Carbohydrate (g)	Fat (g)	Cholesterol (mg)	Sodium (mg)
Meat and meat products *(continued)*								
Cooked ham (8 slices per 8-oz pkg)								
Regular	2 slices	57	105	10	2	6	32	751
Extra lean	2 slices	57	75	11	1	3	27	815
Pork, fresh, cooked								
Chop, loin (cut 3 per lb with bone)								
Broiled								
Lean and fat	3.1 oz	87	275	24	0	19	84	61
Ham (leg), roasted Lean and fat, piece, 2½ by 2½ by ¾ in	3 oz	85	250	21	0	18	79	50
Rib, roasted Lean and fat, piece, 2½ by ¾ in	3 oz	85	270	21	0	20	69	37
Shoulder cut, braised Lean and fat, 3 pieces, 2½ by 2½ by ¼ in	3 oz	85	295	23	0	22	93	75
Sausages								
Bologna	2 slices	57	180	7	2	16	31	581
Frankfurter	1 frank	45	145	5	1	13	23	504
Pork link	1 link	13	50	3	Tr	4	11	168
Salami								
Cooked type, slice (8 per 8-oz pkg)	2 slices	57	145	8	1	11	37	607
Veal, medium fat, cooked, bone removed								
Cutlet, 4⅛ by 2¼ by ½ in, braised or broiled	3 oz	85	185	23	0	9	109	56
Rib, 2 pieces, 4⅛ by 2¼ by ¼ in, roasted	3 oz	85	230	23	0	14	109	57
Mixed dishes and fast foods								
Mixed dishes								
Beef and vegetable stew, from home recipe	1 cup	245	220	16	15	11	71	292
Beef potpie, from home recipe, baked, piece, ⅓ of 9-in diam pie	1 piece	210	515	21	39	30	42	596
Chicken á la king, cooked, from home recipe	1 cup	245	470	27	12	34	221	760

Food item	Serving size	Grams	Calories	Protein (g)	Carbohydrate (g)	Fat (g)	Cholesterol (mg)	Sodium (mg)
Mixed dishes and fast foods (*continued*)								
Chicken and noodles, cooked, from home recipe	1 cup	240	365	22	26	18	103	600
Chicken chow mein								
Canned	1 cup	250	95	7	18	Tr	8	725
From home recipe	1 cup	250	255	31	10	10	75	718
Chicken potpie, from home recipe, baked, piece, ⅓ of 9-in diam pie	1 piece	232	545	23	42	31	56	594
Chili con carne with beans, canned	1 cup	255	340	19	31	16	28	1354
Chop suey with beef and pork, from home recipe	1 cup	250	300	26	13	17	68	1053
Macaroni (enriched) and cheese								
Canned	1 cup	240	230	9	26	10	24	730
From home recipe[u]	1 cup	200	430	17	40	22	44	1086
Spaghetti (enriched) in tomato sauce with cheese								
Canned	1 cup	250	190	6	39	2	3	955
From home recipe[u]	1 cup	250	260	9	37	9	8	955
Spaghetti (enriched) with meatballs and tomato sauce								
From home recipe	1 cup	248	330	19	39	12	89	1009
Poultry and poultry products								
Chicken								
Fried, flesh, with skin[v]								
Batter dipped								
Breast, ½ breast (5.6 oz with bones)	4.9 oz	140	365	35	13	18	119	385
Drumstick (3.4 oz with bones)	2.5 oz	72	195	16	6	11	62	194
Flour coated								
Breast, ½ breast (4.2 oz with bones)	3.5 oz	98	220	31	2	9	87	74
Drumstick (2.6 oz with bones)	1.7 oz	49	120	13	1	7	44	44
Roasted, flesh only								
Breast, ½ breast (4.2 oz with bones and skin)	3.0 oz	86	140	27	0	3	73	64

[u]Made with margarine.

[v]Fried in vegetable shortening.

Food item	Serving size	Grams	Calories	Protein (g)	Carbohydrate (g)	Fat (g)	Cholesterol (mg)	Sodium (mg)
Poultry and poultry products *(continued)*								
Drumstick (2.9 oz with bones and skin)	1.6 oz	44	75	12	0	2	41	42
Turkey, roasted, flesh only								
Dark meat, piece, 2½ by 1⅝ by ¼ in	4 pieces	85	160	24	0	6	72	67
Light meat, piece, 4 by 2 by ¼ in	2 pieces	85	135	25	0	3	59	54
Light and dark meat								
Chopped or diced	1 cup	140	240	41	0	7	106	98
Pieces (1 slice white meat, 4 by 2 by ¼ in and 2 slices dark meat, 2½ by 1⅝ by ¼ in)	3 pieces	85	145	25	0	4	65	60
Soups, sauces, and gravies								
Soups								
Canned, condensed								
Prepared with equal volume of milk								
Clam chowder, New England	1 cup	248	165	9	17	7	22	992
Cream of chicken	1 cup	248	190	7	15	11	27	1047
Cream of mushroom	1 cup	248	205	6	15	14	20	1076
Tomato	1 cup	248	160	6	22	6	17	932
Prepared with equal volume of water								
Bean with bacon	1 cup	253	170	8	23	6	3	951
Beef noodle	1 cup	244	85	5	9	3	5	952
Chicken noodle	1 cup	241	75	4	9	2	7	1106
Chicken rice	1 cup	241	60	4	7	2	7	815
Clam chowder, Manhattan	1 cup	244	80	4	12	2	2	1808
Cream of chicken	1 cup	244	115	3	9	7	10	986
Cream of mushroom	1 cup	244	130	2	9	9	2	1032
Minestrone	1 cup	241	80	4	11	3	2	911
Pea, green	1 cup	250	165	9	27	3	0	988
Tomato	1 cup	244	85	2	17	2	0	871
Vegetable beef	1 cup	244	80	6	10	2	5	956

Food item	Serving size	Grams	Calories	Protein (g)	Carbohydrate (g)	Fat (g)	Cholesterol (mg)	Sodium (mg)
Soups, sauces, and gravies (*continued*)								
Sauces								
From dry mix								
Cheese, prepared with milk	1 cup	279	305	16	23	17	53	1565
Hollandaise, prepared with water	1 cup	259	240	5	14	20	52	1564
Gravies								
Canned								
Beef	1 cup	233	125	9	11	5	7	1305
Chicken	1 cup	238	190	5	13	14	5	1373
Mushroom	1 cup	238	120	3	13	6	0	1357
Sugars and sweets								
Candy								
Caramels, plain or chocolate	1 oz	28	115	1	22	3	1	64
Chocolate								
Milk, plain	1 oz	28	145	2	16	9	6	23
Milk, with almonds	1 oz	28	150	3	15	10	5	23
Milk, with peanuts	1 oz	28	155	4	13	11	5	19
Milk, with rice cereal	1 oz	28	140	2	18	7	6	46
Fudge, chocolate, plain	1 oz	28	115	1	21	3	1	54
Gum drops	1 oz	28	100	Tr	25	Tr	0	10
Hard candy	1 oz	28	110	0	28	0	0	7
Jelly beans	1 oz	28	105	Tr	26	Tr	0	7
Marshmallows	1 oz	28	90	1	23	0	0	25
Custard, baked	1 cup	265	305	14	29	15	278	209
Honey, strained or extracted	1 cup	339	1030	1	279	0	0	17
	1 tbsp	21	65	Tr	17	0	0	1
Jams and preserves	1 tbsp	20	55	Tr	14	Tr	0	2
	1 packet	14	40	Tr	10	Tr	0	2
Jellies	1 tbsp	18	50	Tr	13	Tr	0	5
	1 packet	14	40	Tr	10	Tr	0	4
Popsicle, 3-fl-oz size	1 popsicle	95	70	0	18	0	0	11
Puddings								
Canned								
Chocolate	5-oz can	142	205	3	30	11	1	285
Tapioca	5-oz can	142	160	3	28	5	Tr	252
Vanilla	5-oz can	142	220	2	33	10	1	305
Dry mix, prepared with whole milk								
Chocolate								
Instant	½ cup	130	155	4	27	4	14	440
Regular (cooked)	½ cup	130	150	4	25	4	15	167
Rice	½ cup	132	155	4	27	4	15	140
Tapioca	½ cup	130	145	4	25	4	15	152

Food item	Serving size	Grams	Calories	Protein (g)	Carbohydrate (g)	Fat (g)	Cholesterol (mg)	Sodium (mg)
Sugars and sweets (*continued*)								
Vanilla								
Instant	½ cup	130	150	4	27	4	15	375
Regular (cooked)	½ cup	130	145	4	25	4	15	178
Sugars								
Brown, pressed down	1 cup	220	820	0	212	0	0	97
White, granulated	1 cup	200	770	0	199	0	0	5
	1 tbsp	12	45	0	12	0	0	Tr
	1 packet	6	25	0	6	0	0	Tr
Syrups								
Chocolate-flavored syrup or topping								
Thin type	2 tbsp	38	85	1	22	Tr	0	36
Fudge type	2 tbsp	38	125	2	21	5	0	42
Vegetables and vegetable products								
Asparagus, green, cooked, drained								
From raw, cuts and tips	1 cup	180	45	5	8	1	0	7
From frozen, cuts and tips	1 cup	180	50	5	9	1	0	7
Beans								
Lima, immature seeds, frozen, cooked, drained, thick-seeded types (Ford hooks)	1 cup	170	170	10	32	1	0	90
Beets, cooked, drained, diced or sliced	1 cup	170	55	2	11	Tr	0	83
Black-eyed peas, immature seeds, cooked and drained, from raw	1 cup	165	180	13	30	1	0	7
Broccoli, raw	1 spear	151	40	4	8	1	0	41
Spears, cut into ½-in pieces	1 cup	155	45	5	9	Tr	0	17
Brussels sprouts, cooked, drained, from raw, 7–8 sprouts, 1¼ to 1½-in diam	1 cup	155	60	4	13	1	0	33
Cabbage, common varieties, raw, coarsely shredded or sliced	1 cup	70	15	1	4	Tr	0	13
Carrots, Raw, without crowns and tips, scraped, whole, 7½ by 1⅛ in, or strips, 2½ to 3 in long	1 carrot or 18 strips	72	30	1	7	Tr	0	25

FOOD ITEM	SERVING SIZE	GRAMS	CALORIES	PROTEIN (G)	CARBOHYDRATE (G)	FAT (G)	CHOLESTEROL (MG)	SODIUM (MG)
Vegetables and vegetable products *(continued)*								
Carrots								
Cooked, sliced, drained, from raw	1 cup	156	70	2	16	Tr	0	103
Cauliflower								
Raw (flowerets)	1 cup	100	25	2	5	Tr	0	15
Cooked, drained From raw (flowerets)	1 cup	125	30	2	6	Tr	0	8
Celery, pascal type, raw								
Stalk, large outer, 8 by 1½ in (at root end)	1 stalk	40	5	Tr	1	Tr	0	35
Corn, sweet, cooked, drained								
From raw, ear 5 by 1¾ in	1 ear	77	85	3	19	1	0	13
From frozen	1 ear	63	60	2	14	Tr	0	3
Cucumber, with peel, slices, ⅛ in thick (large, 2⅛-in diam; small, 1¾-in diam)	6 large or 8 small slices	28	5	Tr	1	Tr	0	1
Eggplant, cooked, steamed	1 cup	96	25	1	6	Tr	0	3
Lettuce, raw								
Butterhead, as Boston types:								
Head, 5-in diam	1 head	163	20	2	4	Tr	0	8
Leaves	1 outer or 2 inner leaves	15	Tr	Tr	Tr	Tr	0	1
Crisphead, as iceberg								
Pieces, chopped or shredded	1 cup	55	5	1	1	Tr	0	5
Loose leaf (bunching varieties including romaine or cos), chopped or shredded pieces	1 cup	56	10	1	2	Tr	0	5
Mushrooms								
Raw, sliced or chopped	1 cup	70	20	1	3	Tr	0	
Cooked, drained	1 cup	156	40	3	8	1	0	3
Onions								
Raw, chopped	1 cup	160	55	2	12	Tr	0	3
Cooked (whole or sliced), drained	1 cup	210	60	2	13	Tr	0	17
Peas, edible pod, cooked, drained	1 cup	160	65	5	11	Tr	0	6

Food item	Serving size	Grams	Calories	Protein (g)	Carbohydrate (g)	Fat (g)	Cholesterol (mg)	Sodium (mg)
Vegetables and vegetable products (*continued*)								
Peas, green								
Canned, drained solids	1 cup	170	115	8	21	1	0	372[w]
Frozen, cooked, drained	1 cup	160	125	8	23	Tr	0	139
Potatoes, cooked								
Baked (about 2 per lb, raw)								
With skin	1 potato	202	220	5	51	Tr	0	16
Flesh only	1 potato	156	145	3	34	Tr	0	8
Boiled (about 3 per 1b, raw)								
Peeled after boiling	1 potato	136	120	3	27	Tr	0	5
Peeled before boiling	1 potato	135	115	2	27	Tr	0	7
French fried, strip, 2 to 3½ in long, frozen								
Oven heated	10 strips	50	110	2	17	4	0	16
Fried in vegetable oil	10 strips	50	160	2	20	8	0	108
Potato products, prepared								
Au gratin								
From dry mix	1 cup	245	230	6	31	10	12	1076
From home recipe	1 cup	245	325	12	28	19	56	1061
Hashed brown, from frozen	1 cup	156	340	5	44	18	0	53
Mashed								
From home recipe								
Milk added	1 cup	210	160	4	37	1	4	636
Milk and margarine added	1 cup	210	225	4	35	9	4	620
Potato salad, made with mayonnaise	1 cup	250	360	7	28	21	170	1323
Scalloped								
From dry mix	1 cup	245	230	5	31	11	27	835
From home recipe	1 cup	245	210	7	26	9	29	821
Potato chips	10 chips	20	105	1	10	7	0	94
Pumpkin, cooked from raw, mashed	1 cup	245	50	2	12	Tr	0	2
Radishes, raw, stem ends, rootlets cut off	4 radishes	18	5	Tr	1	Tr	0	4
Sauerkraut, canned, solids and liquid	1 cup	236	45	2	10	Tr	0	1560

[w]For regular pack; special dietary pack contains 3 mg sodium.

Food Item	Serving Size	Grams	Calories	Protein (g)	Carbohydrate (g)	Fat (g)	Cholesterol (mg)	Sodium (mg)
Vegetables and vegetable product *(continued)*								
Spinach								
Raw, chopped	1 cup	55	10	2	2	Tr	0	43
Cooked, drained								
From raw	1 cup	180	40	5	7	Tr	0	126
From frozen (leaf)	1 cup	190	55	6	10	Tr	0	163
Sweet potatoes								
Cooked (raw, 5 by 2 in; about 2½ per lb)								
Baked in skin, peeled	1 potato	114	115	2	28	Tr	0	11
Boiled, without skin	1 potato	151	160	2	37	Tr	0	20
Tomatoes								
Raw, 2⅗-in diam (3 per 12-oz pkg)	1 tomato	123	25	1	5	Tr	0	10
Tomato juice, canned	1 cup	244	40	2	10	Tr	0	881[x]
Tomato products, canned								
Paste	1 cup	262	220	10	49	2	0	170[y]
Sauce	1 cup	245	75	3	18	Tr	0	1482[z]
Vegetable juice cocktail, canned	1 cup	242	45	2	11	Tr	0	883
Miscellaneous items								
Catsup	1 cup	273	290	5	69	1	0	2845
	1 tbsp	15	15	Tr	4	Tr	0	156
Chili powder	1 tsp	2.6	10	Tr	1	Tr	0	26
Mustard, prepared, yellow	1 tsp or individual packet	5	5	Tr	Tr	Tr	0	63
Olives, canned								
Green	4 medium or 3 extra large	13	15	Tr	Tr	2	0	312
Ripe, Mission, pitted	3 small or 2 large	9	15	Tr	Tr	2	0	68
Pickles, cucumber								
Dill	1 pickle	65	5	Tr	1	Tr	0	928
Sweet	1 pickle	15	20	Tr	5	Tr	0	107
Salt	1 tsp	5.5	0	0	0	0	0	2132

[x]For added salt, if none is added, sodium content is 24 mg.

[y]With no added salt; if salt is added, sodium content is 2070 mg.

[z]With no added salt; if salt is added, sodium content is 998 mg.

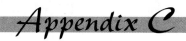

Nutritional Information for Selected Fast-Food Restaurants

ITEM	SERVING (OZ)	(G)	CALORIES	PROTEIN (G)	CARBO-HYDRATE (G)	TOTAL FAT (G)	DIETARY FIBER (G)	CHOLESTEROL (MG)	SODIUM (MG)
Restaurant: Arby's									
Regular Roast Beef	5	147	353	22.2	31.6	14.8	1	39	588
Beef 'N Cheddar	7	197	455	25.7	27.7	26.8	1	63	955
Chicken Breast Sandwich	7	184	493	23.0	47.9	25.0	1	91	1019
Roast Chicken Club	8	234	610	31.0	40.0	33.0	1	80	1500
Turkey Deluxe	7	197	375	23.8	32.5	16.6	2	39	1047
Ham 'N Cheese	6	156	292	22.9	19.2	13.7	1	45	1350
Super Roast Beef	8	234	501	25.1	50.4	22.1	1	40	798
French Fries	3	71	246	2.1	29.8	13.2	2	0	114
Restaurant: Burger King									
Whopper/Everything	10	270	628	27.0	46.0	36.0	2	90	880
Whopper/Cheese	10	294	706	32.0	47.0	43.0	2	113	1164
Hamburger	4	108	272	15.0	29.0	12.0	1	37	509
Cheeseburger	4	121	318	17.0	30.0	15.0	1	48	651
Bacon Double Cheeseburger	6	160	515	33.0	27.0	31.0	1	104	728
Hamburger Deluxe	5	138	344	15.0	30.0	17.0	1	41	486
Cheeseburger Deluxe	5	151	390	17.0	31.0	20.0	2	52	628
Ocean Catch Filet	7	194	488	19.0	45.0	25.0	2	77	592
Chicken Specialty Sandwich	8	229	685	26.0	56.0	40.0	2	82	1423
Chicken Tenders™	3	90	236	20.0	10.0	10.0	1	47	636
French Fries	4	111	341	3.0	24.0	13.0	3	14	160
Onion Rings	3	86	302	4.0	28.0	16.0	2	0	665
Breakfast Croissan'wich/ Bacon	4	118	355	14.0	20.0	24.0	1	249	762
Breakfast Croissan'wich/ Sausage	6	159	538	20.0	20.0	40.0	1	293	1042
Breakfast Croissan'wich/ Ham/Egg/Cheese	5	144	346	19.0	19.0	21.0	1	241	962
Breakfast Bagel Sandwich/ Bacon	6	169	438	20.0	46.0	20.0	2	274	905
Breakfast Bagel Sandwich/ Sausage/Egg/Cheese	7	210	626	27.0	49.0	36.0	2	318	1137
Breakfast Bagel Sandwich/ Ham/Egg/Cheese	7	196	418	23.0	46.0	15.0	2	287	1130
Scrambled Egg Platter	7	211	549	17.0	44.0	30.0	3	370	808
Scrambled Egg Platter/ Sausage	9	260	768	26.0	47.0	53.0	3	412	1271
Scrambled Egg Platter/ Bacon	8	221	610	21.0	44.0	39.0	3	373	1043

Information for all restaurants, except Jack in the Box, from Ross Laboratories, Columbus, OH, 43216, from *Dietetic Currents*, 18:4 (1991). Information for Jack in the Box from M. A. Boyle and G. Zyla. *Personal Nutrition*, 2 ed., St. Paul, MN, West Publishing, 1992.

ITEM	SERVING (OZ)	(G)	CALORIES	PROTEIN (G)	CARBO-HYDRATE (G)	TOTAL FAT (G)	DIETARY FIBER (G)	CHOLESTEROL (MG)	SODIUM (MG)
Restaurant: Burger King (*continued*)									
French Toast Sticks	5	141	538	10.0	53.0	32.0	2	80	537
Great Danish	3	71	500	5.0	40.0	36.0	3	6	288
Vanilla Shake	10	284	334	9.0	51.0	10.0	0	39	205
Chocolate Shake	10	284	326	9.0	49.0	10.0	1	33	202
Apple Pie	4	125	311	3.0	44.0	14.0	2	4	412
Chicken Salad	9	258	142	20.0	8.0	4.0	2	50	440
Chef Salad	10	273	178	17.0	7.0	9.0	2	120	570
Garden Salad	8	223	95	6.0	8.0	5.0	2	15	125
Side Salad	5	135	25	1.0	5.0	0.0	2	0	20
Thousand Island Dressing	2	63	290	1.0	15.0	26.0	0	36	470
Bleu Cheese Dressing	2	59	300	3.0	2.0	32.0	0	40	600
Reduced Calorie Italian	2	59	170	0.0	3.0	18.0	0	3	762
French Dressing	2	64	290	0.0	23.0	22.0	1	2	400
Bacon Bits	0.1	3	16	1.0	0.0	1.0	0	5	1
Croutons	0.3	7	31	1.0	5.0	1.0	0	0	90
Restaurant: Dairy Queen									
Cone, Small	3	85	140	3.0	22.0	4.0	0	10	45
Cone, Regular	5	142	240	6.0	38.0	7.0	0	15	80
Cone, Large	8	213	340	9.0	57.0	10.0	0	25	115
Cone, Small, Chocolate-Dipped	3	92	190	3.0	25.0	9.0	2	10	55
Cone, Regular, Chocolate-Dipped	6	156	340	6.0	42.0	16.0	3	20	100
Cone, Large, Chocolate-Dipped	8	234	510	9.0	64.0	24.0	4	30	145
Chocolate Sundae, Small	4	106	190	3.0	33.0	4.0	1	10	75
Chocolate Sundae, Regular	6	177	310	5.0	56.0	8.0	1	20	120
Chocolate Sundae, Large	9	248	440	8.0	78.0	10.0	2	30	165
Chocolate Shake, Small	9	241	409	8.0	69.0	11.0	1	30	150
Chocolate Shake, Regular	15	418	710	14.0	120.0	19.0	2	50	260
Chocolate Shake, Large	17	489	831	16.0	140.0	22.0	2	60	304
Chocolate Malt, Small	9	241	438	8.0	77.0	10.0	2	30	150
Chocolate Malt, Regular	15	418	760	14.0	134.0	18.0	3	50	260
Chocolate Malt, Large	17	489	889	16.0	157.0	21.0	3	60	304
Float	14	397	410	5.0	82.0	7.0	0	20	85
Peanut Buster Parfait	11	305	740	16.0	94.0	34.0	6	30	250
Parfait	10	283	430	8.0	76.0	8.0	1	30	140
Freeze	14	397	500	9.0	89.0	12.0	0	30	180
Mr Misty, Small	9	248	190	0.0	48.0	0.0	0	0	10
Mr Misty, Regular	12	330	250	0.0	63.0	0.0	0	0	10
Mr Misty, Large	16	439	340	0.0	84.0	0.0	0	0	10
Mr Misty Kiss	3	89	70	0.0	17.0	0.0	0	0	10
Mr Misty Freeze	15	411	500	9.0	91.0	12.0	0	30	140
Mr Misty Float	15	411	390	5.0	74.0	7.0	0	20	95
Buster Bar	5	149	448	10.0	41.0	29.0	6	1 0	175
Fudge Nut Bar	5	142	406	8.0	40.0	25.0	2	10	167
Dilly Bar	3	85	210	3.0	21.0	13.0	1	10	50
DQ Sandwich	2	60	140	3.0	24.0	4.0	0	5	40
Chipper Sandwich	4	113	318	5.0	56.0	7.0	0	13	170

ITEM	SERVING (OZ)	(G)	CALORIES	PROTEIN (G)	CARBO-HYDRATE (G)	TOTAL FAT (G)	DIETARY FIBER (G)	CHOLESTEROL (MG)	SODIUM (MG)
Restaurant: Dairy Queen *(continued)*									
Heath Blizzard, Regular	14	404	800	15.0	125.0	24.0	3	65	325
Single Hamburger	5	148	360	21.0	33.0	16.0	1	45	630
Double Hamburger	7	210	530	36.0	33.0	28.0	1	85	660
Triple Hamburger	10	272	710	51.0	33.0	45.0	1	135	690
Single Hamburger/Cheese	6	162	410	24.0	33.0	20.0	1	50	790
Double Hamburger/Cheese	8	239	650	43.0	34.0	37.0	1	95	980
Triple Hamburger/Cheese	11	301	820	58.0	34.0	50.0	1	145	1010
Hot Dog	4	100	280	11.0	21.0	16.0	1	45	830
Hot Dog/Chili	5	128	320	13.0	23.0	20.0	1	55	985
Hot Dog/Cheese	4	114	330	15.0	21.0	21.0	1	55	990
Super Hot Dog	6	175	520	17.0	44.0	27.0	1	80	1365
Super Hot Dog/Chili	8	218	570	21.0	47.0	32.0	2	100	1595
Super Hot Dog/Cheese	7	196	580	22.0	45.0	34.0	1	100	1605
Fish Filet	6	177	430	20.0	45.0	18.0	1	40	674
Fish Filet/Cheese	7	191	483	23.0	46.0	22.0	1	49	870
Chicken Breast Filet	7	202	608	27.0	46.0	34.0	2	78	725
Chicken Breast Filet/Cheese	8	216	661	30.0	47.0	38.0	2	87	921
All White Chicken Nuggets	4	99	276	16.0	13.0	18.0	1	39	505
BBQ Nugget Sauce	1	28	41	0.0	9.0	0.7	0	0	130
French Fries, Small	3	71	200	2.0	25.0	10.0	2	10	115
French Fries, Large	4	113	320	3.0	40.0	16.0	3	15	185
Onion Rings	3	85	280	4.0	31.0	16.0	3	15	140
Restaurant: Domino's Pizza (2 slices of each pizza)									
Cheese Pizza	6	168	376	21.6	56.3	10.0	6	19	483
Pepperoni Pizza	7	187	460	24.1	55.6	17.5	5	28	825
Sausage/Mushroom Pizza	7	200	430	24.2	55.3	15.8	8	28	552
Veggie Pizza	9	261	498	31.0	60.0	18.5	8	36	1035
Deluxe Pizza	8	234	498	26.7	59.2	20.4	7	40	954
Double Cheese/Pepperoni Pizza	8	227	545	32.1	55.2	25.3	8	48	1042
Ham Pizza	7	186	417	23.2	58.0	11.0	2	26	805
Restaurant: Jack in the Box									
Breakfast Jack Sandwich	4	126	307	18	30	13	< 1	203	871
Canadian Crescent	5	134	472	19	25	31	< 1	226	851
Sausage Crescent	6	156	584	22	28	43	< 1	187	1012
Supreme Crescent	5	146	547	20	27	40	< 1	178	1053
Pancakes Breakfast Platter	8	231	612	15	87	22	< 1	99	888
Scrambled Egg Breakfast Platter	9	249	662	24	52	40	< 1	354	1188
Hamburger	3	98	276	13	30	12	< 1	29	521
Cheeseburger	4	113	323	16	32	15	< 1	42	749
Jumbo Jack	7	205	485	26	38	26	< 1	64	905
Jumbo Jack w/Cheese	9	246	630	32	45	35	< 1	110	1665
Bacon Cheeseburger Supreme	8	231	724	34	44	46	< 1	70	1307
Swiss and Baconburger	8	231	643	33	31	43	< 1	99	1354
Ham and Swiss Burger	7	203	638	36	37	39	< 1	117	1330
Chicken Supreme	8	228	601	31	39	36	< 1	60	1582

Item	Serving (oz)	(g)	Calories	Protein (g)	Carbo-hydrate (g)	Total Fat (g)	Dietary Fiber (g)	Cholesterol (mg)	Sodium (mg)
Restaurant: Jack in the Box *(continued)*									
Double Cheeseburger	5	149	467	21	33	27	—	72	842
Tacos									
Regular	3	81	191	8	16	11	< 1	21	460
Super	5	135	288	12	21	17	< 1	—	—
French Fries	2	68	221	2	27	12	< 1	8	164
Hash Brown Potatoes	2	62	116	2	11	7	< 1	3	211
Onion Rings	4	108	382	5	39	23	< 1	27	407
Milkshakes									
Chocolate	11	322	330	11	55	7	0	25	270
Strawberry	12	328	320	10	55	7	0	25	240
Vanilla	11	317	320	10	57	6	0	25	230
Apple Turnover	4	119	410	4	45	24	< 1	15	350
Restaurant: Kentucky Fried Chicken									
Nuggets	1	16	46	2.8	2.2	2.9	0	12	140
Barbeque Sauce	1	28	35	0.3	7.1	0.6	0	0	450
Sweet and Sour Sauce	1	28	58	0.1	13.0	0.6	0	0	148
Chicken Littles Sandwich	2	47	169	5.7	13.8	10.1	0	18	331
Buttermilk Biscuit	2	65	235	4.5	28.0	11.9	1	1	655
Mashed Potatoes/Gravy	4	98	71	2.4	11.9	1.6	1	0	339
French Fries, Regular	3	77	244	3.2	31.1	11.9	2	2	139
Corn-on-the-cob	5	143	176	5.1	31.9	3.1	7	0	21
Coleslaw	3	91	119	1.5	13.3	6.6	1	5	197
Original Recipe Chicken									
Wing	2	55	178	12.2	6.0	11.7	0	64	372
Breast	4	115	283	27.5	8.8	15.3	0	93	672
Drumstick	2	57	146	13.1	4.2	8.5	0	67	275
Thigh	4	104	294	17.9	11.1	19.7	1	123	619
Extra Crispy Chicken									
Wing	2	65	254	12.4	9.3	18.6	0	67	422
Breast	5	135	342	33.0	11.7	19.7	1	114	790
Drumstick	2	69	204	13.6	6.1	13.9	0	71	324
Thigh	4	119	406	20.0	14.4	29.8	1	129	688
Restaurant: Long John Silver's Seafood Shoppe									
Three-piece Fish Light/ Paprika (Baked)	5	134	120	28.0	1.0	1.0	0	110	120
Three-piece Fish/Lemon Crumb (Baked)	5	141	150	29.0	4.0	1.0	0	110	370
Three-piece Fish/Scampi Sauce (Baked)	5	148	170	28.0	2.0	5.0	0	110	270
Shrimp/Scampi Sauce (Baked)	5	148	120	15.0	2.0	5.0	0	205	610
Chicken Light/Herbs (Baked)	4	117	140	25.0	1.0	4.0	0	70	670
Rice Pilaf	5	142	210	5.0	43.0	2.0	1	0	570
Green Beans	4	113	30	1.0	6.0	1.0	3	5	540
Garden Vegetables	4	113	120	4.0	16.0	6.0	5	5	95
Coleslaw	3	98	140	1.0	20.0	6.0	1	15	260
Breadstick	1	34	110	3.0	18.0	3.0	1	0	120
Small Salad	2	54	8	1.0	2.0	0.0	1	0	0

ITEM	SERVING (OZ)	(G)	CALORIES	PROTEIN (G)	CARBO-HYDRATE (G)	TOTAL FAT (G)	DIETARY FIBER (G)	CHOLESTEROL (MG)	SODIUM (MG)
Restaurant: McDonald's									
Egg McMuffin	5	138	290	18.2	28.1	11.2	1	226	740
Hotcakes/Butter/Syrup	6	176	410	8.2	74.4	9.2	2	21	640
Scrambled Eggs	4	100	140	12.4	1.2	9.8	0	399	290
Pork Sausage	2	48	180	8.4	0.0	16.3	0	48	350
English Muffin/Butter	2	59	170	5.4	26.7	4.6	1	9	270
Hashbrown Potatoes	2	53	130	1.4	14.9	7.3	2	9	330
Biscuit/Biscuit Spread	3	75	260	4.6	31.9	12.7	1	1	730
Biscuit/Sausage	4	123	440	13.0	31.9	29.0	1	49	1080
Biscuit/Sausage/Egg	6	180	520	19.9	32.6	34.5	1	275	1250
Biscuit/Bacon/Egg/Cheese	6	156	440	17.5	33.3	26.4	1	253	1230
Sausage McMuffin	4	117	370	16.5	27.3	21.9	1	64	830
Sausage McMuffin/Cheese	6	167	440	22.6	27.9	26.8	1	263	980
Apple Danish	4	115	390	5.8	51.2	17.9	2	25	370
Iced Cheese Danish	4	110	390	7.4	42.3	21.8	1	47	420
Cinnamon Raisin Danish	4	110	440	6.4	57.5	21.0	2	34	430
Raspberry Danish	4	117	410	6.1	61.5	15.9	2	26	310
Apple Bran Muffin	3	85	190	5.0	46.0	0.0	2	0	230
Blueberry Muffin	3	85	170	3.0	40.0	0.0	1	0	220
Chicken McNuggets	4	113	290	19.0	16.5	16.3	1	65	520
Hot Mustard Sauce	1	30	70	0.5	8.2	3.6	0	5	250
Barbeque Sauce	1	32	50	0.3	12.1	0.5	0	0	340
Sweet and Sour Sauce	1	32	60	0.2	13.8	0.2	0	0	190
Hamburger	4	102	260	12.3	30.6	9.5	1	37	500
Cheeseburger	4	116	310	15.0	31.2	13.8	1	53	750
McLean Deluxe	7	203	310	20.0	34.0	10.0	2	37	650
Quarter Pounder	6	166	410	23.1	34.0	20.7	1	86	660
Quarter Pounder/Cheese	7	194	520	28.5	35.1	29.2	1	118	1150
Big Mac	8	215	560	25.2	42.5	32.4	1	103	950
Filet-O-Fish	5	142	440	13.8	37.9	26.1	1	50	1030
McD.L.T.	8	234	580	26.3	36.0	36.8	2	109	990
McChicken	7	190	490	19.2	39.8	28.6	1	43	780
Chef Salad	10	283	230	20.5	7.5	13.3	2	128	490
Garden Salad	8	213	110	7.1	6.2	6.6	2	83	160
Chicken Salad Oriental	9	244	140	23.1	5.0	3.4	2	78	230
Side Salad	4	115	60	3.7	3.3	3.3	1	41	85
Bleu Cheese Dressing	1	14	70	0.5	1.2	6.9	0	6	150
French Dressing	1	14	58	0.1	2.7	5.2	0	0	180
Ranch Dressing	1	14	83	0.2	1.3	8.6	0	5	130
1000 Island Dressing	1	14	78	0.2	2.4	7.5	0	8	100
Lite Vinaigrette Dressing	1	14	15	0.2	2.0	0.5	0	0	75
Oriental Dressing	1	14	24	0.2	5.8	0.1	0	0	180
Red French Reduced Calorie Dressing	1	14	40	0.1	5.2	1.9	0	0	110
Caesar Dressing	1	14	60	0.4	0.6	6.1	0	7	170
Peppercorn Dressing	1	14	80	0.2	0.5	8.7	0	7	85
French Fries, Small	2	68	220	3.1	25.6	12.0	2	9	110
French Fries, Medium	3	97	320	4.4	36.3	17.1	3	12	150
French Fries, Large	4	122	400	5.6	45.9	21.6	3	16	200
Apple Pie	3	83	260	2.2	30.0	14.8	2	6	240

Item	Serving (oz)	(g)	Calories	Protein (g)	Carbo-hydrate (g)	Total Fat (g)	Dietary Fiber (g)	Cholesterol (mg)	Sodium (mg)
Restaurant: McDonald's *(continued)*									
Vanilla Low-fat Milk Shake	11	293	290	10.8	60.0	1.3	0	10	170
Chocolate Low-fat Milk Shake	11	293	320	11.0	66.0	1.7	1	10	240
Strawberry Low-fat Milk Shake	11	293	320	10.7	67.0	1.3	0	10	170
Soft Serve Cone	3	86	140	3.9	21.9	4.5	0	16	70
Strawberry Sundae	6	171	210	5.7	49.2	1.1	1	5	95
Hot Fudge Sundae	6	169	240	7.3	50.5	3.2	1	6	170
Hot Caramel Sundae	6	174	270	6.6	59.3	2.8	0	13	180
McDonaldland Cookies	2	56	290	4.2	47.1	9.2	1	0	300
Chocolaty Chip Cookies	2	56	330	4.2	41.9	15.6	0	4	280
Restaurant: Pizza Hut									
Pan Pizza, 2 slices									
Cheese	7	205	492	30.0	57.0	18.0	5	34	940
Pepperoni	8	211	540	29.0	62.0	22.0	5	42	1127
Supreme	9	255	589	32.0	53.0	30.0	7	48	1363
Super Supreme	9	257	563	33.0	53.0	26.0	6	55	1447
Thin 'n Crispy Pizza 2 slices									
Cheese	5	148	398	28.0	37.0	17.0	4	33	867
Pepperoni	5	146	413	26.0	20.0	20.0	4	46	986
Supreme	7	200	459	28.0	41.0	22.0	5	42	1328
Super Supreme	7	203	463	29.0	44.0	21.0	5	56	1336
Hand-Tossed Pizza 2 slices									
Cheese	8	220	518	34.0	55.0	20.0	7	55	1276
Pepperoni	7	197	500	28.0	50.0	23.0	6	50	1267
Supreme	8	239	540	32.0	50.0	26.0	7	55	1470
Super Supreme	9	243	556	33.0	54.0	25.0	7	54	1648
Personal Pan Pizza 1 pizza									
Pepperoni	9	256	675	37.0	76.0	29.0	8	53	1335
Supreme	9	264	647	33.0	76.0	28.0	9	49	1313
Restaurant: Taco Bell									
Bean Burrito/Red Sauce	7	191	356	13.1	54.4	10.2	5	9	888
Beef Burrito/Red Sauce	7	191	403	22.5	39.1	17.3	3	57	1051
Burrito Supreme/Red Sauce	9	241	413	18.0	46.6	17.6	4	33	921
Double Beef Burrito Supreme/Red Sauce	9	255	457	23.7	41.7	21.8		57	1053
Tostada/Red Sauce	6	156	243	9.5	26.6	11.1	6	16	596
Enchirito/Red Sauce	8	213	382	19.8	30.9	19.7	4	54	1243
Pintos and Cheese/Red Sauce	5	128	191	9.0	19.0	8.7	4	16	642
Nachos	4	106	346	7.5	37.5	18.5	4	9	399
Nachos Bellgrande	10	287	649	21.6	60.6	35.3	7	36	997
Taco	28	778	183	10.3	11.0	10.8	1	32	276
Taco Bellgrande	6	163	355	18.3	17.7	23.1	2	56	472
Taco Light	6	170	410	19.0	18.1	28.8	2	56	594
Soft Taco	3	92	228	11.8	17.9	11.9	1	32	516

Item	Serving (oz)	(g)	Calories	Protein (g)	Carbohydrate (g)	Total Fat (g)	Dietary Fiber (g)	Cholesterol (mg)	Sodium (mg)
Restaurant: Taco Bell (*continued*)									
Soft Taco Supreme	4	124	275	12.6	19.1	16.3	1	32	516
Taco Salad/Salsa	21	595	941	36.0	63.1	61.3	10	80	1662
Taco Salad/Salsa without Shell	19	530	520	30.6	30.0	31.4	6	80	1431
Taco Salad without Shell	19	530	520	29.5	26.3	31.3	6	80	1056
Mexican Pizza	8	223	575	21.3	39.7	36.8	6	52	1031
Taco Sauce	< 1	< 1	2	0.1	0.4	0.0	0	0	126
Hot Taco Sauce	< 1	< 1	3	0.1	0.3	0.1	0	0	82
Jalapeno Peppers	5	100	20	1.0	4.0	0.2	1	0	1370
Steak Fajita	5	135	234	14.6	19.5	10.9	1	14	485
Chicken Fajita	5	135	226	13.6	19.8	10.2	1	44	619
Sour Cream	1	21	46	0.6	0.9	4.4	0	16	10
Pico De Gallo	1	28	8	0.3	1.1	0.2	0	1	88
Guacamole	1	21	34	0.4	3.0	2.3	1	0	113
Meximelt	4	106	266	12.9	18.7	15.4	1	38	689
Restaurant: Wendy's									
Junior Hamburger	3	104	260	15.0	32.0	9.0	1	35	570
Junior Cheeseburger	3	116	300	18.0	33.0	13.0	1	35	770
Small Hamburger	4	111	260	15.0	33.0	9.0	1	34	570
Small Cheeseburger	4	125	310	18.0	33.0	13.0	1	34	770
Chicken Sandwich	8	219	430	26.0	41.0	19.0	2	60	725
Big Classic/Cheese	10	295	640	30.0	46.0	38.0	4	100	1370
Plain Single	4	126	340	24.0	30.0	15.0	1	65	500
Single/Everything	8	210	420	25.0	35.0	21.0	1	70	890
Plain Single/Cheese	5	137	410	25.0	29.0	22.0	1	80	710
Garden Salad (Take-Out)	10	227	102	7.0	9.0	5.0	4	0	110
Chef Salad (Take-Out)	12	331	180	15.0	10.0	9.0	4	120	140
New Chili	9	256	220	21.0	23.0	7.0	7	45	750
Taco Salad	28	791	660	40.0	46.0	37.0	9	35	1110
French Fries, Small	3	91	240	3.0	33.0	12.0	2	15	145
Baked Potatoes									
Plain	9	250	250	6	52	< 1	5	0	60
W/bacon and cheese	12	350	570	19	57	30	5	22	1180
W/broccoli and cheese	13	365	500	13	54	25	5	22	430
W/cheese	12	350	590	17	55	34	5	22	450
W/chili and cheese	14	400	510	22	63	20	8	22	610
W/sour cream and chives	11	310	460	7	53	24	5	15	230

Appendix D

American College of Sports Medicine Position Statements

Increasing numbers of persons are becoming involved in endurance training activities and thus, the need for guidelines for exercise prescription is apparent. Based on the existing evidence concerning exercise prescription for healthy adults and the need for guidelines, the American College of Sports Medicine (ACSM) makes the following recommendations for the quantity and quality of training for developing and maintaining cardiorespiratory fitness, body composition, and muscular strength and endurance in the healthy adult:

1. **Frequency of training:** 3–5 d·wk^{-1}.

2. **Intensity of training:** 60–90% of maximum heart rate (HR$_{max}$), or 50–85% of maximum oxygen uptake ($\overset{\circ}{V}O_{2max}$) or HR$_{max}$ reserve.*

3. **Duration of training:** 20–60 min of continuous aerobic activity. Duration is dependent on the intensity of the activity, thus lower intensity activity should be conducted over a longer period of time. Because of the importance of the "total fitness" effect and the fact that it is more readily attained in longer duration programs, and because of the potential hazards and compliance problems associated with high intensity activity, lower to moderate intensity activity of longer duration is recommended for the non-athletic adult.

4. **Mode of activity:** Any activity that uses large muscle groups, that can be maintained continuously, and is rhythmical and aerobic in nature, e.g. walking-hiking, running-jogging, cycling-bicycling, cross-country skiing, dancing, rope skipping, stair climbing, swimming, skating, and various endurance game activities.

5. **Resistance training:** Strength training of a moderate intensity, sufficient to develop and maintain fat free weight (FFW), should be an integral part of an adult fitness procram. One set of 8–12 repetitions of eight to ten exercises that condition the major muscle groups at least 2 d·wk is the recommended minimum.

*Maximum heart rate reserve is calculated from the difference between resting and maximum heart rate. To estimate training intensity, a percentage of this value is added to the resting heart rate and is expressed as a percentate of HR$_{max}$ reserve.

Source: Copyright American College of Sports Medicine 1990: Position Stand, "The Recommended Quantity and Quality of Exercise for Developing and Maintaining Cardiorespiratory and Muscular Fitness in Healthy Adults," *Med. Sci. Sports Exerc.* 22:2 (1990): pp. 529–533.

Rationale and Research Background

Introduction The questions, "How much exercise is enough," and "What type of exercise is best for developing and maintaining fitness?" are frequently asked. It is recognized that the term "physical fitness" is composed of a variety of characteristics included in the broad categories of cardiovascular-respiratory fitness, body composition, muscular strength and endurance, and flexibility. In this context fitness is defined as the ability to perform moderate to vigorous levels of physical activity without undue fatigue and the capability of maintaining such ability throughout life. It is also recognized that the adaptive response to training is complex and includes peripheral, central, structural, and functional factors. Although many such variables and their adaptive response to training have been documented, the lack of sufficient indepth and comparative data relative to frequency, intensity, and duration of training make them inadequate to use as comparative models. Thus, in respect to the above, questions, fitness is limited mainly to changes in $\overset{\circ}{V}O_{2max}$, muscular strength and endurance, and body composition, which includes total body mass, fat weight (FW), and FFW. Further, the rationale and research background used for this position stand will be divided into programs for cardiorespiratory fitness and weight control and programs for muscular strength and endurance.

Fitness versus Health Benefits of Exercise Since the original position statement was published in 1978, an important distinction has been made between physical activity as it relates to health versus fitness. It has been pointed out that the quantity and quality of exercise needed to attain health-related benefits may differ from what is recommended for fitness benefits. It is now clear that lower levels of physical activity than recommended by this position statement may reduce the risk for certain chronic degenerative diseases and yet may not be of sufficient quantity or quality to improve $\overset{\circ}{V}O_{2max}$. ACSM recognizes the potential health benefits of regular exercise performed more frequently and for a longer duration, but at lower intensities than prescribed in this position statement. ACSM will address the issue conceming the proper amount of physical activity necessary to derive health benefits in another statement.

Need for Standardization of Procedures and Reporting Results Despite an abundance of information available concerning the training of the human organism, the lack of standardization of testing protocols and procedures, of methodology in relation to training procedures and experimental design, and of a preciseness in the documentation and reporting of the quantity and quality of training prescribed make interpretation difficult. Interpretation and comparison of results are also dependent on the initial level of fitness, length of time of the training experiment, and specificity of the testing and training. For example, data from training studies using subjects with varied levels of $\overset{\circ}{V}O_{2max}$, total body mass, and FW have found changes to occur in relation to their initial values; i.e., the lower the initial $\overset{\circ}{V}O_{2max}$ the larger the percentage of improvement found, and the higher the FW the greater the reduction. Also, data evaluating trainability with age, comparison of the different magnitudes and quantities of effort, and comparison of the trainability of men and women may have been influenced by the initial fitness levels.

In view of the fact that improvement in the fitness variables discussed in this position statement continues over many months of training, it is reasonable to believe that short-term studies conducted over a few weeks have certain limitations. Middle-aged sedentary and older participants may take several weeks to adapt to the initial rigors of training, and thus need a longer adaptation period to get the full benefit from a program. For example, Seals et al. exercise trained 60–69-yr-olds for 12 months. Their subjects showed a 12% improvement in $\overset{\circ}{V}O_{2max}$ after 6 months of moderate intensity walking training. A further 18% increase in $\overset{\circ}{V}O_{2max}$ occurred during the next 6 months of training when jogging was introduced. How long a training experiment should be conducted is difficult to determine, but 15–20 wk may be a good minimum standard. Although it is difficult to control exercise training experiments for more than 1 yr, there is a need to study this effect. As stated earlier, lower doses of exercise may improve $\overset{\circ}{V}O_{2max}$ and control or maintain body composition, but at a slower rate. Although most of the information concerning training described in this position statement has been conducted on men, the available evidence indicates that women tend to adapt to endurance training in the same manner as men.

Exercise Prescription for Cardiorespiratory Fitness and Weight Control

Exercise prescription is based upon the frequency, intensity, and duration of training, the mode of activity (aerobic in nature, e.g. listed under No. 4 on previous page), and the initial level of fitness. In evaluating these factors, the following observations have been derived from studies conducted for up to 6–12 months with endurance training programs.

Improvement in $\overset{\circ}{V}O_{2max}$ is directly related to frequency, intensity, and duration of training. Depending upon the quantity and quality of training, improvement in $\overset{\circ}{V}O_{2max}$ ranges from 5 to 30%. These studies show that a minimum increase in $\overset{\circ}{V}O_{2max}$ of 15% is generally attained in programs that meet the above stated guidelines. Although changes in $\overset{\circ}{V}O_{2max}$ greater than 30% have been shown, they are usually associated with large total body mass and FW loss, in cardiac patients, or in persons with a very low initial level of fitness. Also, as a result of leg fatigue or a lack of motivation, persons with low initial fitness may have spuriously low initial $\overset{\circ}{V}O_{2max}$ values. Klissouras and Bouchard have shown that human variation in the trainability of $\overset{\circ}{V}O_{2max}$ is important and related to current phenotype level. That is, there is a genetically determined pretraining status of the trait and capacity to adapt to physical training. Thus, physiological results should be interpreted with respect to both genetic variation and the quality and quantity of training performed.

Intensity-Duration Intensity and duration of training are interrelated, with total amount of work accomplished being an important factor in improvement in fitness. Although more comprehensive inquiry is necessary, present evidence suggests that, when exercise is performed above the minimum intensity threshold, the total amount of work accomplished is an important factor in fitness development and maintenance. That is, improvement will be similar for activities performed at a lower intensity-longer duration compared to higher intensity-shorter duration if the total energy costs of the activities are equal. Higher intensity exercise is associated with greater cardiovascular risk, orthopedic injury, and lower compliance to training than lower intensity exercise. Therefore, programs emphasizing low to moderate intensity training with longer duration are recommended for most adults.

The minimal training intensity threshold for improvement in $\overset{\circ}{V}O_{2max}$ is approximately 60% of the HR_{max} (50% of $\overset{\circ}{V}O_{2max}$ or HR_{max} reserve). The 50% of HR_{max} reserve represents a heart rate of approximately 130–135 beats·min^{-1} for young persons. As a result of the age-related change in maximum heart rate, the absolute heart rate to achieve this threshold is inversely related to age and can be as low as 105–115 beats·min^{-1}, for older persons. Patients who are taking beta-adrenergic blocking drugs may have significantly lower heart rate values. Initial level of fitness is an other important consideration in prescribing exercise. The person with a low fitness level can achieve a significant training effect with a sustained training heart rate as low as 40–50% of HR_{max} reserve, while persons with higher fitness levels require a higher training stimulus.

Classification of Exercise Intensity The classification of exercise intensity and its standardization for exercise prescription based on a 20–60 min training session has been confusing, misinterpreted, and often taken out of context. The most quoted exercise classification system is based on the energy expenditure (kcal·min^{-1}·kg^{-1}) of industrial tasks. The original data for this classification system were published by Christensen in 1953 and were based on the energy expenditure of working in the steel mill for an 8-h day. The classification of industrial and leisure-time tasks by using absolute values of energy expenditure have been valuable for use in the occupational and nutritional setting. Although this classification system has broad application in medicine and, in particular, making recommendations for weight control and job placement, it has little or no meaning for preventive and rehabilitation exercise training programs. To extrapolate absolute values of energy expenditure for completing an industrial task based on an 8-h work day to 20–60 min regimens of exercise training does not make sense. For example, walking and jogging/running can be accomplished at a wide range of speeds; thus, the relative intensity becomes important under these conditions. Because the endurance training regimens recommended by ACSM for nonathletic adults are geared for 60 min or less of physical activity, the system of classification of exercise training intensity shown in Table D-1 is recommended. The use of a realistic time period for training and an individual's relative exercise intensity makes this system amenable to young, middle-aged, and elderly participants, as well as patients with a limited exercise capacity.

Table D.1 ✦ Classification of Intensity of Exercise Based on 20–60 min of Endurance Training

RELATIVE INTENSITY (%)

HR_{max}*	$\overset{\circ}{V}O_{2max}$* or HR_{max} reserve	Rating of Perceived Exertion	Classification of Intensity
< 35%	< 30%	< 10	Very light
35–59%	30–49%	10–11	Light
60–79%	50–74%	12–13	Moderate (somewhat hard)
80–89%	75–84%	14–16	Heavy
≥ 90%	≥ 85%	> 16	Very heavy

Source: M.L. Pollack and J.H. Wilmore. *Exercise in Health and Disease: Evaluation and Prescription for Prevention and Rehabilitation*, 2nd Ed. Philadelphia: W.B. Saunders, 1990. Published with permission.

*HR_{max} = maximum heart rate; $\overset{\circ}{V}O_{2max}$ = maximum oxygen uptake.

Table D-1 also describes the relationship between relative intensity based on percent HR_{max}, percentage of HR_{max} reserve or percentage of $\overset{\circ}{V}O_{2max}$, and the rating of perceived exertion (RPE). The use of heart rate as an estimate of intensity of training is the common standard.

The use of RPE has become a valid tool in the monitoring of intensity in exercise training programs. It is generally considered an adjunct to heart rate in monitoring relative exercise intensity, but once the relationship between heart rate and RPE is known, RPE can be used in place of heart rate. This would not be the case in certain patient populations where a more precise knowledge of heart rate may be critical to the safety of the program.

Frequency The amount of improvement in $\overset{\circ}{V}O_{2max}$ tends to plateau when frequency of training is increased above 3 d·wk^{-1}. The value of the added improvement found with training more than 5 d·wk^{-1} is small to not apparent in regard to improvement in $\overset{\circ}{V}O_{2max}$. Training of less than 2 d·wk^{-1} does not generally show a meaningful change in $\overset{\circ}{V}O_{2max}$.

Mode If frequency, intensity, and duration of training are similar (total kcal expenditure), the training adaptations appear to be independent of the mode of aerobic activity. Therefore, a variety of endurance activities, e.g., those listed above, may be used to derive the same training effect.

Endurance activities that require running and jumping are considered high impact types of activity and generally cause significantly more debilitating injuries to beginning as well as long-term exercisers than do low impact and non-weight bearing type activities. This is particularly evident in the elderly. Beginning joggers have increased foot, leg, and knee injuries when training is performed more than 3 d·wk^{-1} and longer than 30 min duration per exercise session. High intensity interval training (run-walk) compared to continuous jogging training was also associated with a higher incidence of injury. Thus, caution should be taken when recommending the type of activity and exercise prescription for the beginning exerciser. Orthopedic injuries as related to overuse increase linearly in runners/joggers when performing these activities. Thus, there is

a need for more inquiry into the effect that different types of activities and the quantity and quality of training has on injuries over short-term and long-term participation.

An activity such as weight training should not be considered as a means of training for developing $\overset{\circ}{V}O_{2max}$, but it has significant value for increasing muscular strength and endurance and FFW. Studies evaluating circuit weight training (weight training conducted almost continuously with moderate weights, using 10–15 repetitions per exercise session with 15–30 s rest between bouts of activity) show an average improvement in $\overset{\circ}{V}O_{2max}$ of 6%. Thus, circuit weight training is not recommended as the only activity used in exercise programs for developing $\overset{\circ}{V}O_{2max}$.

Age Age in itself does not appear to be a deterrent to endurance training. Although some earlier studies showed a lower training effect with middle-aged or elderly participants, more recent studies show the relative change in $\overset{\circ}{V}O_{2max}$ to be similar to younger age groups. Although more investigation is necessary concerning the rate of improvement in $\overset{\circ}{V}O_{2max}$ with training at various ages, at present it appears that elderly participants need longer periods of time to adapt. Earlier studies showing moderate to no improvement in $\overset{\circ}{V}O_{2max}$ were conducted over a short time span, or exercise was conducted at a moderate to low intensity, thus making the interpretation of the results difficult.

Although $\overset{\circ}{V}O_{2max}$ decreases with age and total body mass and FW increases with age, evidence suggests that this trend can be altered with endurance training. A 9% reduction in $\overset{\circ}{V}O_{2max}$ per decade for sedentary adults after age 25 has been shown, but for active individuals the reduction may be less than 5% per decade. Ten or more year follow-up studies where participants continued training at a similar level showed maintenance of cardiorespiratory fitness. A cross-sectional study of older competitive runners showed progressively lower values in $\overset{\circ}{V}O_{2max}$ from the fourth to seventh decades of life, but also showed less training in the older groups. More recent 10-yr follow-up data on these same athletes (50–82 yr of age) showed $\overset{\circ}{V}O_{2max}$ to be unchanged when training quantity and quality remained unchanged. Thus, life-style plays a significant role in the maintenance of fitness. More inquiry into the relationship of long-term training (quantity and quality), for both competitors and noncompetitors, and physiological function with increasing age is necessary before more definitive statements can be made.

Maintenance of Training Effect In order to maintain the training effect, exercise must be continued on a regular basis. A significant reduction in cardiorespiratory fitness occurs after 2 wk of detraining, with participants returning to near pretraining levels of fitness after 10 wk to 8 months of detraining. A loss of 50% of their initial improvement in $\overset{\circ}{V}O_{2max}$ has been shown after 4–12 wk of detraining. Those individuals who have undergone years of continuous training maintain some benefits for longer periods of detraining than subjects from short-term training studies. While stopping training shows dramatic reductions in $\overset{\circ}{V}O_{2max}$, reduced training shows modest to no reductions for periods of 5–15 wk. Hickson et al., in a series of experiments where frequency, duration, or intensity of training were manipulated, found that, if intensity of training remained unchanged, $\overset{\circ}{V}O_{2max}$ was maintained for up to 15 wk when frequency and duration of training were reduced by as much as ⅔. When frequency and duration of training remained constant and intensity of training was reduced by ⅓ or ⅔, $\dot{V}O_{2max}$ was significantly reduced. Similar findings were found in regards to reduced strength training exercise. When strength training exercise was reduced from 3 or 2 d·wk-1 to at least 1 d·wk-1, strength was maintained for 12 wk of reduced training. Thus, it appears that missing an exercise session periodically or reducing training for up to 15 wk will not adversely effect $\dot{V}O_{2max}$ or muscular strength and endurance as long as training intensity is maintained.

Even though many new studies have given added insight into the proper amount of exercise, investigation is necessary to evaluate the rate of increase and decrease of fitness when varying training loads and reduction in training in relation to level of fitness, age, and length of time in training. Also, more information is needed to better identify the minimal level of exercise necessary to maintain fitness.

Weight Control and Body Composition Although there is variability in human response to body composition change with exercise, total body mass and FW are generally reduced with endurance training programs, while FFW remains constant or increases slightly. For example, Wilmore reported the results of 32 studies that met the criteria for developing cardiorespiratory fitness that are outlined in this position stand and found an average loss in total body mass of 1.5 kg and percent fat of 2.2%. Weight loss programs using dietary manipulation that result in a more dramatic decrease in total body mass show reductions in both FW and FFW. When these programs are conducted in conjunction with exercise training, FFW loss is more modest than in programs using diet alone. Programs that are conducted at least 3 d·wk-1, of at least 20 min duration, and of sufficient intensity to expend approximately 300 kcal per exercise session (75 kg person)* are suggested as a threshold level for total body mass and FW loss. An expenditure of 200 kcal per session has also been shown to be useful in weight reduction if the exercise frequency is at least 4 d·wk-1. If the primary purpose of the training program is for weight loss, then regimens of greater frequency and duration of training and low to moderate intensity are recommended. Programs with less participation generally show little or no change in body composition. Significant increases in $\dot{V}O_{2max}$ have been shown with 10–15 min of high intensity training; thus, if total body mass and FW reduction are not considerations, then shorter duration, higher intensity programs may be recommended for healthy individuals at low risk for cardiovascular disease and orthopedic injury.

Exercise Prescription for Muscular Strength and Endurance

The addition of resistance/strength training to the position statement results from the need for a well-rounded program that exercises all the major muscle groups of the body. Thus, the inclusion of resistance training in adult fitness programs should be effective in the development and maintenance of

*Haskell and Haskell et al. have suggested the use of 4 kcal kg⁻¹ of body weight of energy expenditure per day for a minimum standard for use in exercise programs.

FFW. The effect of exercise training is specific to the area of the body being trained. For example, training the legs will have little or no effect on the arms, shoulders, and trunk muscles. A 10-yr follow-up of master runners who continued their training regimen, but did no upper body exercise, showed maintenance of $\dot{V}O_{2max}$ and a 2-kg reduction in FFW. Their leg circumference remained unchanged, but arm circumference was significantly lower. These data indicate a loss of muscle mass in the untrained areas. Three of the athletes who practiced weight training exercise for the upper body and trunk muscles maintained their FFW. A comprehensive review by Sale carefully documents available information on specificity of training.

Specificity of training was further addressed by Graves et al. Using a bilateral knee extension exercise, they trained four groups: group A, first ½ of the range of motion; group B, second ½ of the range of motion; group AB, full range of motion; and a control group that did not train. The results clearly showed that the training result was specific to the range of motion trained, with group AB getting the best full range effect. Thus, resistance training should be performed through a full range of motion for maximum benefit.

Muscular strength and endurance are developed by the overload principle, i.e., by increasing more than normal the resistance to movement or frequency and duration of activity. Muscular strength is best developed by using heavy weights (that require maximum or nearly maximum tension development) with few repetitions, and muscular endurance is best developed by using lighter weights with a greater number of repetitions. To some extent, both muscular strength and endurance are developed under each condition, but each system favors a more specific type of development. Thus, to elicit improvement in both muscular strength and endurance, most experts recommend 8–12 repetitions per bout of exercise.

Any magnitude of overload will result in strength development, but higher intensity effort at or near maximal effort will give a significantly greater effect. The intensity of resistance training can be manipulated by varying the weight load, repetitions, rest interval between exercises, and number of sets completed. Caution is advised for training that emphasizes lengthening (eccentric) contractions, compared to shortening (concentric) or isometric contractions, as the potential for skeletal muscle soreness and injury is accentuated.

Muscular strength and endurance can be developed by means of static (isometric) or dynamic (isotonic or isokinetic) exercises. Although each type of training has its favorable and weak points, for healthy adults, dynamic resistance exercises are recommended. Resistance training for the average participant should be rhythmical, performed at a moderate to slow speed, move through a full range of motion, and not impede normal forced breathing. Heavy resistance exercise can cause a dramatic acute increase in both systolic and diastolic blood pressure.

The expected improvement in strength from resistance training is difficult to assess because increases in strength are affected by the participants' initial level of strength and their potential for improvement. For example, Mueller and Rohmert found increases in strength ranging from 2 to 9% per week depending on initial strength levels. Although the literature reflects a wide range of improvement in strength with resistance training programs, the average improvement for sedentary young and middle-aged men and women for up to 6 months of training is 25–30%. Fleck and Kraemer, in a review of 13 studies representing various forms of isotonic training, showed an average improvement in bench press strength of 23.3% when subjects were tested on the equipment with which they were trained and 16.5% when tested on special isotonic or isokinetic ergometers (six studies). Fleck and Kraemer also reported an average increase in leg strength of 26.6% when subjects were tested with the equipment that they trained on (six studies) and 21.2% when tested with special isotonic or isokinetic ergometers (five studies). Results of improvement in strength resulting from isometric training have been of the same magnitude as found with isotonic training.

In light of the information reported above, the following guidelines for resistance training are recommended for the average healthy adult. A minimum of 8–10 exercises involving the major muscle groups should be performed a minimum of two times per week. A minimum of one set of 8–12 repetitions to near fatigue should be completed. These minimal standards for resistance training are based on two factors. First, the time it takes to complete a comprehensive, well-rounded exercise program is important. Programs lasting more than 60 min per session are associated with higher dropout rates. Second, although greater frequencies of training and additional sets or combinations of sets and repetitions elicit larger strength gains, the magnitude of difference is usually small. For example, Braith et al. compared training 2 d·wk^{-1} with 3 d·wk^{-1} for 18 wk. The subjects performed one set of 7–10 repetitions to fatigue. The 2 d·wk^{-1} group showed a 21% increase in strength compared to 28% in the 3 d·wk^{-1} group. In other words, 75% of what could be attained in a 3 d·wk^{-1} program was attained in 2 d·wk^{-1}. Also, the 21% improvement in strength found by the 2 d·wk^{-1} regimen is 70–80% of the improvement reported by other programs using additional frequencies of training and combinations of sets and repetitions. Graves et al., Gettman et al., Hurley et al. and Braith et al. found that programs using one set to fatigue showed a greater than 25% increase in strength. Although resistance training equipment may provide a better graduated and quantitative stimulus for overload than traditional calisthenic exercises, calisthenics and other resistance types of exercise can still be effective in improving and maintaining strength.

Summary

The combination of frequency, intensity, and duration of chronic exercise has been found to be effective for producing a training effect. The interaction of these factors provide the overload stimulus. In general, the lower the stimulus the lower the training effect, and the greater the stimulus the greater the effect. As a result of specificity of training and the need for maintaining muscular strength and endurance, and flexibility of the major muscle groups, a well-rounded training program including resistance training and flexibility exercises is recommended. Although age in itself is not a limiting factor to exercise training, a more gradual approach in applying the prescription at older ages seems prudent. It has also been shown that endurance training of fewer than 2 d·wk^{-1}, at less than 50% of maximum oxygen uptake and for less than 10 min·d^{-1}, is inadequate for developing and maintaining fitness for healthy adults.

In the interpretation of this position statement, it must be recognized that the recommendations should be used in the context of participants' needs, goals, and initial abilities. In this regard, a sliding scale as to the amount of time allotted and intensity of effort should be carefully gauged for both the cardiorespiratory and muscular strength and endurance components of the program. An appropriate warm-up and cool-down, which would include flexibility exercises, is also recommended. The important factor is to design a program for the individual to provide the proper amount of physical activity to attain maximal benefit at the lowest risk. Emphasis should be placed on factors that result in permanent life-style change and encourage a lifetime of physical activity.

PROPER AND IMPROPER WEIGHT LOSS PROGRAMS

Millions of individuals are involved in weight reduction programs. With the number of undesirable weight loss programs available and a general misconception by many about weight loss, the need for guidelines for proper weight loss programs is apparent.

Based on the existing evidence concerning the effects of weight loss on health status, physiologic processes, and body composition parameters, the American College of Sports Medicine makes the following statements and recommendations for weight loss programs.

For the purposes of this position stand, body weight will be represented by two components, fat and fat-free (water, electrolytes, minerals, glycogen stores, muscular tissue, bone, etc.):

1. Prolonged fasting and diet programs that severely restrict caloric intake are scientifically undesirable and can be medically dangerous.

2. Fasting and diet programs that severely restrict caloric intake result in the loss of large amounts of water, electrolytes, minerals, glycogen stores, and other fat-free tissue (including proteins within fat-free tissues), with minimal amounts of fat loss.

3. Mild calorie restriction (500–1000 kcal less than the usual daily intake) results in a smaller loss of water, electrolytes, minerals, and other fat-free tissue and is less likely to cause malnutrition.

4. Dynamic exercise of large muscles helps to maintain fat-free tissue, including muscle mass and bone density, and results in losses of body weight. Weight loss resulting from an increase in energy expenditure is primarily in the form of fat weight.

5. A nutritionally sound diet resulting in mild calorie restriction coupled with an endurance exercise program along with behavioral modification of existing eating habits is recommended for weight reduction. The rate of sustained weight loss should not exceed 1 kg (2 lb) per week.

6. To maintain proper weight control and optimal body fat levels, a lifetime commitment to proper eating habits and regular physical activity is required.

Research Background for the Position Stand

Each year millions of individuals undertake weight loss programs for a variety of reasons. It is well known that obesity is associated with a number of health-related problems. These problems include impairment of cardiac function due to an increase in the work of the heart and to left ventricular dysfunction; hypertension; diabetes; renal disease; gall bladder disease; respiratory dysfunction; joint diseases and gout; endometrial cancer; abnormal plasma lipid and lipoprotein concentrations; problems in the administration of anesthetics during surgery; and impairment of physical working capacity. As a result, weight reduction is frequently advised by physicians for medical reasons. In addition, there are a vast number of individuals who are on weight reduction programs for aesthetic reasons.

It is estimated that 60–70 million American adults and at least 10 million American teenagers are overfat. Because millions of Americans have adopted unsupervised weight loss programs, it is the opinion of the American College of Sports Medicine that guidelines are needed for safe and effective weight loss programs. This position stand deals with desirable and undesirable weight loss programs. Desirable weight loss programs are defined as those that are nutritionally sound and result in maximal losses in fat weight and minimal losses of fat-free tissue. Undesirable weight loss programs are defined as those that are not nutritionally sound, that result in large losses of fat-free tissue, that pose potential serious medical complications, and that cannot be followed for long-term weight maintenance.

Therefore, a desirable weight loss program is one that:

1. Provides a caloric intake not lower than 1200 kcal·d^{-1} for normal adults in order to get a proper blend of foods to meet nutritional requirements. (Note: this requirement may change for children, older individuals, athletes, etc.)

2. Includes foods acceptable to the dieter from the viewpoints of socio-cultural background, usual habits, taste, cost, and ease in acquisition and preparation.

3. Provides a negative caloric balance (not to exceed 500–1000 kcal·d^{-1} lower than recommended), resulting in gradual weight loss without metabolic derangements. Maximal weight loss should be 1 kg·wk^{-1}.

4. Includes the use of behavior modification techniques to identify and eliminate dieting habits that contribute to improper nutrition.

5. Includes an endurance exercise program of at least 3 d/wk, 20–30 min in duration, at a minimum intensity of 60% of maximum heart rate (refer to ACSM Position Stand on the Recommended Quantity and Quality of Exercise for Developing and Maintaining Fitness in Healthy Adults, *Med. Sci. Sports Exerc.* 22:2, pp. 529–533, 1990).

6. Provides that the new eating and physical activity habits can be continued for life in order to maintain the achieved lower body weight.

1. Since the early work of Keys et al. and Bloom, which indicated that marked reduction in caloric intake or fasting (starvation or semistarvation) rapidly reduced body weight, numerous fasting, modified fasting, and fad diet and weight loss programs have emerged. While these programs promise and generally cause rapid weight loss, they are associated with significant medical risks.

The medical risks associated with these types of diet and weight loss programs are numerous. Blood glucose concentrations have been shown to be markedly reduced in obese subjects who undergo fasting. Further, in obese non-diabetic subjects, fasting may result in impairment of glucose tolerance. Ketonuria begins within a few hours after fasting or low-carbohydrate diets are begun and hyperuricemia is common among subjects who fast to reduce body weight. Fasting also results in high serum uric acid levels with decreased urinary output. Fasting and low-calorie diets also result in urinary nitrogen loss and a significant decrease in fat-free tissue. In comparison to ingestion of a normal diet, fasting substantially elevates urinary excretion of potassium. This, coupled with the aforementioned nitrogen loss, suggests that the potassium loss is due to a loss of lean tissue. Other electrolytes, including sodium, calcium, magnesium, and phosphate, have been shown to be elevated in urine during prolonged fasting. Reductions in blood volume and body fluids are also common with fasting and fad diets. This can be associated with weakness and fainting. Congestive heart failure and sudden death have been reported in subjects who fasted or markedly restricted their caloric intake. Myocardial atrophy appears to contribute to sudden death. Sudden death may also occur during refeeding. Untreated fasting also has been reported to reduce serum iron binding capacity, resulting in anemia. Liver glycogen levels are depleted with fasting and liver function and gastrointestinal tract abnormalities are associated with fasting. While fasting and calorically restricted diets have been shown to lower serum cholesterol levels, a large portion of the cholesterol reduction is a result of lowered HDL-cholesterol levels. Other risks associated with fasting and low-calorie diets include lactic acidosis, alopecia, hypoalaninemia, edema, anuria, hypotension, elevated serum bilirubin, nausea and vomiting, alterations in thyroxine metabolism, impaired serum triglyceride removal and production, and death.

2. The major objective of any weight reduction program is to lose body fat while maintaining fat-free tissue. The vast majority of research reveals that starvation and low-calorie diets result in large losses of water, electrolytes, and other fat-free tissue. One of the best controlled experiments was conducted from 1944 to 1946 at the Laboratory of Physiological Hygiene at the University of Minnesota. In this study subjects had their base-line caloric intake cut by 45% and body weight and body composition changes were followed for 24 wk. During the first 12 wk of semistarvation, body weight declined by 25.4 lb (11.5 kg) with only an 11.6-lb (5.3 kg) decline in body fat. During the second 12-

wk period, body weight declined an additional 9.1 lb (4.1 kg) with only a 6.1-lb (2.8 kg) decrease in body fat. These data clearly demonstrate that fat-free tissue significantly contributes to weight loss from semistarvation. Similar results have been reported by several other investigators. Buskirk et al. reported that the 13.5-kg weight loss in six subjects on a low-calorie mixed diet averaged 76% fat and 24% fat-free tissue. Similarly, Passmore et al. reported results of 78% of weight loss (15.3 kg) as fat and 22% as fat-free tissue in seven women who consumed a 400-kcal·d-1 diet for 45 d. Yang and Van Itallie followed weight loss and body composition changes for the first 5 d of a weight loss program involving subjects consuming either an 800-kcal mixed diet, an 800-kcal ketogenic diet, or undergoing starvation. Subjects on the mixed diet lost 1.3 kg of weight (59% fat loss, 3.4% protein loss, 37.6% water loss), subjects on the ketogenic diet lost 2.3 kg of weight (33.2% fat, 3.8% protein, 63.0% water), and subjects on starvation regimens lost 3.8 kg of weight (32.3% fat, 6.5% protein, 61.2% water). Grande and Grande et al. reported similar findings with a 1000-kcal carbohydrate diet. It was further reported that water restriction combined with 1000-kcal·d-1 of carbohydrate resulted in greater water loss and less fat loss.

Recently, there has been some renewed speculation about the efficacy of the very-low-calorie diet (VLCD). Krotkiewski and associates studied the effects on body weight and body composition after 3 wk on the so-called Cambridge diet. Two groups of obese middle-aged women were studied. One group had a VLCD only, while the second group had a VLCD combined with a 55-min/d, 3-d/wk exercise program. The VLCD-only group lost 6.2 kg in 3 wk, of which only 2.6 kg was fat loss, while the VLCD-plus-exercise group lost 6.8 kg in 3 wk with only a 1.9-kg body fat loss. Thus it can be seen that VLCD results in undesirable losses of body fat, and the addition of the normally protective effect of chronic exercise to VLCD does not reduce the catabolism of fat-free tissue. Further, with VLCD, a large reduction (29%) in HDL-cholesterol is seen.

3. Even mild calorie restriction (reduction of 500–1000 kcal·d-1 from base-line caloric intake), when used alone as a tool for weight loss, results in the loss of moderate amounts of water and other fat-free tissue. In a study by Goldman et al., 15 female subjects consumed a low-calorie mixed diet for 7–8 wk. Weight loss during this period averaged 6.43 kg (0.85 kg·wk-1), 88.6% of which was fat. The remaining 11.4% represented water and other fat-free tissue. Zuti and Golding examined the effect of 500 kcal·d-1 calorie restriction on body composition changes in adult females. Over a 16-wk period the women lost approximately 5.2 kg; however, 1.1 kg of the weight loss (21 %) was due to a loss of water and other fat-free tissue. More recently, Weltman et al. examined the effects of 500 kcal·d-1 calorie restriction (from base-line levels) on body composition changes in sedentary middle-aged males. Over a 10-wk period subjects lost 5.95 kg, 4.03 kg (68%) of which was fat loss and 1.92 kg (32%) was loss of water and other fat-free tissue. Further, with calorie restriction only, these subjects exhibited a decrease in HDL-cholesterol. In the same study, the two other groups who exercised and/or dieted and exercised were able to maintain their HDL-cholesterol levels. Similar results for females have been presented by

Thompson et al. It should be noted that the decrease seen in HDL-cholesterol with weight loss may be an acute effect. There are data that indicate that stable weight loss has a beneficial effect on HDL-cholesterol.

Further, an additional problem associated with calorie restriction alone for effective weight loss is the fact that it is associated with a reduction in basal metabolic rate. Apparently exercise combined with calorie restriction can counter this response.

4. There are several studies that indicate that exercise helps maintain fat-free tissue while promoting fat loss. Total body weight and fat weight are generally reduced with endurance training programs while fat-free weight remains constant or increases slightly. Programs conducted at least 3 d/wk, of at least 20-min duration, and of sufficient intensity and duration to expend at least 300 kcal per exercise session have been suggested as a threshold level for total body weight and fat weight reduction. Increasing caloric expenditure above 300 kcal per exercise session and increasing the frequency of exercise sessions will enhance fat weight loss while sparing fat-free tissue. Leon et al. had six obese male subjects walk vigorously for 90 min, 5 d/wk for 16 wk. Work output progressed weekly to an energy expenditure of 1000–1200 kcal/session. At the end of 16 wk, subjects averaged 5.7 kg of weight loss with a 5.9-kg loss of fat weight and a 0.2-kg gain in fat-free tissue. Similarly, Zuti and Golding followed the progress of adult women who expended 500 kcal/exercise session 5 d/wk for 16 wk of exercise. At the end of 16 wk the women lost 5.8 kg of fat and gained 0.9 kg of fat-free tissue.

5. Review of the literature cited above strongly indicates that optimal body composition changes occur with a combination of calorie restriction (while on a well-balanced diet) plus exercise. This combination promotes loss of fat weight while sparing fat-free tissue. Data of Zuti and Golding and Weltman et al. support this contention. Calorie restriction of 500 kcal·d-1 combined with 3–5 d of exercise requiring 300–500 kcal per exercise session results in favorable changes in body composition. Therefore, the optimal rate of weight loss should be between 0.45–1 kg (1–2 lb) per wk. This seems especially relevant in light of the data which indicates that rapid weight loss due to low caloric intake can be associated with sudden death. In order to institute a desirable pattern of calorie restriction plus exercise, behavior modification techniques should be incorporated to identify and eliminate habits contributing to obesity and/or overfatness.

6. The problem with losing weight is that, although many individuals succeed in doing so, they invariably put the weight on again. The goal of an effective weight loss regimen is not merely to lose weight. Weight control requires a lifelong commitment, an understanding of our eating habits and a willingness to change them. Frequent exercise is necessary, and accomplishment must be reinforced to sustain motivation. Crash dieting and other promised weight loss cures are ineffective.

References for both ACSM position statements are available from ACSM and are included in the Instructor's Manual for this textbook.

Absolute VO₂ Expressing the volume of oxygen consumption in the units of liters of oxygen consumed per minute (l/min).

Acute Disease or pain characterized by sudden onset and a short, severe course.

Adenosine diphosphate (ADP) A substrate present in muscle tissue that combines with phosphate to form ATP for muscle contractions.

Adenosine triphosphate (ATP) The basic substrate used by the muscle to provide energy for muscle contractions.

Adipose tissue Fatty tissue.

Aerobic metabolism The process of breaking down energy nutrients such as carbohydrates and fats in the presence of oxygen in order to yield energy in the form of ATP.

Aerobics Activity performed in the presence of oxygen, using fat as the major source of fuel.

Afterburn The period of time following exercise when resting metabolism remains elevated.

Amenorrhea Loss of at least three consecutive menstrual cycles when they are otherwise expected to occur.

Amino acids The basic component of most proteins.

Amphetamines Drugs that stimulate the central nervous system increasing heart rate, blood pressure, and other body processes.

Anabolic steroids Drugs that are derivatives of the male sex hormone testosterone that are sometimes illegally used by those desiring to increase their body size, speed, or strength.

Anaerobic metabolism The process of breaking down carbohydrates (glucose or glycogen) in the absence of oxygen in order to yield energy in the form of ATP.

Anaerobics High-intensity activity, such as sprinting, that is performed in the absence of oxygen using glucose as the major source of fuel.

Anemia Occurs when the hemoglobin level falls below the normal reference range for individuals of the same sex and age.

Angina pectoris Chest pain caused by restricted blood flow to the heart.

Anorexia nervosa An eating disorder that involves lack or loss of appetite to the point of self-starvation and dangerous weight loss.

Appetite The desire to eat; pleasant sensations aroused by the thoughts of the taste and enjoyment of food.

Atherosclerosis A condition in which plaque has formed and blocks the passage of blood through a blood vessel.

Autogenic training A relaxation technique in which you imagine your arms and legs are heavy, warm, and tingly.

Ballistic stretching Flexibility exercises employing bouncing and jerking movements at the extreme range of motion or point of discomfort.

Basal metabolism The energy expended (calories burned), measured by oxygen consumption, during a resting state over a 24-hour period.

Bioavailability Synonymous with absorbability; refers to the individual differences in ease of absorption of nutrients.

Blood lipid analysis Examination and study of the fats present in the blood.

Body cathexis Physical self-esteem, how highly you regard your physical self.

Body composition The relationship between your fat weight and your lean body mass.

Body mass index (BMI) A method of determining overweight and obesity by dividing body weight (in kilograms) by height (in meters) squared; this method is considered superior to height/weight table ranges.

Body scanning A relaxation technique in which you identify a part of your body that feels relaxed and transport that feeling to another part of your body.

Bulimia An eating disorder found most often in women involving eating binges followed by self-induced vomiting or the use of laxatives to expel the unwanted food.

Caffeine A stimulant drug present in coffee, tea, and colas and other soft drinks that have not been decaffeinated.

Carbohydrate loading (supercompensation) An attempt to reduce carbohydrate intake to near zero for two to three days (depletion stage) before resorting to a high-carbohydrate diet for three to four days (loading phase) to raise glycogen stores in skeletal muscle and the liver to increase energy levels on the day of competition.

Carcinogens Agents (toxins, chemicals, and so forth) that can cause cancer.

Cardiac output The volume of blood pumped by the heart per minute; usually expressed in units of liters per minute (l/min).

Cardiorespiratory endurance The ability of the heart, blood vessels, and lungs to deliver oxygen to the exercising muscles in amounts sufficient to meet the demands of the workload.

Cardiorespiratory system Joint functioning of the respiratory system (the lungs and airway passages) and the circulatory system (the heart and blood vessels).

Cartilage Fibrous connective tissue between the surfaces of movable and immovable joints.

Cholesterol One of the sterols, or fat-like chemical substances manufactured in the body and consumed from foods of animal origins only; high intake is associated with elevated blood cholesterol levels and heart disease.

Chronic Disease or pain of slow onset and long duration.

Cirrhosis A scarring of cells of the liver that is associated with the excessive use of alcohol.

Citric acid energy cycle The aerobic energy pathway fueled primarily by fat, small quantities of glucose fragments, and certain amino acids.

Cocaine A drug that stimulates the central nervous system and that can cause tremors, rapid heart beat, and harmful psychological effects.

Collagen The connective tissue portion of the true skin and of other organs.

Complete protein Food source containing all essential amino acids in the correct proportions.

Complex carbohydrates (polysaccharides) Starch and fiber; chains of sugar molecules (three or more) found in fruits, vegetables, and grains.

Cooldown The use of 3 to 10 minutes of very light exercise movements at the end of a vigorous workout designed to cool the body slowly to near normal core temperature.

Coronary heart disease (CHD) A condition in which the heart is supplied with insufficient blood due to clogging of coronary arteries.

Cortical bone A very dense, ivorylike bone that forms an outer shell that protects and encompasses trabecular bone; it also composes the shafts of all long bones in the body.

Counterirritants Medication, heat, cold, electricity, and so forth used to eliminate pain and inflammation.

Creatine phosphate (CP) A substrate present in muscle tissue that is broken down into its component parts (creatine and phosphate) in order to provide phosphates for the production of ATP.

Cross training The practice of alternating exercise choices throughout the week to avoid overuse injuries from repetitive movements.

Delayed onset muscle soreness (DOMS) Muscle soreness that typically occurs 12 to 24 hours after a high-intensity exercise session.

Depleted iron stores The initial state of iron depletion whereby you become vulnerable to low iron stores but you do not experience any adverse physiological effects.

Diabetes mellitus A disease caused by insufficient production of insulin by the endocrine portion of the pancreas; **Type I** (insulin dependent) or **Type II** (noninsulin dependent).

Diastolic blood pressure The force of the blood against the arterial walls when the heart is relaxed.

Dietary fiber The undigestible portion of food after it is exposed to the body's enzymes.

Drug abuse The use of an illegal drug or the use of a legal drug for purposes other than those it was intended for.

Drug misuse The inappropriate use of a legal drug.

Drug use The proper use of a drug.

Dysmenorrhea Painful menstrual cycles.

ECG See **Electrocardiogram.**

Electrical impedance A quick, accurate means of determining an individual's percent of body fat that uses electrodes attached to wrists and ankles to electronically determine the percent.

Electrocardiogram (ECG) A tracing of the electrical currents involved in the cycles of a heart beat.

Electrolytes Chemical compounds (sodium, potassium, and chlorine) in solution in the human body capable of producing electric current; important in the prevention of cramps, heat exhaustion, and heat stroke.

Electrotherapy The use of electricity (infrared radiation therapy, shortwave and microwave diathermies, and ultrasound therapy) in the treatment of disease or injury.

Endurance The ability to work a long time without experiencing fatigue or exhaustion.

Essential amino acids Amino acids that cannot be manufactured by the body and therefore must be acquired from food sources.

Essential fat The amount of fat required for normal physiological functioning.

Eumenorrhea Regularly occurring menstrual cycles.

Eustress Stress that results in personal growth or development and, therefore, the person experiencing it is better for having been stressed.

Fast-twitch (FI) fibers The type of muscle fiber used in anaerobic, power sports, which are metabolically equipped to meet the demands of short duration, high-intensity activities.

Fast-twitch, glycolytic muscle fiber White muscle fiber used in anaerobic activity that contracts rapidly and explosively but tires quickly because it has a poor blood supply.

Fast-twitch, oxidative, glycolytic fiber An intermediate fiber that can be used in both anaerobic and aerobic activity.

Fat weight The weight of your body fat.

Ferritin A protein-rich compound that contains iron and constitutes the form in which iron is stored in the liver, the spleen, and the bone marrow.

Fight-or-flight response A physiological reaction to a threatening stressor; another name for **stress reactivity**.

Flexibility The range of motion around a joint or the ability to move limbs gracefully and efficiently.

Frostbite Destruction of tissue by freezing.

Glucagon A natural hormone secreted by the pancreas that stimulates the metabolism of sugar; it is secreted when blood sugar is too low, a condition that causes the release of liver glycogen and its transformation into glucose.

Glucostatic theory A theory about hunger regulation suggesting that blood-glucose levels determine whether one is hungry or satiated through the exhaustion of liver glycogen.

Glycogen The stored form of carbohydrate in the muscles and liver.

Glycolysis energy cycle The anaerobic energy pathway fueled primarily by glucose.

Graded exercise test (stress test) Test designed to monitor the electrical activity of the heart; it is performed by walking on a treadmill that is slowly being elevated to increase the work load.

Harvard step test Test designed to measure cardiorespiratory endurance (aerobic fitness).

Health The total of your physical, social, emotional, mental, and spiritual status.

Heat exhaustion (heat prostration) Collapse due to loss of fluid and salts caused by oversweating.

Heat stroke Severe, sustained rise in fever due to the failure of the body-heat-regulating mechanism after a prolonged period of elevated temperature.

Heme iron The form of iron found in most meats, fish, and poultry; has a high rate of absorption.

Hemodilution An increase in the plasma volume (fluid portion of blood) that exceeds the increase in the total amount of hemoglobin produced, creating symptoms of anemia.

Hemoglobin An iron-containing protein responsible for carrying oxygen throughout the bloodstream to body tissues, such as muscle, where it is used to provide energy for all forms of physical work.

High biological value A protein source such as meat that contains all eight essential amino acids in the correct proportions.

High-density lipoproteins (HDL) Fatty particles in the blood that pick up unused cholesterol and transport it for processing and elimination from the body.

Hunger A physiological response of the body involving unpleasant sensations indicating a need for food.

Hydrostatic weighing An accurate method of measuring body fat by submerging an individual in water.

Hyperplasia New fat cell formation.

Hypertension High blood pressure; usually greater than 140 systolic blood pressure and/or greater than 90 diastolic blood pressure.

Hypertrophy An increase in the size of the muscle.

Hypervitaminosis The toxic side effects that result from the consumption of excess vitamins.

Hypothalamus gland A portion of the brain that regulates body temperature and other functions; thought to be important in the regulation of food intake.

Hypothermia Subnormal body temperature.

Incomplete protein Food sources that do not containing all essential amino acids or contain several in incorrect proportions.

Insulin A natural hormone produced in the pancreas gland that aids in the digestion of sugars and other carbohydrates; it is secreted when blood sugar is too high.

Invisible fat Hidden fat in food that cannot be seen, such as the fat in dairy products, egg yolks, and meat.

Iron-deficiency anemia A condition that occurs when the red blood cells do not contain enough hemoglobin and consequently do not deliver enough oxygen to the tissues.

Iron deficiency without anemia The second phase of iron depletion where some adverse physiological effects occur, such as chronic fatigue, decreased physical work capacity, and diminished productivity due to a reduced hemoglobin level.

Ischemia A condition of localized diminished blood supply.

Isokinetic contraction Muscular movement that involves both muscle shortening and lengthening during the positive and negative phase.

Isometric contraction Force applied to an immovable object that does not result in muscle shortening.

Isotonic contraction Shortening of the muscle in the positive phase and lengthening during the negative phase of an action.

Jogging Running at a 9-minute-per-mile pace or slower.

Kilocalorie A large calorie, equal to one thousand small calories; one kilocalorie is the amount of heat required to raise the temperature of one kilogram (about one quart) of water one degree Celsius.

Lactovegetarian An individual who eats fruits, vegetables, grains, and dairy products, and avoids meat products.

Lean body mass The nonfatty component of your body.

Ligament Fibrous bands or folds that support organs, hold bones together, or attach muscles to bones.

Lipoproteins Fatty particles that can collect on the walls of the blood vessels.

Lipostatic theory A theory about hunger-control suggesting that the size of fat stores signal us to eat.

Locus of control The degree to which you believe you are in control of events in your life.

Low biological value A protein source such as corn and wheat that does not contains all eight essential amino acids or contains some in low proportions.

Low-density lipoproteins (LDL) Fatty particles in the blood that carry cholesterol to cells throughout the body.

Maximal oxygen consumption (VO₂) The optimal capacity of the heart to pump blood, of the lungs to fill with larger volumes of air, and of the muscle cells to use the oxygen and remove waste products that are produced during the process of aerobic metabolism.

Megavitamin intake Consuming 10 to 100 times the RDA for a particular vitamin.

Metabolic rate Amount of calories burned at rest.

Metabolic specificity Training a specific energy system (citric acid cycle or glycolysis cycle).

Metabolism The sum of energy expended in carrying on the normal body processes: converting nutrients into tissue, muscle contraction, and maintenance of the body's chemical machinery.

Metastasis The process in which cancerous cells from one part of the body travel to other parts of the body.

Monounsaturated fat Fat containing one double bond between carbons, found in foods such as avocados, cashews, and peanut and olive oils.

Muscle extensibility The ability of muscle tissue to stretch.

Muscle fibers Bundles of tissue composed of cells.

Muscular endurance A muscle's ability to continue submaximal contractions against resistance.

Muscular strength The amount of force a muscle can exert for one repetition.

Myofibrils Thin protein filaments that interact and slide by one another during a muscular contraction.

Myoglobin Another iron-containing protein that helps transport oxygen directly into the muscle for the production of energy.

Negative phase of muscular contraction The phase of a weight-training exercise when weight is returned to the starting position and muscle lengthening occurs.

Neuromuscular specificity Training a specific muscle group.

Nonessential amino acids Amino acids that can be manufactured by the body if they cannot be acquired from food sources.

Nonessential nutrients Nutrients the body can manufacture in sufficient quantities without there being any of that substance in your diet.

Nonheme iron The form of iron found in most plant sources of iron; has a much lower absorption rate than heme iron does.

Norepinephrine An end product of some of the secretions of the adrenal gland; influences nervous system activity, constricts blood vessels, and increases blood pressure.

Nutrition density Foods that are high in nutrients and low in calories.

Nutrition pyramid New dietary guidelines emphasizing fruits, vegetables, and grains and deemphasizing meats, dairy products, sweets, fats, and oils.

Occluded Clogged arteries that no longer allow the normal amount of blood to pass through them.

Oligomenorrhea Reduced, scanty, or irregular menstruation.

1.5 mile test Field test designed to measure cardiorespiratory endurance (aerobic fitness).

1 RM The maximum amount of weight that can be lifted at one time.

Osteoporosis An abnormal decalcification of bones causing loss of bone density.

Ovolactovegetarian An individual who eats fruits, vegetables, grains, dairy products, and eggs but avoids meat products.

Oxygen debt The difference between the exact amount of oxygen needed for an exercise task and the amount actually taken in.

Oxygen-transport system The ability of the body to take in and use oxygen at the tissue level during physical activity.

Percent body fat The percentage of your body weight made up of fat.

Pica A craving for nonfood substances which occurs as a symptom of iron-deficiency anemia.

Plaque A collection of blood fats and other substances that combine to clog blood vessels.

Polyunsaturated fat Fat containing two or more double bonds between carbons; found heavily in vegetable oils, nuts (such as almonds, pecans, walnuts, and filberts), fish, and margarine.

Positive phase of muscular contraction The phase of a weight-training exercise when weight is brought toward the body and muscle shortening occurs.

Postexercise peril Illness, dizziness, nausea, and sudden death following vigorous exercise, particularly when a cooldown period is not used.

Preconditioning period A period of several weeks taken to prepare the body slowly for maximum effort testing or engagement in a vigorous activity or sport.

Progressive relaxation A relaxation technique in which you contract, then relax, muscle groups throughout the body.

Progressive resistance exercise (PRE) A method of slowly increasing the amount of resistance to be overcome and/or the number of repetitions each workout.

Pronate Rolling the foot inward when it is pushing off.

Proprioceptive neuromuscular facilitation (PNF) stretching A two-person stretching technique involving the application of steady pressure by a partner at the extreme range of motion for a particular exercise and steady resistance to the pressure.

Protein sparing Consuming sufficient amounts of dietary carbohydrate and fat on a daily basis to prevent the conversion of dietary and lean muscle protein to glucose.

Psychosomatic Illnesses or diseases that are either worsened or develop in the first place because of the body changes resulting from an interpretation of thoughts.

Purinegic theory A theory about hunger suggesting that the circulating levels of purines, molecules found in DNA and RNA, govern hunger.

Reference daily intake (RDI) Previously referred to as the U.S. Recommended Dietary Allowances, the new nutrition labels use RDI to identify the levels of nutrients that satisfy or exceed the needs of most healthy people in the United States for one day.

Relative VO$_2$ Expressing the volume of oxygen consumption in the units of milliliters of oxygen per kilogram of body weight per minute (ml/kg $\times$ min^{-1}).

Repetitions The number of times a specific exercise is completed.

Rest interval Amount of time taken between sets.

Running Running faster than 9 minutes per mile.

Saturated fat Fat that contains glycerol and saturated fatty acids, found in high quantities in animal products (such as meat, milk, butter, and cheese) and in low quantities in vegetable products; high intake is associated with elevated blood cholesterol levels.

Sciatica Pain along the course of the great sciatic nerve (hip, thigh, leg, foot).

Selective awareness A means of managing stress by consciously focusing on the positive aspects of a situation or person.

Self-esteem The amount of regard you hold for yourself; the amount of value you place on yourself.

Set A group of repetitions for a particular exercise.

Set point A theory postulating that each individual has an ideal weight (the set point) and that the body will attempt to maintain this weight against pressure to change it.

Simple carbohydrates (monosaccharides and disaccharides) Sugars; chains of sugar molecules (one or two) found in concentrated sugar and the sugar that occurs naturally in food.

Sit-and-reach test A test designed to measure the flexibility of the lower-back and hamstring muscles.

Slow-twitch (SI) fibers The type of muscle fiber used in endurance sports, which are equipped metabolically to meet the demands of aerobic activities of long duration.

Slow-twitch, oxidative muscle fiber Red muscle fiber used in aerobic activity that contracts and tires slowly.

Social isolation The lack of other people with whom to discuss important matters relevant to your life.

Soft tissue Tissue other than bone.

Static stretching Flexibility exercises in which a position is held steady for a designated period of time at the extreme range of motion.

Storage fat Fat that is stored in the adipose tissue.

Stress The combination of a stressor and stress reactivity.

Stress reactivity The physical reaction to a stressor that results in increased muscle tension, heart rate, blood pressure, and so forth.

Stressor A stimulus that has the potential to elicit stress reactivity.

Stroke volume The amount of blood pumped per beat of the heart; usually expressed in units of milliliters per beat (ml/beat).

Subcutaneous fat The layer of adipose tissue directly beneath the skin.

Supinate Rocking the foot to the outside when it is pushing off.

Systolic blood pressure The force of the blood against the arterial blood-vessel walls when the left ventricle contracts and blood is pumped out of the heart.

Tendon A fibrous band into which some muscles narrow down for attachment to a bone.

Thermotherapy The application of heat.

Trabecular bone The interior of the bone which looks like a dense lacy crystal network and makes up part of the body's calcium bank.

Transferrin Another protein-rich compound that transports iron in the bloodstream.

Triglyceride The fatty substance in lipoproteins.

Type A behavior pattern A constellation of behaviors that makes individuals susceptible to coronary heart disease.

Type B behavior pattern A combination of behaviors that seem to protect people from contracting coronary heart disease: i.e., lack of hostility, anger, aggression; cooperativeness, focusing on one task at a time.

United States recommended dietary allowances (U.S. RDA) A simplified RDA appearing on food labels showing the percent of the RDA by serving and other valuable nutritional information.

Vasodilation Increase or opening of the blood vessels.

Vegan A strict vegetarian who consumes only fruits, vegetables, and grains.

Vertebrae The 33 bones of the spinal column, some of which are normally fused together (sacral and the coccygeal vertebrae).

Visible fat Fat content of food that can be seen, such as the fat in butter and oils.

Warmup The preparation of the body for vigorous activity through stretching, calisthenics, running, and specific sport movements designed to raise core temperature.

Wellness Having the components of health balanced and at sufficient levels.